# EVALUATION OF THE PATIENT WITH HEART DISEASE

## Integrating the Physical Exam & Echocardiography

Editors

**Carlos A. Roldan**, M.D., F.A.C.C.

*Associate Professor of Medicine*
*Department of Internal Medicine*
*University of New Mexico School of Medicine*
*Director of Echocardiography Laboratory*
*Department of Internal Medicine*
*Veterans Affairs Medical Center*
*Albuquerque, New Mexico*


**Jonathan Abrams**, M.D., F.A.C.C..

*Professor of Medicine*
*Cardiology Division*
*University of New Mexico School of Medicine*
*Staff Cardiologist*
*Department of Internal Medicine*
*University Hospital*
*Albuquerque, New Mexico*

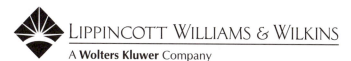

LIPPINCOTT WILLIAMS & WILKINS
A **Wolters Kluwer** Company
Philadelphia · Baltimore · New York · London
Buenos Aires · Hong Kong · Sydney · Tokyo

*Acquisitions Editor:* Ruth W. Weinberg
*Developmental Editor:* Tanya Lazar
*Production Editor:* Tom Wang
*Manufacturing Manager:* Tim Reynolds
*Cover Designer:* Diana Andrews
*Compositor:* Lippincott Williams & Williams Desktop Division
*Printer:* Maple Press

**© 2002 by LIPPINCOTT WILLIAMS & WILKINS**
**530 Walnut Street**
**Philadelphia, PA 19106 USA**
**LWW.com**

Printed in the USA

**Library of Congress Cataloging-in-Publication Data**

Evaluation of the patient with heart disease : integrating the physical exam & echocardiography / edited by Carlos A. Roldan and Jonathan Abrams.
     p. ; cm.
   Includes bibliograpical references and index.
   ISBN 0-7817-2479-1 (alk. paper)
   1. Heart—Diseases—Diagnosis. 2. Echocardiography. 3. Physical diagnosis.
I. Roldan, Carlos A. II. Abrams, Jonathan.
   [DNLM: 1. Heart Diseases—diagnosis. 2. Echocardiography. 3. Physical Examination—methods. WG 210 E92 2002]
RC683.E84 2002
616.1"2075—dc21

2001050470

10   9   8   7   6   5   4   3   2   1

# EVALUATION OF THE PATIENT WITH HEART DISEASE

*To my wife Patricia, my daughters Paola and Pamela, and my sons Carlos and Pablo Roldan,*
*for their love, support, and inspiration.*

CAR

# Contents

# Contributing Authors

**Jonathan Abrams, M.D. F.A.C.C.** *Professor of Medicine, Cardiology Division, University of New Mexico School of Medicine; and Staff Cardiologist, Department of Internal Medicine, University Hospital, Albuquerque, New Mexico*

**Phoebe A. Ashley, M.D.** *Assistant Professor of Medicine, Department of Internal Medicine, University of New Mexico School of Medicine; and Staff Cardiologist, Department of Internal Medicine, Veterans Affairs Medical Center, Albuquerque, New Mexico*

**Gerald A. Charlton, M.D. F.A.C.C.** *Assistant Professor of Medicine, Department of Internal Medicine, University of New Mexico School of Medicine; and Staff Cardiologist, Department of Internal Medicine, Veterans Affairs Medical Center, Albuquerque, New Mexico*

**Michael A. Chizner, M.D., F.A.C.P., F.A.C.C.** *Clinical Professor, Department of Medicine, University of Miami School of Medicine, Miami, Florida; Clinical Professor, Department of Medicine, University of Florida College of Medicine, Gainesville, Florida; and Chief Medical Director, The Heart Center of Excellence, North Broward Hospital, Fort Lauderdale, Florida*

**Michael H. Crawford, M.D., F.A.C.C.** *Professor, Department of Internal Medicine, Mayo Medical School, Rochester, Minnesota; and Consultant, Department of Cardiovascular Diseases, Mayo Clinic Scottsdale, Scottsdale, Arizona*

**Edward A. Gill, M.D.** *Associate Professor of Medicine, Department of Internal Medicine, University of Washington School of Medicine; and Director of Echocardiography Laboratory, Cardiology Division, Harborview Medical Center, Seattle, Washington*

**M. Beth Goens, M.D.** *Assistant Professor of Medicine, Department of Pediatrics, University of New Mexico School of Medicine; and Director of Echocardiography, Department of Pediatrics, University of New Mexico Health Sciences Center, Albuquerque, New Mexico*

**Robert R. Phillips, M.D.** *Staff Cardiologist, Idaho Cardiology Associates, Boise, Idaho*

**Carlos A. Roldan, M.D., F.A.C.C.** *Associate Professor of Medicine, Department of Internal Medicine, University of New Mexico School of Medicine; and Director of Echocardiography Laboratory, Department of Internal Medicine, Veterans Affairs Medical Center, Albuquerque, New Mexico*

**Bruce K. Shively, M.D.** *Associate Professor, Cardiology Division, Oregon Health Sciences University; and Co-Director, Echocardiographic Laboratory, Oregon Health and Science University Hospital, Portland, Oregon*

**David Spodick, M.D., D.Sc., F.A.C.C.** *Professor, Department of Medicine, University of Massachusetts Medical School; and Director of Cardiovascular Fellowship Training, Department of Cardiovascular Medicine, Saint Vincent Hospital at Worcester Medical Center, Worcester, Massachusetts*

**Robert A. Taylor, M.D., F.A.C.C.** *Assistant Professor of Medicine, Department of Internal Medicine, University of New Mexico School of Medicine; and Staff Cardiologist, Department of Internal Medicine, University of New Mexico Health Sciences Center, Albuquerque, New Mexico*

**Kirsten Tolstrup, M.D.** *Assistant Professor of Medicine, Department of Internal Medicine, University of California Los Angeles; and Staff Cardiologist, Department of Internal Medicine, Cedars-Sinai Medical Center, Los Angeles, California*

# Foreword

Physician skills in physical diagnosis have deteriorated during the last thirty years. No longer can the average cardiologist predict the valve area of a patient with mitral stenosis following a period of careful auscultation. Indeed, many primary care physicians today still experience difficulty hearing diastolic murmurs. Dr. Roldan and Dr. Abrams are attempting to remedy this deplorable situation with their new book, **Evaluation of the Patient with Heart Disease: Integrating the Physical Exam & Echocardiography**.

This text is not just a simple review of various aspects of the cardiovascular physical examination. Indeed, it is much more. The need for careful integration of physical findings and the results of an echocardiographic study make this text a "must read" for all cardiologists, noncardiologist physicians, medical students, residents in internal medicine and family practice, and mid-level providers. A simple clinical example will prove this point. If all elderly patients with a systolic ejection murmur underwent an echocardiographic examination in order to quantitate the degree of aortic stenosis, the cost each year to our health care system in the United States would be huge. However, universal use of echocardiography for such patients is not necessary if the practitioner realizes that most of these systolic murmurs represent benign aortic sclerosis. A semi-quantitative estimate of the aortic valve area can be obtained by timing the duration of the systolic ejection murmur with respect to the second heart sound. When the murmur fills 2/3 or less of systole, the aortic valve gradient, and hence, the severity of the aortic stenosis is modest. Such patients do not require an echocardiographic examination. Once the systolic ejection murmur fills more than 2/3 of systole, however, an echocardiographic study is indicated in order to quantitate the severity of the aortic stenotic lesion.

This text is filled with clinically relevant, important lessons like the one just given. Students of clinical medicine will benefit greatly from a thorough reading of this book. The principles learned from this text should improve the quality of medical care delivered by anyone who takes to heart the message of Dr. Roldan, Dr. Abrams, and their collaborators.

*Joseph S. Alpert, M.D.*
*Robert S. and Irene P. Flinn Professor of Medicine*
*Head*
*Department of Medicine*
*University of Arizona College of Medicine*
*Tucson, Arizona*

# Preface

The cardiovascular physical examination remains the oldest diagnostic tool (aside from the patient history) in the evaluation of real or suspected heart disease. Physicians in earlier eras often had highly proficient skills in the cardiac physical exam; many observations made by outstanding clinicians accurately predicted subsequent discoveries made with echocardiography or cardiac catheterization. In recent years, however, the "master clinician," skilled in cardiac physical diagnosis has become a disappearing breed. Medical students, housestaff, and many recently trained physicians have only rudimentary skills and knowledge of the cardiovascular exam. This book will guide the interested reader to an enhanced knowledge and understanding of cardiac physical diagnosis, and provides concordant discussions of the echocardiogram and its correlation with the physical exam. This integrative approach to the history, physical exam, and echocardiography is ideal for the evaluation of patients with suspected or known heart disease. A clear understanding of the diagnostic value and limitations of the physical exam and echocardiography will aid in the determination of the best diagnostic and therapeutic approach to patients with cardiac disorders.

Color-Doppler echocardiography is not only sensitive for the detection of heart disease, but it is also accurate in the assessment of the severity of cardiac disease, defining prognosis, and helping to define appropriate therapy. Transesophageal echocardiography (TEE), stress and contrast echocardiography, harmonic imaging, and three-dimensional echo, have all increased the applications of echocardiography for the detection of heart disease. Yet, echocardiography has limitations. It is technically inadequate for interpretation in at least 5% to 10% of patients. The sensitivity, specificity, and predictive accuracy of the ultrasound technique varies according to the echocardiographic modality utilized, and even for each type of heart disease. Echocardiography can miss, misclassify, underestimate or overestimate the severity of heart disease.

In spite of these limitations, because of its safety, overall accuracy, and easy availability, echocardiography has become routine in the evaluation of patients with suspected or known heart disease. However, in this era of cost containment, and despite the many positive attributes of echocardiography, a careful history and physical examination continue to be the primary screening methods in the assessment of individuals with suspected or known heart disease. Clinical data, then, should determine the need for echocardiography.

The cardiovascular physical examination is an important screening method for the detection of valvular, myocardial, and pericardial diseases. The experienced clinician, knowledgeable in conducting and interpreting the cardiac physical exam, can often predict the results of the echocardiogram. Both the presence and severity of valvular abnormalities are usually detectable by the physician. However, in the setting of left or right ventricular systolic dysfunction, the cardiac exam is often altered, such that the information obtainable on palpation and auscultation is diminished, often considerably. In patients with COPD or obesity and in those who are muscular or large breasted, the cardiac exam may be quite limited.

Despite the importance of the physical exam, and although the teaching and application of this technique should be encouraged, only a few textbooks on cardiovascular physical diagnosis are currently available. This contrasts with the many (and increasing number) of textbooks in echocardiography oriented to the education of cardiology fellows, practicing cardiologists, experts in echocardiography, and researchers. This is a paradox since the majority of patients undergoing echocardiography are referred by non-cardiologists. Such practitioners frequently have a limited understanding of the implications of positive or negative echocardiographic findings. This can lead to misinterpretation of results and omission or overuse of further work-up and cardiology consultations.

This text should enable the physician to correlate better and more accurately the echocardiographic findings with the physical exam. The purpose of this book is to provide the non-cardiologist physician or practitioner (medical students, mid-level providers, residents, practicing primary care providers) as well as cardiologists in training and practicing general cardiologists, with an integrative approach to the diagnostic utility and limitations of the physical exam and echocardiography. This book, in contrast to many currently available textbooks, provides disease-specific diagnostic criteria plus parameters of disease severity, and it includes Class I indications for echocardiography according to ACC/AHA guidelines. The text emphasizes the limitations of both the physical exam and echocardiography.

The contents of the book encompass the most prevalent and important heart diseases in an adult population, for which the physical exam and echocardiography are of primary and complementary diagnostic value. The fifteen chapters include much of adult structural cardiac disease. For each chapter, a detailed discussion of echocardiography follows a thorough review of the pertinent physical examination findings. Each chapter is illustrated with tables and figures and concludes with a summary statement or tables defining the diagnostic value and limitations of the physical exam and the echocardiogram.

We believe our text will reinforce the view that the physical exam remains of important diagnostic utility in the assessment of patients with suspected or known heart disease as well as allow a more appropriate utilization of echocardiography. This, in turn, should lead to a better understanding and integration of echocardiographic findings to clinical data. We hope this text will contribute to better and more cost-effective patient care.

*Carlos A. Roldan, M.D.*
*Jonathan Abrams, M.D.*

# Acknowledgments

Our sincere appreciation to all the contributors of this book. Their outstanding work will help make this book a valuable educational tool.

We thank the cardiac sonographers of the echocardiography laboratory of the Albuquerque Veterans Affairs Medical Center, Aggie Schaeffer and Frank T. Gurule, for their expert technical assistance in obtaining echocardiographic illustrations.

Our sincere appreciation to Jim Janis of Medical Media of the Albuquerque Veterans Affairs Medical Center for his expert technical assistance in the preparation of the illustrations for this book.

Finally, thanks to Sophie Gutierrez and Anne-Marie Collins-Hornyak for their secretarial and editorial assisstance.

# 1

# The Normal Cardiovascular Physical Examination

Jonathan Abrams

*Cardiology Division, University of New Mexico School of Medicine; and
Department of Internal Medicine, University Hospital, Albuquerque, New Mexico*

The cardiac physical examination is a useful and often important aspect of the evaluation of individuals with suspected or known cardiovascular disease. Furthermore, a careful examination occasionally can detect significant abnormalities in apparently normal people not suspected of having a cardiac problem (e.g., atrial or ventricular septal defect, hypertrophic cardiomyopathy, significant valve disease).

Assessment of cardiac size and function by physical examination requires knowledge and skill. The physician should approach the patient in a systematic fashion that has long been validated by experience (but not randomized clinical trials).

This chapter outlines the cardinal features of the cardiac examination. In this era of high-tech medicine (including echo Doppler), intelligent use of eyes, hands, and ears can provide valuable information about our patients and a real sense of satisfaction of a job well done.

## PERTINENT FEATURES OF CARDIAC SOUND

Several features of cardiac sound require analysis during auscultation. *Loudness* of sound is a subjective judgment and is closely related to the amplitude or intensity of sound waves. The *pitch* of a heart sound or murmur relates to the underlying *frequency*. Low-frequency sounds are low pitched (25 to 150 Hz), whereas high-frequency sounds are high pitched. The audible range of cardiac sound is approximately 30 to 80 Hz; the optimal range of auditory acuity is 1,000 to 2,000 Hz, higher than the range of most cardiac sound. Very-low-frequency events (<25 Hz) are inaudible but often may be palpable; this explains the occasional finding of palpable atrial and ventricular filling sounds ($S_4$ and $S_3$).

### Theory of Heart Sound Production

Cardiac sound represents vibrations of cardiac structures (muscle, valves) and blood

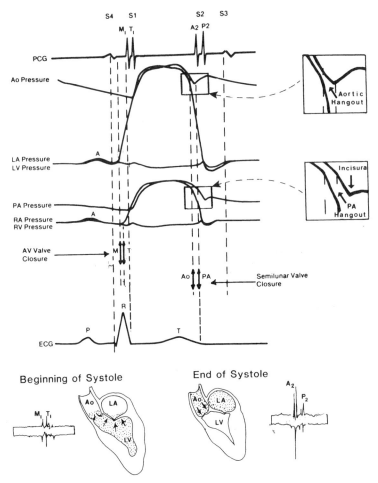

**FIG. 1.1.** Relationship of heart sounds to intracardiac pressures and valve motion. Note that pressure crossover between the atria and the ventricles, as well as between the ventricles and the great vessels, always precedes the resultant cardiac sound. Actual valve closure is either synchronous with or immediately precedes the related heart sound. See text for further discussion. (Abrams J. The First Heart Sound. PC, 1981;7:21–43. Adapted in part from Luisada A, MacCanon DM; and modified from Abrams J. Prim Cardiol 1982.)

within the heart. These vibrations are produced by acceleration or deceleration of the blood mass during the cardiac cycle. Tensing of closed valves results from rapidly increasing pressure gradients producing sound vibrations. Pressure "crossover" initiating $S_1$ or $S_2$ (e.g., left atrial–left ventricular [LA-LV], aorta–LV) always precedes the heart sound itself (Fig. 1.1). Thus, valve leaflets are still in motion at the precise point of pressure crossover.

### Cardiac Cycle

#### *Systole*

Electrical activation of the ventricles is initiated by the QRS of the electrocardiogram (ECG). Depolarization of the LV begins before the right ventricle (RV). The rapidly rising pressure in each ventricle helps close the two atrioventricular (AV) valves, resulting in the first heart sound ($S_1$). However, because the LV has a far greater muscle mass and must develop a peak systolic pressure four to five times greater than the RV, it takes longer for LV isovolumic pressure to open the aortic valve than for RV pressure to open the pulmonary valve (isovolumic contraction time). Thus, pulmonary valve opening and ejection of the aortic blood begin before the aortic valve opens (Fig. 1.1).

### *Diastole*

During inspiration, aortic valve closure ($A_2$) occurs before pulmonary valve closure ($P_2$), but during expiration the two valves normally close simultaneously. Pressure continues to fall in both ventricles after semilunar valve closure (isovolumic relaxation); the AV valves open passively (and silently) in early diastole when ventricular pressure drops below that in the corresponding atrium. The mitral valve opens before the tricuspid valve (Fig. 1.1).

Rapid ventricular filling follows the maximal opening excursion of the mitral and tricuspid valves in diastole and may result in the third heart sound ($S_3$). Approximately 70% to 80% of the ventricular end-diastolic volume is achieved during early and mid diastole, well before atrial contraction. The AV valves drift back toward their respective atria with a closing motion in mid diastole. Following the P wave, the atria contract and the AV valves reopen, resulting in augmentation of blood flow to the ventricles in late diastole ($S_4$). At end-diastole, the AV valves again begin a closing movement. The mitral and tricuspid valves close completely with the onset of ventricular contraction. Ventricular–atrial pressure crossover, however, precedes actual AV valve closure (Fig. 1.1).

### Stethoscope and Its Proper Uses

The stethoscope consists of a dual *chest piece* with a valve that allows switching from bell to diaphragm, *binaural connectors,* and *earpieces.* The component parts should be well made, durable, without air leaks, and easy to use.

### *Bell*

The bell (Fig. 1.2) is used primarily for detection of low-frequency sound (30 to 150 Hz). *Lower frequencies are attenuated, and higher frequencies are accentuated as increased pressure is applied to the bell.* Firm pressure with the bell stretches the skin of the chest wall, which then transmits higher-frequency sound vibrations; the bell then performs similarly to the diaphragm of the stethoscope. *Practical Point: To emphasize detection of low-frequency sounds (e.g., $S_3$, $S_4$, mitral rumble), the lightest possible contact pressure should be used with the bell.*

The bell should have a large diameter (at least 1 inch). A detachable rubber ring is highly desirable for use in conjunction with the bell (Fig. 1.2). This allows for light skin contact pressure, minimizes air leaks, increases the diameter of the bell, and does not get cold.

### *Diaphragm*

The diaphragm is the high-frequency component of the chest piece. A proper diaphragm

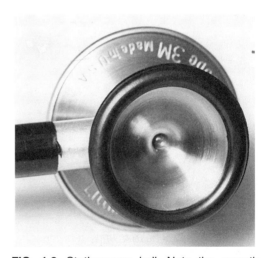

**FIG. 1.2.** Stethoscope bell. Note the smooth rubber rim attached to the metallic bell. It is advisable to use a rubber ring with the stethoscope bell in order to provide a skin seal with light stethoscope pressure, thus increasing the ability to hear low-frequency cardiac sound.

should filter out low frequencies (<300 Hz); often, it will amplify high-pitched cardiac sound. As with the bell, increasing pressure tightens the skin and allows transmission of higher-frequency sound.

### *Identification of Systole and Diastole*

Proper identification of the two phases of the cardiac cycle usually is not difficult. During tachycardia, however, diastole shortens more than systole and, with rapid heart rates, it may be difficult to distinguish between the two. *Practical Point: Use the carotid pulse and apical impulse to identify the phases of the cardiac cycle. The carotid upstroke and*

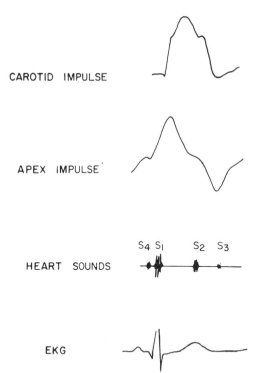

**FIG. 1.3.** Timing of heart sounds. It is important to use simultaneous palpation of the carotid arterial pulse or apical impulse when listening to the heart sounds. Note that $S_1$ immediately precedes the upstroke of the carotid pulse and is virtually simultaneous with the earliest palpable precordial activity. $S_2$ marks the end of systole and follows the palpable carotid and apical impulse.

*the beginning outward thrust of the initial apex beat immediately follow $S_1$. $S_2$ occurs shortly after the carotid and apical impulses are felt (Fig. 1.3).*

### *Helpful Hints on Stethoscope Use*

#### *"Inching"*

Levine and Harvey popularized this valuable technique in which the stethoscope is slowly moved or inched from a site on the chest where systole and diastole are identified clearly to other precordial locations where it is more difficult to determine which sound is systolic or diastolic. It usually is best to begin auscultation at the base where systole and diastole usually are most easily identified.

#### *Selective Listening*

Selective listening is the hallmark of accurate and meaningful cardiac auscultation. The importance of focusing on only one part of the cardiac cycle at a time during auscultation has been stressed by Dr. W. Proctor Harvey. For instance, when early systole is analyzed, only the acoustic events around $S_1$ are auscultated. The rest of systole and all of diastole are consciously excluded. Systole and diastole should each be divided into early and late phases and each segment focused upon in turn. Heart sounds should be assessed first, followed by attention to heart murmurs. With this approach, little will be missed. *Practical Point: Intense concentration is the key to competent cardiac auscultation.*

## CARDIAC EXAMINATION

### Arterial Pulse

Examination of the arterial pulse often reveals valuable information about the cardiovascular system. In certain conditions, such as aortic valve disease, hypertrophic cardiomyopathy, and pericardial tamponade, accurate assessment of pulse contour and amplitude can be of great importance in making a proper diagnosis.

### Normal Physiology

The arterial pulse wave is related to many physiologic factors, including LV stroke volume and ejection velocity and compliance of the arterial system. The relative distensibility or "stiffness" of the arterial system affects both the contour and velocity of the arterial pulse.

The first portion of the central aortic pulse wave (Fig. 1.4) reflects peak velocity of blood ejected during early systole, which is "stored" in the central aorta. The mid to late systolic portion of the normal pulse wave is produced by blood moving from the central aorta *to* the periphery simultaneous with a reflection of the pulse wave returning *from* the arteries of the upper body. With aging or decreased compliance of the arterial tree, the later portion of the pulse wave is accentuated, and the pulse contour becomes somewhat more sustained.

Diastole is initiated by an abrupt negative wave called the dicrotic notch (Fig. 1.4). The nadir coincides precisely with aortic leaflet closure and the aortic component of $S_2$ ($A_2$). *Practical Point: The dicrotic notch normally is not felt.*

### Pulse Wave Alteration in the Periphery

The normal pulse contour becomes altered with increasing distance from the aortic valve, being characterized by a greater amplitude and velocity and a lower dicrotic notch. These changes become progressively more pronounced distally (Fig. 1.5). *Practical Point: The peripheral arteries (e.g., radial, femoral) should not be used to routinely assess the arterial pulse contour. Normal physiologic pulse wave alteration in distal vessels may mask important diagnostic information present in the proximal vessels.*

### Pulse Wave Alterations with Decreased Vascular Compliance

In states of increased vascular resistance or stiffness, such as occurs with atherosclerosis, hypertension, and vasoconstriction, the relatively noncompliant arterial tree contributes to increased pulse wave velocity. This increase results in a pulse contour with a rapid upstroke and greater amplitude. *Practical Point: In older subjects, hypertensive patients, or those with diffuse vascular disease, information obtained from examina-*

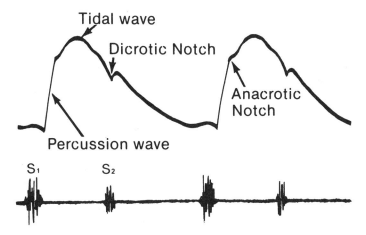

**FIG. 1.4.** Normal arterial pulse. Note the rapid upstroke, the rounded summit or peak, and the falloff in late systole. Normally, only the systolic peak is palpable; diastolic events are not felt. The dicrotic notch times precisely with $S_2$ and is coincident with aortic and pulmonic valve closure. The terms percussion wave, tidal wave, and anacrotic notch are discussed in the text. (The Arterial Pulse. PC, 1982;8:138–158.)

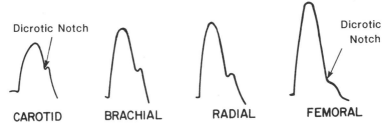

**FIG. 1.5.** Arterial pulse contour alteration in the peripheral circulation. As the distance increases from the peripheral artery to the central aorta, the amplitude and upstroke velocity of the pulse contour also increase and the dicrotic notch becomes lower. The higher systolic pressure in peripheral arteries is one reason why the arterial pulse is best evaluated at the carotid artery rather than distally. (The Arterial Pulse. PC, 1982;8:138–158.)

*tion of the arterial pulse is less reliable. Conversely, with intense arterial vasoconstriction, the palpable pulse volume may appear to be reduced when, in fact, the ejected stroke volume is normal.*

### *Examination*

#### *Technique*

Both the patient and the physician should be relaxed. The subject's head and thorax should be slightly elevated at 15 to 30 degrees. Either the thumb or the first two fingers are used to feel the arterial pulse; the finger pads usually are quite sensitive for optimal palpation. Gentle but firm pressure is necessary, with the thumb or finger placed directly on the summit of the vessel. To obtain maximal information, the palpating pressure should be varied. Surprisingly light pressure may be needed once direct contact with the blood vessel has been established. The normal pulse has a brief crest that is slightly sustained and somewhat rounded (Fig. 1.4).

#### *Which Artery to Palpate?*

In a complete cardiovascular examination, all accessible arterial pulses should be assessed. It is important to compare bilateral vessels. A missing or extremely weak pulse may have major significance, suggesting atherosclerosis, embolic occlusion, dissection, vascular compression, or a congenital anom-

aly. In any patient with hypertension or in infants with heart failure, the radial or brachial artery and the femoral artery *must be palpated simultaneously* to exclude coarctation of the aorta. Normally, the femoral pulsation immediately precedes the radial pulse; in coarctation, the femoral arterial pulse is distinctly delayed and reduced in volume when compared to the arm pulses.

#### *Use the Carotid Artery*

The carotid arterial pulse provides the most accurate evaluation of arterial pulse volume and contour because it is the largest palpable proximal vessel, is the closest accessible artery to the aortic valve, and its contour closely resembles the directly recorded central aortic pulse. On the other hand, distal vessels may be affected by typical waveform alterations that occur in peripheral arteries (Fig. 1.5). Thus, diagnostic abnormalities of the central arterial pulse may be attenuated or disappear in the peripheral circulation.

When examining the carotid artery, careful attention should be paid to the lower half of the neck. The adjacent sternocleidomastoid muscle should be under no tension, and pressure should not be placed on the carotid sinus itself.

#### *Characteristics to Assess*

The characteristics to assess are *cardiac rhythm, pulse volume* (generally related to the size of the stroke volume), *pulse amplitude,* and *pulse contour,* with special attention to the crest or peak of the pulse and rate of rise of ejection (early systole).

Occasionally one can feel a shudder or thrill in the carotid pulse representing a palpable bruit or transmitted murmur. Localized atherosclerosis or abnormalities of the LV outflow tract account for most carotid thrills. A hyperkinetic circulation, often found in normal children or patients with aortic regurgitation, may produce a slight "buzz" to the carotid pulse.

In older subjects or those in whom there is suspicion of peripheral vascular disease, both the carotid and femoral arteries should be routinely auscultated and palpated.

### Jugular Venous Pulse

Careful observation of the venous pulse can lead to valuable information about cardiac events. Unfortunately, examination of the neck veins often is viewed with anxiety and dismay; the terminology appears arcane, the task obscure.

### *Normal Physiology*

Although the venous system contains about 70% to 80% of the circulating blood volume, it maintains a very low intravascular pressure (3 to 7 mm Hg). Thus, venous compliance is high, that is, veins are extremely distensible. During diastole, the jugular veins directly reflect RV filling pressure; during systole, right atrial (RA) pressure. Thus, analysis of the jugular venous pulse provides considerable information about right-sided cardiac physiology.

### *Waveforms*

There are two visible peaks or waves and two visible descents or troughs in the normal jugular venous pulse (Fig. 1.6). The A wave is followed by the X descent, and the V wave is followed by the Y descent. When the jugular pulse or RA pressure is recorded, a C wave usually is present, interrupting the X descent.

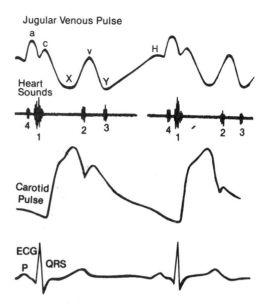

**FIG. 1.6.** Normal jugular venous pulse. Note the biphasic venous waveform with a large A wave immediately preceding the carotid upstroke and roughly coinciding with $S_1$, and a smaller V wave that peaks almost coincident with $S_2$. The jugular X descent occurs during systole and in some individuals may be quite prominent. The Y descent occurs during early diastole; the nadir of the Y descent times with $S_3$. The C wave and H wave are not visible to the eye but are often recordable in venous pulse tracings. (The Jugular Venous Pulse. PC, 1982;8:33–44.)

The physiologic bases of these waves and descents is as follows.

*A Wave.* This wave directly reflects RA contraction, which results in retrograde blood flow into the superior vena cava and jugular veins. The jugular venous A wave follows the P wave of the ECG, precedes the upstroke of the carotid pulse, and is almost synchronous with $S_1$.

*X Descent.* The early portion of the X descent results from RA relaxation during atrial diastole. The later and dominant portion reflects the fall in RA pressure during early RV systole, as the tricuspid valve ring is pulled caudally by the contracting RV ("descent of the base").

The X descent is often the most prominent motion of the normal jugular venous pulse. It begins *during systole* and ends just before $S_2$.

*C Wave.* This positive wave has caused enormous controversy and confusion over the years. *Practical Point: Because the C wave usually is not visible as a separate waveform and has no importance in the examination of the jugular venous pulse, it should be disregarded.*

*V Wave.* The V wave is the second major positive wave. It begins in late systole and ends in early diastole. The V wave results from continued venous inflow into the RA during ventricular systole while the tricuspid valve is closed. It is roughly synchronous with the carotid pulse and peaks just after $S_2$.

*Y Descent.* The Y descent is the negative deflection of RA pressure that occurs when the tricuspid valve opens in early diastole. It begins and ends during diastole.

*Practical Point: In normal persons, the RA A wave is larger than the V wave, and the X descent is more prominent than the Y descent. When the neck veins are examined, in the normal subject and most conditions, a larger A than V wave will be seen (Fig. 1.6).*

### Respiratory Influences

Inspiration may result in increased visibility of the venous pulse. During inspiration, the velocity of venous flow and the return to the right heart increases. RA and RV contraction become more vigorous (Starling effect), exaggerating the X and Y descents. Although mean venous pressure falls slightly, the waveforms are accentuated during inspiration.

### *Examination*

#### *Anatomy*

The venous pulse is visible but not palpable. The external jugular veins course vertically over the sternocleidomastoid muscle posterior and lateral to the internal jugular vein. Discrete external venous pulsations usually are seen more easily than the internal jugular system (Fig. 1.7); however, when visible, assessment of the internal jugular veins

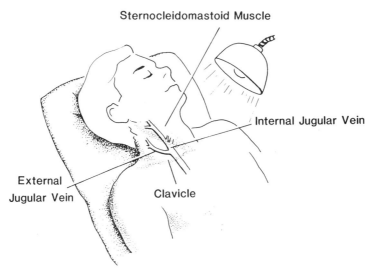

Sternocleidomastoid Muscle

Internal Jugular Vein

External Jugular Vein

Clavicle

**FIG. 1.7.** Important landmarks of the venous pulse. The external jugular veins are easily seen lateral to the sternocleidomastoid muscles, extending vertically upward toward the back of the ear. The internal jugular veins are of small amplitude and undulant in nature. They usually are not well seen in individuals with a normal venous pulse but may be prominent when the jugular venous pressure is elevated or when prominent V waves are present. The ideal patient position consists of modest elevation of the thorax and head. It is important for the patient to be relaxed with no tension on the neck muscles. Tangential lighting is helpful to accentuate the jugular veins.

is *preferable* to the external jugular veins. The right side of the neck usually is better than the left for examination of the jugular venous pulse.

### Patient Position

The patient should be reclining and comfortable without excessive tension on the tissues of the neck (Fig. 1.7). Often, it is helpful to elevate the chin and slightly rotate the head to the left, gently stretching the skin of the right lower neck and supraclavicular area. Natural light is desirable for inspection of the venous pulsations, although a flashlight or bedside lamp can be beneficial to cast a shadow on the venous pulsations occurring in the lower neck.

### Estimating Venous Pressure

Optimal positioning of the neck and thorax is essential for analysis of venous pressure and waveforms. The examiner first should estimate whether the venous pressure is normal or elevated and then position the patient accordingly.

*Normal Venous Pressure.* In most patients without elevation of venous pressure, the supine or 15- to 30-degree position is best. The patient's head and neck must be positioned so that the venous waveforms are clearly identifiable. The height of the venous column at the peak of the A and V waves generally is taken as an indication of the venous pressure, although the actual mean jugular venous pressure will be slightly lower.

The sternal angle (of Louis), found at the junction of the manubrium and sternum at the level of the second rib, is used as the standard reference point for determining venous pressure noninvasively. In the supine position, the RA is 5 to 7 cm below this point. Conventional wisdom has held that the RA is approximately 5 cm below the sternal angle at *any* body position; therefore, the height of the mean jugular venous pulse was determined by measuring the distance from the angle of Louis to the estimated level of the venous column and adding 5 cm to give an approximation of the mean RA pressure. However, this "golden rule" is erroneous. Although it is true that when patients are lying flat, the RA pressure is approximately 5 cm below the sternum, as soon as the thorax is elevated to 30 degrees or more, the relationship between the RA and the sternal angle is altered such that the physician should add *10 cm* to the height of the venous column from the sternal angle to obtain an estimate of the peak venous pressure. Thus, if the mean venous column is 3 cm above the sternal angle with the chest at 45 degrees, the estimated venous pressure is 13 cm $H_2O$, which is elevated.

One should make a diagnosis of an *elevated* mean jugular venous pressure when the thorax is positioned at 30 degrees or greater from the horizontal and the mean peak of the venous column is clearly 2 to 3 cm $H_2O$ or more above the sternal angle of Louis. In the supine position, however, or with only a pillow under the patient's head, the venous column can be up to 2 to 3 cm above the sternal landmark and still be normal.

*Elevated Venous Pressure.* In conditions where the venous pressure is very high, pulsations may not be seen until the patient is sitting up, and even then the waves may be invisible. Careful inspection of the upper neck beneath the angle of the jaw is important. The external jugular veins also should be analyzed when increased levels of venous pressure are suggested. In severe tricuspid insufficiency, the ear lobes and soft tissues of the upper neck may move gently laterally with each V wave.

*Practical Point: Adequate visualization of the jugular venous pressure is difficult, if not impossible, in many persons, particularly obese subjects or patients with short, thick necks. Nevertheless, with care and attention to detail, the venous pulse can be identified in the majority of subjects.*

### Timing of Venous Waves

Timing the venous pulse is best assessed by palpating the left carotid pulse simultaneously with visual inspection of the right-sided jugular veins. This approach relies on the dominance of the jugular A wave, which will be seen as a flickering pulsation just *before* the carotid artery pulse is felt. *Practical Point: Identification of the jugular A wave preceding the palpable carotid pulse usually is all that is necessary for accurate identification of the venous pulse waves.*

### Hepatojugular Reflux (Abdominal Compression Test)

This technique, popularized by Ewy, uses sustained pressure applied to the right upper quadrant of the abdomen. The hepatojugular reflux test is a useful diagnostic maneuver when the jugular venous pulse is borderline elevated or when latent RV failure or silent tricuspid regurgitation is suspected. Abdominal compression forces venous blood into the thorax. A failing or dilated RV may not be able to receive the augmented venous return to the right heart without a rise in mean venous pressure. In normal persons, prolonged (60 seconds) abdominal pressure will not elevate the venous pressure or will cause only a slight (1 cm) elevation that is not sustained. In congestive heart failure or tricuspid regurgitation, this maneuver will result in elevation of the venous pressure >1 cm that persists throughout the time the pressure is applied. The hepatojugular reflux test then is said to be positive (Fig. 1.8).

*Technique.* In the abdominal compression test, the patient is positioned so that the upper level of the venous column is at mid-neck level. Gentle but firm compression of the right upper quadrant with an open-fingered hand is applied for 10 to 20 seconds. If there is significant tenderness or discomfort over the liver, the pressure can be applied elsewhere in the abdomen with similar results.

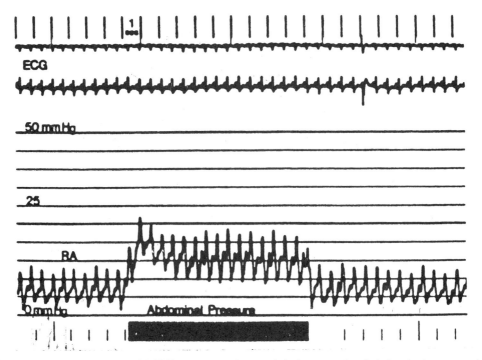

**FIG. 1.8.** Elevation in right atrial (RA) pressure observed during sustained abdominal pressure in a patient with mild congestive heart failure. (Courtesy of Gordon Ewy, M.D.)

**TABLE 1.1.** *Differentiation of jugular venous pulsations from carotid arterial pulse*

|  | Internal jugular vein | Carotid artery |
|---|---|---|
| Location | Low in neck; lateral | Deep in neck; medial |
| Contour | Double peaked | Single peaked |
| Character | Undulant, not palpable | Forceful, brisk, easily felt |
| Inspiration | A and V waves often more visible, although mean pressure decreases | No change |
| Upright position | Decrease in mean pressure | No change |
| Compressibility | Readily obliterated by gentle pressure 3–4 cm above clavicle | Cannot compress easily |
| Abdominal compression | May see transient increase in pressure | No effect |

A positive test indicates incipient or actual RV failure (Fig. 1.8). In isolated LV failure, the response will be normal. Patients with hypervolemia or fluid overload will have a positive test.

### Differentiation of Jugular and Carotid Pulses

In most instances, careful examination of the neck pulses should prevent confusing venous with carotid artery activity. In severe tricuspid regurgitation, however, venous pulsations may be palpable and visible from the foot of the bed and be confused with the arterial pulsations of severe aortic regurgitation. Table 1.1 lists the features that allow proper identification of the venous and arterial pulses in the neck.

### Precordial Impulse

Precordial palpation enables the physician to detect cardiac activity on the chest wall. In the normal individual, cardiac motion is represented by the *apex beat* or *apical impulse,* produced by contraction of the LV free wall and septum. When cardiac hypertrophy or dilatation is present, abnormal systolic and diastolic events emanating from the LV or RV may be detected on palpation.

### Normal Precordial Activity

The palpable apical impulse in a normal subject is produced by anterior movement of the LV during early systole (Fig. 1.9). As intraventricular pressure rises, the LV rotates in a counterclockwise direction on its long axis as the cardiac apex lifts and makes contact with the left anterior chest wall. Following aortic valve opening, the LV chamber moves away from the chest wall after the first half of ejection, and the ventricle continues to decrease in size until systole is completed. Thus, the impulse felt or recorded on the precordium consists of an early outward thrust followed by retraction during the last part of

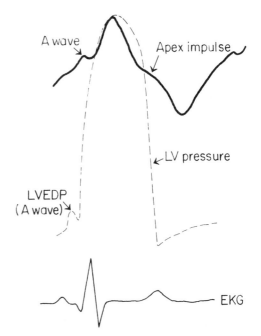

**FIG. 1.9.** Relationships of the normal apical impulse to left ventricular pressure. LVEDP, left ventricular end-diastolic pressure. (From Abrams J. Precordial motion. In: Horwitz LD, Groves BM, eds. Signs and symptoms in cardiology. Philadelphia: JB Lippincott, 1985, with permission.)

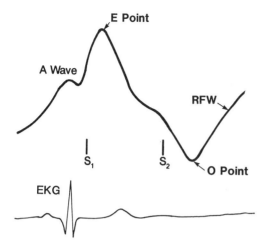

**FIG. 1.10.** Normal precordial impulse. Note that the outward motion occurs entirely within the first half of systole. The left ventricle retracts from the chest wall as it becomes smaller during late systole. The palpable apical impulse is brief. Normally, the A wave and diastolic events are not palpable. RFW, rapid filling wave.

systole. *Practical Point: Normal palpable cardiac activity occurs only during the first half of systole.* Diastolic events, such as those produced by rapid LV filling ($S_3$) or LA contraction ($S_4$), normally are not palpable, but with alterations in LV diastolic volume, pressure, or compliance, these events may be palpable (Fig. 1.10). The characteristics of the normal precordial impulse are listed in Table 1.2.

### Right Ventricular Activity

Although the RV, located just beneath the sternum and left third to fifth ribs, is closer to

**TABLE 1.2.** *Normal supine apical impulse*

- Gentle, nonsustained tap
- Early systolic anterior motion that ends before the last third of systole
- Located within 10 cm of the mid-sternal line in the fourth or fifth left intercostal space
- A palpable area <2 to 2.5 cm$^2$ and detectable in only one intercostal space
- Right ventricular motion normally not palpable
- May be completely absent in older persons

the chest wall than the LV, RV activity normally is not felt. In normal children and young adults or thin subjects who have a narrow anteroposterior (AP) thoracic diameter, gentle RV activity occasionally may be felt.

### *Examination of the Precordium*

The subject should be lying comfortably in the supine position or with the thorax elevated no more than 30 degrees (Fig. 1.11). *Practical Point: Patients with suspect or definite cardiovascular disease should be routinely examined both in the supine and left lateral decubitus position. The subject should be instructed to turn on his or her left side at a 45- to 60-degree angle to the examining table and elevate the left arm above the head so that the physician may have unobstructed access to the left precordium (Fig. 1.12).*

### *Inspection*

This may be more helpful after preliminary palpation has identified the site of the apex or other impulses, if present. Retraction movements may be more obvious to the eye than outward motion and can be quite prominent

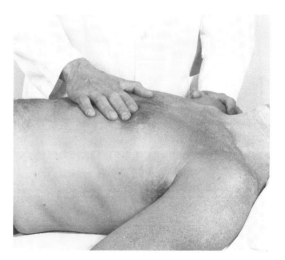

**FIG. 1.11.** Palpation of the apex, supine position.

with severe LV or RV enlargement. Tangential lighting may accentuate visible movements on the chest wall.

### Palpation

The examiner should be standing comfortably at the patient's right side. Both the palm of the hand and the ventral surface of the proximal metacarpals and fingers may be used for palpation. Varying pressure should be applied once the precordial impulse is identified. High-frequency sounds, such as increased $S_1$, opening snap, or transmitted thrill, are best detected with firm application of the hand to the chest. However, the subtle low-frequency motion of a palpable $S_3$ or $S_4$ or double systolic apical impulse will be felt only with light pressure.

Timing of precordial events is best carried out using simultaneous palpation of the carotid arterial pulse with the left hand (Fig. 1.4). Some find that concomitant auscultation of $S_1$ and $S_2$ is useful for timing purposes.

### Right Ventricle

The patient is supine. Held end-expiration is optimal for the RV examination. Firm pressure using the palm or heel of the hand with the wrist cocked upward is advisable (Fig. 1.13). The lower sternum and adjacent third through fifth ribs and left interspaces should be examined in this manner. *Movement of the examining hand and fingers should be carefully sought, as the typical low-amplitude RV activity often is better seen than felt.*

Some experts suggest exploring the subxiphoid or epigastric region with the extended fingers oriented superiorly. The patient should be instructed to hold the breath in end-inspiration while the descending RV is carefully palpated. This technique is particularly useful in patients with an increased AP diameter, chronic obstructive pulmonary disease, obesity, or muscular chest in whom a parasternal impulse cannot be felt.

### Characteristics of the Normal Apical Impulse

Characteristics Of the normal apical impulse are given in Table 1.2 and Fig. 1.10. In

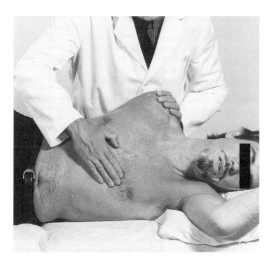

**FIG. 1.12.** Palpation of the apical impulse, left lateral decubitus position. This maneuver should be used in any patient with suspected left ventricular disease. The patient should be turned 45 to 60 degrees onto the left side with the left arm extended above the head. (From Abrams J. Precordial palpation. In: Horwitz LD, Groves BM, eds. Signs and symptoms in cardiology. Philadelphia: JB Lippincott, 1985, with permission.)

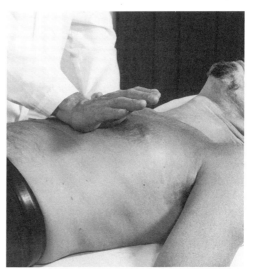

**FIG. 1.13.** Precordial palpation for detection of parasternal or right ventricular activity. Use firm downward pressure with the heel of the hand while the patient's breath is held in end-expiration.

normal subjects, the apical impulse in the supine position or at 30-degree elevation produces a gentle outward motion that usually is felt in only one interspace. This anterior movement is brief and nonsustained, pulling away from the examining fingers by mid systole. It occupies a maximal area of 2 to 2.5 cm (no larger than a quarter) and is located in the fourth or fifth left interspace at or inside the mid-clavicular line. It usually is within 7 to 8 cm from the left sternal edge and should not be located >10 cm to the left of the mid-sternal line. In tall, thin persons, the apex beat can be distal (sixth interspace) and more medial than usual. When there is intrathoracic disease or a short stocky body habitus, the apex beat may be displaced leftward. It has been suggested that an apical impulse of 3 cm in area or greater in the left lateral position is specific for LV enlargement. In the supine position, the palpable apical impulse should be no larger than a nickel (2 to 3 cm) and should be felt in only one intercostal space.

*Right Ventricular Activity.* In the normal subject, parasternal activity usually is not detectable except in young or thin persons. In such cases, a gentle shock or tap at the lower left sternal border may be felt. Forceful, sustained, or high-amplitude parasternal motion is always an abnormal finding. Occasionally a pulmonary artery impulse in the second to third left interspace adjacent to the sternum may be detected.

*Other Palpable Events.* In a subject with suspected cardiac disease, the examiner should explore the entire precordium with firm pressure of the hand and proximal fingers, analyzing the aortic, pulmonic, lower sternal, and apical regions. In such a fashion, the unexpected vascular impulse, such as a dilated or aneurysmal ascending aorta or pulmonary artery, may be detected. If a patient has coronary artery disease, particularly previous myocardial infarction, careful examination for an ectopic impulse should be carried out (see Chapter 3). This typically occurs medial and superior to the apical impulse. Use of the entire palm and proximal metacarpals will help detect the diffuse lift of a very large LV

or RV. On occasion, the entire anterior precordium will move in systole. This technique also is suited for the detection of thrills and palpable heart sounds.

### Percussion

Under ordinary circumstances, percussion is not a useful procedure. However, when the point of maximal impulse (PMI) cannot be identified in the supine or left decubitus position, this technique may help establish the presence or absence of cardiomegaly and detect the approximate left border of the heart.

### Variations of the Apex Beat

#### Absent Apical Impulse

It is not commonly realized that many older subjects (over age 50) do not have palpable cardiac activity when they are examined in the supine position. Whenever an apical impulse cannot be felt in the supine position, the left heart border should be percussed, and the patient should be carefully examined in the left lateral decubitus position (Fig. 1.12). The latter is a much more valuable maneuver than percussion. In most adults, LV activity can be detected when the subject is turned onto the left side, particularly in expiration. Often the PMI then may be detectable when the patient is again turned supine. In some normal adults, an apical impulse will not be detectable in either position.

### What to Look For

Assessment of the apical cardiac impulse should include analysis of the following parameters: (i) location, (ii) duration, (iii) size, (iv) force, and (v) contour. In addition, visual inspection of the chest for the presence of prominent retraction waves, as well as systolic and diastolic events, should be carried out.

#### Characteristics of the Apical Impulse

*Location.* Identify the site of impulse on the thorax with respect to both the longitudinal and horizontal axes of the patient. Note in which intercostal space the PMI or apex beat is located; occasionally a large heart will result in detectable precordial activity in two or even three intercostal spaces. Localize the apical impulse with reference to the mid-clavicular line, distance from the mid sternum, or relationship to the left anterior axillary line.

*Duration.* The duration of the systolic outward motion probably is the most important feature of the precordial examination. *Practical Point: Although cardiomegaly or hypertrophy can exist in the presence of a brief "normal" outward movement, or even when the PMI is absent, a truly sustained LV impulse in the supine or 30-degree elevation position is distinctly abnormal* (Fig. 1.14C). Such findings suggest a pressure overloaded ventricle (e.g., aortic stenosis, hypertension), depressed LV ejection fraction, or a substantially dilated LV cavity.

*The critical point to assess is whether or not the impulse "stays up" into the second half of systole.* Proper timing of the apex beat using simultaneous auscultation of $S_1$ and $S_2$ is essential in making this observation.

*Size.* If the apical impulse is larger than normal, it is useful to note the area of contact with the chest. Any impulse >2 to 2.5 cm in the supine position or >3 cm in the left decubitus position represents cardiac enlargement.

*Force or Amplitude.* Is the apex beat a soft, unimpressive impulse, or does it lift the examining fingers off the chest wall? Is the anterior or outward excursion greater than normal, consistent with a hyperdynamic or hyperkinetic PMI? An increase in force is consistent with LV hypertrophy and preserved systolic function. Assessment of the force of contraction is the most subjective and least quantifiable aspect of precordial examination.

*Contour.* The normal apical impulse consists of a brief, nonsustained anterior motion in early systole (Figs. 1.10 and 1.14A). A sustained LV beat is the most common abnormality of contour, but occasionally other patterns are noted.

A double systolic impulse may be seen in hypertrophic obstructive cardiomyopathy and occasionally in some patients with severe LV dyssynergy or an LV aneurysm in coronary artery disease.

*Palpable Fourth Heart Sound.* Presystolic distention commonly is found in the left lateral position in patients who have decreased LV compliance, such as coronary artery disease, hypertensive heart disease, or aortic valve disease (Fig. 1.15). A palpable A wave reflects high LV end-diastolic pressure and decreased LV compliance. It is an important observation, as it suggests the presence of LV

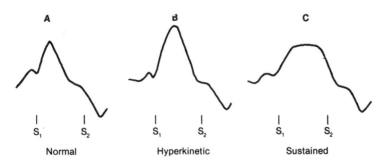

| A | B | C |
| S₁  S₂ | S₁  S₂ | S₁  S₂ |
| Normal | Hyperkinetic | Sustained |

**FIG. 1.14.** Precordial motion patterns. **A:** Normal left ventricular impulse. The outward motion is brief and low amplitude. **B:** Hyperdynamic impulse. Note that the duration of the impulse is unchanged from normal, but the amplitude is greater. This is a common finding in individuals with hyperkinetic states or volume/diastolic overload, such as mitral or aortic regurgitation. Often, the site of the apical impulse in such individuals will be displaced laterally and downward. **C:** Sustained left ventricular impulse. This finding is characteristic of a left ventricular chamber that is substantially dilated, usually but not always with depression of systolic dysfunction. The point of maximum impulse (PMI) is almost always displaced to the left and inferiorly at this stage, and the force of apical impulse is often increased. This type of impulse often is called a left ventricular heave.

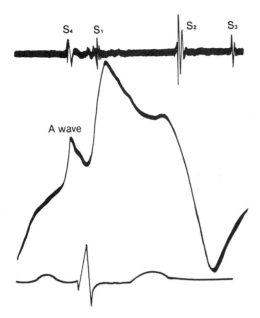

$S_4$   $S_1$      $S_2$   $S_3$

A wave

**FIG. 1.15.** Palpable atrial sound. Careful examination of the left ventricular apex beat may reveal that a very loud $S_4$ is associated with a palpable presystolic impulse. This is more likely to be found when patients are turned into the left lateral decubitus position. *Practical Point: The presence of a palpable $S_4$ indicates that the atrial sound is pathologic.* (Abrams J. The third and fourth heart sounds. Primary Cardiology, 1982;156–168.)

hypertrophy and increased chamber stiffness. Audibility of the $S_4$ does not correlate with palpability; presystolic distention may be detectable when the $S_4$ is quite soft. Occasionally one is not able to hear an $S_4$, although it is clearly palpable.

*Palpable Third Heart Sound.* The third sound is less often palpable than an $S_4$. It is found most often in severe mitral regurgitation or a markedly dilated cardiomyopathic ventricle. As with the $S_4$, palpation of the LV $S_3$ is greatly enhanced in the left decubitus position. The $S_3$ will be noted as a brief outward motion occurring in early diastole that gently taps the examiner's finger pads.

*Parasternal or Right Ventricular Impulses.* All of the above (palpable $S_3$ and $S_4$) also apply to the evaluation of RV or parasternal activity. However, the low-amplitude impulse produced

by RV hypertrophy or dilation usually is more difficult to evaluate than LV apical activity. Nevertheless, an increase in amplitude or sustained parasternal motion usually is discernible with careful examination technique.

RV abnormalities are only detectable in the supine position. Firm downward pressure with the hand on the lower left sternal area is necessary; the patient should be alerted that the examiner will be pushing down on the sternum (Fig. 1.13). Because RV activity usually is low amplitude, it will not be detected without such firm compression. Held end-expiration may be very useful in detecting a subtle or slight RV lift.

In adults with RV enlargement from acquired heart disease, pulmonary hypertension invariably is present. A palpable $P_2$ and pulmonary artery impulse in the second or third interspace should be sought in these patients to provide valuable confirmatory evidence for RV hypertrophy.

### First and Second Heart Sounds

#### *First Heart Sound*

In general, abnormalities of $S_1$ do not provide many important clues for cardiac physical diagnosis. Alteration in intensity of $S_1$ is the most useful observation that can aid the clinician.

#### *Normal Physiology*

$S_1$ signals the onset of LV contraction. Pressure within the LV begins to develop just before $S_1$ (Fig. 1.1). LV pressure rises above LA pressure well *before* forward flow across the mitral valve ceases and the valve leaflets have reached their maximally closed position.

Two major, medium- to high-frequency components of $S_1$ usually can be recorded in normal people ("split $S_1$"). The first major component of $S_1$ ($M_1$) is coincident with the maximal closing excursion of the mitral cusps. Echophonocardiograms have confirmed the coincidence of tricuspid valve closure ($T_1$) with the second component of $S_1$.

*Factors Affecting Intensity of the First Heart Sound*

Factors that affect the intensity of $S_1$ are listed in Table 1.3.

*PR Interval.* A shorter PR interval results in late mitral valve closure and a loud $S_1$. When the PR is short, LV pressure is higher at the time of LV–LA pressure crossover, causing a more rapid mitral valve closing motion and an increased intensity of $S_1$. With a long PR, the mitral valve may already be closed or the leaflets are closing, and the first sound is soft.

Maximal (increased) intensity of $S_1$ occurs at a PR interval range from 80 to 140 ms. PR intervals >140 ms (0.15 second) result in a normal $S_1$, and PR intervals >200 ms produce an attenuated or absent $S_1$.

*Left Ventricular Contractility.* In general, the more vigorous the LV contraction, the louder the $S_1$. Depressed LV contractility will result in a decreased intensity of $S_1$.

*How to Listen to the First Heart Sound*

*Timing.* Experienced physicians rarely have difficulty identifying $S_1$ unless there is a rapid heart rate and/or several murmurs are present. Tachycardia shortens diastole relatively more than systole. At heart rates of 120 to 130, systole and diastole are of equal length. If there is any doubt of the proper identification of $S_1$ and $S_2$, $S_1$ should be timed simultaneously with palpation of the carotid pulse or apical impulse (Fig. 1.3).

*Characteristics.* Typically, $S_1$ is of medium to high frequency, although occasionally it is low pitched. Use of the diaphragm or increased pressure with the bell will bring out the crisp, high-frequency vibrations of $S_1$. Splitting of $S_1$ is audible in many, but not all, normal subjects. $S_1$ usually is not prominent at the base and should always be single at the second and third interspaces. *Practical Point: When apparent splitting of $S_1$ is heard at the base, one should suspect the presence of an ejection sound (ES) or early mid-systolic click.*

### Second Heart Sound

Careful and intelligent evaluation of the intensity and splitting characteristics of $S_2$ represents one of the most valuable aspects of cardiac physical diagnosis. Clues to unsuspected or known cardiovascular abnormalities frequently are detected after assessment of $S_2$. The second heart sound is composed of an aortic ($A_2$) and a pulmonic ($P_2$) component. Both $A_2$ and $P_2$ should be separately sought, identified, and analyzed on auscultation.

*Normal Physiology*

The two components of $S_2$ represent vibrations resulting from deceleration of the blood mass at the end of ventricular systole when the semilunar valve cusps coapt and tense to prevent diastolic reflux of blood (Fig. 1.1). $A_2$ and $P_2$ coincide precisely with the respective incisurae in the aorta and pulmonary artery pressure recordings (Fig. 1.1). The incisura represents the peak deceleration of the blood mass and immediately is followed by a rebound of pressure. The relative distensibility or stiffness of the pulmonary and systemic vascular tree provides a partial explanation for differences in the timing of $A_2$ and $P_2$. In the central aorta, resistance is relatively high, compliance is low, and recoil from the ejection of blood into the aorta is brisk. Conse-

**TABLE 1.3.** *Factors affecting intensity of $S_1$*

Loud $S_1$
  Short PR interval (<160 ms)
  Tachycardia or hyperkinetic states
  "Stiff" left ventricle
  Mitral stenosis
  Left atrial myxoma
  Holosystolic mitral valve prolapse
Soft $S_1$
  Long PR interval (>200 ms)
  Depressed left ventricular contractility
  Premature closure of mitral valve (e.g., acute aortic regurgitation)
  Left bundle branch block
  Extracardiac factors (e.g., obesity, muscular chest, chronic obstructive pulmonary disease, large breasts)
  Flail mitral leaflet

quently, $A_2$ and its incisura closely follow the end of LV ejection. In the pulmonary artery, the highly distensible, low-resistance pulmonary vasculature allows for a late recoil following RV ejection. Thus, $P_2$ and the pulmonary artery incisura are somewhat delayed after the end of RV systole.

*Respiratory Effects of the Aortic and Pulmonic Components.* Inspiration normally produces audible separation (inspiratory splitting) of $A_2$ and $P_2$. The classic view of the mechanism of inspiratory splitting of $S_2$ is that increased venous return during inspiration causes a delay in RV systole, whereas LV systole remains unchanged or is somewhat shortened. This difference results in an increase in the $A_2$-$P_2$ interval. During expiration, RV stroke volume diminishes as LV stroke volume increases; the Q-$A_2$ interval lengthens and Q-$P_2$ shortens. Respiratory variation of compliance in the great vessels contributes to the phenomenon of inspiratory splitting.

### How to Listen to the Second Heart Sound

The physician must carefully evaluate the characteristics of *both* $A_2$ and $P_2$ during the routine cardiac examination. Because the major vibrations of $S_2$ are relatively high pitched, firm or increased pressure on the diaphragm of the stethoscope should be used to auscultate $S_2$. During expiration, $S_2$ normally is heard as a single sound. On inspiration, "splitting" or separation of the two components usually can be heard. Most people cannot differentiate two sounds that are only 20 to 25 ms apart. Therefore, if $A_2$ and $P_2$ are separated by 20 ms or less, they will be heard as a single sound. Such a sound is described as *single* or *fused.*

$A_2$ is louder than $P_2$ in normal subjects and in most abnormal states, unless pulmonary hypertension is present or the sound of aortic closure is diminished. *Practical Point: Normally, only $A_2$ is audible at the cardiac apex. $P_2$ normally does not radiate to the apex as a separate, audible sound except in young or thin subjects or with pulmonary hypertension.* The normal $P_2$ is somewhat softer than $A_2$, even at the pulmonary area, and usually is heard over a relatively small area of the chest. $P_2$ is readily detected at the second to fourth left interspaces.

*Second Heart Sound During Respiration.* During inspiration, clear-cut separation of $A_2$ and $P_2$ normally is observed (Fig. 1.16). This splitting is prominent in young subjects but is found less predictably in older age groups. $P_2$ usually becomes maximally delayed in mid to late inspiration. During expiration, the two components of $S_2$ are fused or single. Slow regular respirations are best for auscultation. The upright position often accentuates inspiratory separation of $A_2$ and $P_2$.

As the two components separate, a *ta-dup* cadence is heard in inspiration. The average peak $A_2$-$P_2$ splitting interval is 30 to 40 ms (0.03 to 0.04 second), with a range from 10 to 60 ms. Any interval $<30$ ms is considered "narrow splitting," and the two components of $S_2$ may not be detectable. Detectable expiratory splitting of 40 ms or more usually is abnormal. A subject who has *audible expiratory splitting* of $S_2$ in the supine position should be examined while he or she is sitting or standing. Often $S_2$ will be muffled in expiration but not discretely split. Asking the subject to hold his or her breath in end-expiration may be useful. Younger persons (children and young adults) are more likely to have normal expiratory asynchrony in the supine position and almost always will have prominent inspiratory splitting of $S_2$. In contrast, normal older subjects rarely have audible expiratory splitting but often have no detectable inspiratory splitting (single $S_2$).

*Proper Identification of Systole.* It is best to begin auscultation at the base. The cadence of $S_1$ and $S_2$ is most characteristic at the second to third interspace. Murmurs and other heart sounds usually are more easily sorted out away from the cardiac apex. The inspiratory motion of $A_2$ and $P_2$ should identify definitely which sound is $S_2$. $S_1$ usually is louder at the apex unless the PR interval is long or LV function is deranged.

*Is Splitting of the Second Heart Sound Present?* In patients with rapid heart rates, particularly infants, the two components of $S_2$ may be difficult or impossible to hear. In tachypneic

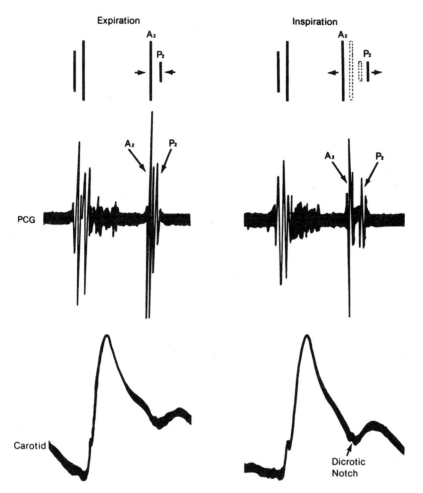

**FIG. 1.16.** Physiologic splitting of $S_2$. Under normal circumstances, $S_2$ in expiration is heard as a single event, but in late inspiration audible splitting of $A_2$ and $P_2$ is noted. The normal range of expiratory splitting is from 10 to 60 ms (average 40 ms). Most examiners cannot acoustically separate sounds that are 20 ms or less apart; thus, a narrow splitting interval will be heard as a fused or single $S_2$. The inspiratory increase consists predominantly of an increase in the total Q-$P_2$ duration, with a small decrease in Q-$A_2$. (The Second Heart Sound. PC 1982;8:35–54.)

patients, the rapid respirations may not allow sufficient time to hear the normal variation in $S_2$, particularly if the respirations are shallow. During sustained arrhythmias, particularly atrial fibrillation or frequent premature ventricular contractions, proper evaluation of respiratory splitting can be difficult.

*Paradoxic Splitting.* The most common causes of reversed or paradoxic splitting of $S_2$ are left bundle branch block (Fig. 1.17), aortic stenosis, and occasionally impaired LV ejec-

tion. Typically, LV systole is prolonged and results in reversed or paradoxic splitting of $S_2$.

### Third and Fourth Heart Sounds

The presence of an $S_3$ or $S_4$ can be extremely important in the evaluation of adults with suspected or known cardiovascular disease. An $S_3$ may be a normal or abnormal finding. An $S_3$ in an adult over 40 may have serious implications about the status of LV

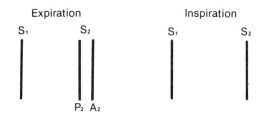

**Paradoxical Splitting of S₂ in LBBB**

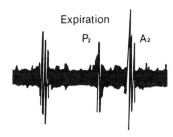

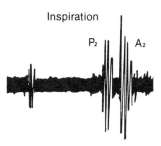

S₂ splitting varies from 0.10 sec (expiration)

**FIG. 1.17.** Reversed or paradoxic splitting of the second heart sound. The usual cause of paradoxic splitting is abnormally delayed left ventricular ejection, such that aortic closure (A₂) follows pulmonic closure (P₂). This commonly results in audible expiratory splitting. During inspiration, the normal delay in the Q-P₂ interval and shortening of Q-A₂ results in P₂ "moving into" A₂, and a single or narrower S₂ occurs. Thus, the normal respiratory pattern is reversed. (The Second Heart Sound. PC 1982;8:35–54.)

function, but this finding in a young subject usually is normal. An audible S₄ generally is present only in abnormal hearts.

### Third Heart Sound

#### Physiology of the Third Heart Sound

The S₃ follows mitral valve opening and the onset of rapid ventricular filling. Rapid deceleration of blood during inflow to the LV is translated into vibratory energy, resulting in the S₃. The relaxing ventricle and increasing diastolic blood volume set the ventricular walls, mitral valve apparatus, and blood mass into vibration.

The intensity of S₃ is increased when early diastolic filling is rapid due to elevated LA pressure and/or blood volume, or when LV distensibility in early diastole is increased. When LV compliance is decreased, the rate of early diastolic filling is decreased. In these situations, S₃ may not be present but an S₄ may be audible.

The physiologic explanation for the presence of an S₃ in normal children and young adults, which is not a normal finding in older subjects, is unclear. An S₃ may be produced in the RV when there is RV dysfunction or excessive flow across the tricuspid valve.

*Terminology.* The S₃ sometimes is called a ventricular gallop, early diastolic gallop or sound, or S₃ gallop. Although the term S₃ or *third heart sound* is preferable, ventricular gallop is acceptable when there is definite underlying heart disease.

#### Clinical Significance of the Third Heart Sound

An S₃ may be present in (i) normal hearts, (ii) diastolic overload states, and (iii) patients who have LV dysfunction, with or without overt congestive heart failure.

An S₃ commonly is found in normal children and young adults. Although not usually present in healthy subjects over 40 years of age, an S₃ occasionally may be found in individuals in their 30s (especially in women) without evidence of cardiac disease. In states such as anemia, thyrotoxicosis, anxiety, exercise, and pregnancy, a physiologic S₃ may become more prominent or appear for the first time. The S₃ is acoustically indistinguishable from a pathologic ventricular gallop. It may be soft or loud and usually will attenuate or disappear when the subject assumes the upright position. Most individuals with a physiologic S₃ are young and may have associated systolic flow murmurs and/or a venous hum. *Practical Point: In children and young adults, it is important to consider the possibility that an S₃ is physiologic and related to increased cardiac output. This will avoid the false diagnosis of cardiac disease.* Occasionally, a physiologic $S_3$ will be sustained in duration and can simulate a short diastolic murmur.

In significant LV systolic dysfunction with or without clinical symptoms of heart failure, the $S_3$ is an important and prognostically serious finding. The intensity of the $S_3$ may vary in relation to the state of cardiac compensation. In general, a persistent $S_3$ implies a poor prognosis. Optimal detection of the $S_3$ is discussed on pages 22–23.

### Fourth Heart Sound

Although there is no disagreement about the mechanism of production of the $S_4$, there has been considerable controversy regarding its true incidence and clinical implications.

### *Physiology of the Fourth Heart Sound*

The $S_4$ is a low-frequency sound following LA systole (Figs. 1.1 and 1.15). Although the $S_4$ also is known as the atrial sound, the $S_4$ is ventricular in origin. The *hemodynamic correlates* of the abnormal $S_4$ include an LV chamber that often is hypertrophied but has little or no increase in LV diameter; normal LV pressure in early diastole with an elevation of *end-diastolic* pressure; impaired velocity of early LV relaxation and diastolic filling; and preserved cardiac output. The LV chamber is stiff and noncompliant.

*Normal Fourth Heart Sound.* An $S_4$ occasionally may be heard when there are no detectable abnormalities of ventricular function other than increased blood flow, as in young subjects or patients with thyrotoxicosis, or in the presumed physiologic loss of LV compliance with aging. Whether a distinct audible $S_4$ is truly normal in older adults remains the subject of controversy.

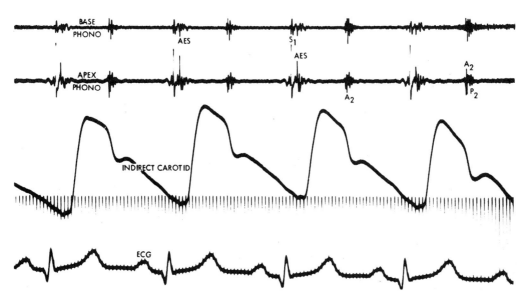

**FIG. 1.18.** Aortic ejection sound. This phonocardiogram and carotid arterial pulse tracing demonstrates a prominent, discrete aortic ejection sound that is better heard and recorded at the apex than at the base. This is characteristic of aortic ejection sounds or clicks. Note the prominent separation of the ejection sound from S₁ by approximately 40 to 50 ms. (From Shaver JA, Griff FW, Leonard JJ. Ejection sounds of left-sided origin. In: Leon DF, Shaver JA, eds. Physiologic principles of heart sounds and murmurs. American Heart Association Monograph No. 46, 1975, with permission.)

*Abnormal Fourth Heart Sound.* In the normal heart, the LV passively receives 70% to 80% of its diastolic filling volume from the LA during early to mid diastole, with a smaller contribution from atrial contraction in late diastole. In myocardial diseases such as hypertrophy and/or dilation, LA contraction becomes responsible for a greater proportion of LV filling. This LA "booster pump" function takes on increasing importance as LV distensibility decreases. LA contraction may provide up to 30% to 40% of LV diastolic filling in some circumstances. Under these conditions, the $S_4$ or atrial gallop may be prominent, and LV end-diastolic pressure is elevated. The $S_4$ often is palpable in these circumstances (Fig. 1.15).

### Clinical Significance

The significance of an $S_4$ remains an unresolved controversy: There is a general consensus that a *very loud* or *palpable $S_4$* is always abnormal and signifies decreased LV compliance.

A prominent $S_4$, often with a palpably increased precordial A wave amplitude, is found commonly in patients with underlying coronary disease, hypertension, aortic stenosis, or hypertrophic cardiomyopathy. The intensity of an $S_4$ varies considerably; when prominent, the $S_4$ may be the loudest heart sound heard at the apex. The common denominator in individuals with a prominent $S_4$ is LV hypertrophy with increased LV end-diastolic pressure and restricted early diastolic filling produced by a stiff LV. The clinical implication of an audible $S_4$ is far different from that of the $S_3$, which often signifies cardiac decompensation, incipient or overt congestive heart failure, and a poor long-term outlook. In general, an $S_4$ implies a less serious alteration in LV function and carries a more benign prognosis than the $S_3$. *Practical Point: The majority of clinicians and investigators believe that the presence of a distinctly audible atrial sound or $S_4$ in an older subject is almost always abnormal and, conversely, that normal persons infrequently have a distinctly audible $S_4$.*

*Summation Gallop and Quadruple Rhythm.* Whenever the PR interval is long and/or the heart rate is rapid, atrial contraction will "move into" the rapid filling phase of diastole. Because diastole shortens more than systole when heart rate increases, passive ventricular filling is superimposed on the augmented flow across the mitral valve due to LA systole. This combination may cause a very loud *summation* gallop ($S_3$ plus $S_4$). Rate slowing with carotid sinus massage is a useful bedside technique to evaluate gallop rhythm during tachycardia or to help analyze other confusing cardiac findings when there is a rapid heart rate.

When both an $S_3$ and $S_4$ are clearly audible, the term *quadruple rhythm* is used. This is commonly found in patients with LV aneurysm, cardiomyopathy, severe LV failure, or LV dilation.

### How to Listen for Third and Fourth Heart Sounds

Proper approach to auscultation of $S_3$ and $S_4$ is given in Table 1.4. The third and fourth heart sounds are low pitched (20 to 60 cycles per second and usually of low intensity. The $S_3$ often has some "duration" or after-vibrations; the $S_4$ is slightly higher pitched and usually is

**TABLE 1.4.** *Proper approach to auscultation of $S_3$ and $S_4$*

| | |
|---|---|
| Stethoscope technique | |
|   Have a quiet room and surroundings | |
|   Routinely use left lateral position | |
|   Identify left ventricular apex impulse | |
|   Use the bell with light pressure | |
|   Use rubber outer ring on bell | |
| Helpful physiologic maneuvers | |
|   *Alterations in venous return* | *Response* |
|   Increase:  Leg elevation | Increase |
|              Coughing |   intensity |
|              Sit-ups | |
|              Abdominal compression | |
|              Valsalva release phase | |
|   Decrease:  Sitting | Decrease |
|              Standing |   intensity |
|              Valsalva strain phase | |
|   Sustained handgrip (isometric) | Increase |
|   If heart rate is rapid, use |   intensity |
|     carotid sinus massage | |

louder. *Both sounds must be actively sought in order to be detected.* They typically sound like a distant thud. The sounds may be palpable, particularly the $S_4$. To optimally hear the $S_3$ and $S_4$, a noise-free room without background vibrations from air conditioning or heating systems is desirable. One should avoid sound artifacts from muscle tremor or interfering noises from clothing or stethoscope tubing. The $S_3$ and $S_4$ often are best heard immediately upon beginning auscultation and may appear to fade away after a short period. Frequently, gallop sounds are heard only immediately after the patient assumes a new position, such as getting onto the examination table or turning over into the left lateral position.

## Timing

The $S_3$ is linked to $S_2$ in timing, whereas the $S_4$ occurs just before $S_1$ (Fig. 1.1). These relationships hold for very slow or very rapid heart rates. The $S_3$ occurs in early diastole. The $S_4$ is presystolic; it follows the P wave by 0.12 to 0.20 seconds.

## Helpful Maneuvers in Auscultation of Third and Fourth Heart Sounds

Maneuvers that alter venous return are useful during auscultation of the low-frequency diastolic filling sounds (Table 1.4). Anything that increases venous return and intracardiac blood volume accentuates the loudness of $S_3$ and $S_4$; conversely, a decrease in cardiac filling will attenuate these sounds. A right-sided $S_3$ or $S_4$ will augment with inspiration. Having the patient assume the upright posture often is helpful; both an $S_3$ and an $S_4$ typically attenuate or disappear. Carotid sinus pressure may be effective in slowing the heart rate when there is difficulty in timing the gallop rhythm. Handgrip exercise may increase the intensity of both $S_3$ and $S_4$.

## Proper Use of the Stethoscope

The $S_3$ and $S_4$ are low-frequency transients that are best and often only heard with the bell of the stethoscope. A large-diameter bell with a rubber outer ring is best (Fig. 1.3). The lightest possible pressure to make a skin seal should be used. As stethoscope pressure is increased to filter out low-frequency vibrations, $S_3$ and $S_4$ will attenuate. A particularly loud $S_3$ or $S_4$ usually has medium- to high-frequency components, may sound more high pitched than usual, and may remain audible even when firm stethoscope pressure is applied.

## Location

LV $S_3$ and $S_4$ are maximal at the apical impulse. The apical impulse should be carefully identified with the examining finger (Fig. 1.10), and then the bell should be placed directly on the apex using light pressure. In patients with emphysema, LV $S_3$ or $S_4$ may be best heard at the subxiphoid area or lower left sternal border. Differentiation from gallops of RV origin in these patients may be difficult.

## Left Lateral Decubitus Position

It is essential to examine any patient suspected of having LV disease in the left oblique or left lateral decubitus position (Fig. 1.12). *Practical Point:* $S_3$ and $S_4$ often are inaudible when the patient is supine and may be heard only in the left lateral position. This maneuver thrusts the apex of the LV close to the chest wall and accentuates audibility of low-pitched diastolic sounds, often increasing the amplitude of both $S_3$ and $S_4$ dramatically. In this position, these low-frequency events may become palpable. Light pressure on the pads of the fingers should be used, with careful attention for a presystolic bulge or an early systolic thrust. Palpable presystolic distention ($S_4$) is much more common than a palpable $S_3$ and is a most important confirmatory finding in patients with a suspected $S_4$.

## Palpable Fourth Heart Sound

Careful palpation of the apical impulse in the left decubitus position may be rewarded by detection of an outward presystolic thrust in patients with a palpable $S_4$ (Figs. 1.11 and 1.16). This motion often is subtle; commonly, it feels as if there is a shelf or notch on the upstroke of the apical impulse.

The palpable A wave occurs just before the maximal outward apical excursion during isovolumic systole. Two fingers should be used for detection of a palpable $S_4$. It is important to feel the apex beat over many cardiac cycles, as the size of maximum impulse may alter slightly with respiration and the low-amplitude A wave may not be palpable with each heart beat. *Practical Point: The finding of a palpable $S_4$ indicates that the associated atrial sound is definitely abnormal.*

### Ejection Sounds

ES are high-frequency transients that occur in early systole immediately following $S_1$ (Fig. 1.18). They also are known as ejection clicks; either term is acceptable. ES occur more frequently than is commonly realized. Unless the observer is aware of the possibility of such acoustic events, the ES easily can be assumed to be a part of $S_1$ and will be completely missed. The finding of an ejection click may be the critical clue that a systolic murmur is truly organic and almost always implies underlying cardiovascular disease.

#### *Pathophysiology of Ejection Sounds*

Two different mechanisms may result in an ES: (i) the "snapping" opening or doming of a stenotic thickened or malformed *pulmonary* or *aortic valve* (Fig. 1.19A), or (ii) a sound transient produced by sudden tensing or reverberation of the proximal *aorta* or *pulmonary artery* at the time of early ejection (vascular or root origin) (Fig. 1.19B). Ejection clicks of valve origin classically are found in congenital aortic and pulmonary artery valve stenosis. Aortic and pulmonary ES of the nonstenotic valve variety invariably are associated with either a dilated aorta or pulmonary artery or a systemic or pulmonary vascular tree with increased systolic pressure and reduced vascular compliance.

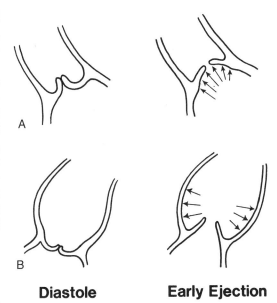

**Diastole          Early Ejection**

**FIG. 1.19.** Origin of ejection sounds. **A:** Ejection sound or click produced by the opening motion of a thickened, often stenotic, aortic or pulmonary valve. **B:** Ejection sound produced by sudden tensing of the proximal aorta or pulmonary artery during early ejection. This usually is associated with a dilated and/or hypertensive great vessel (see text).

#### *Semilunar Valve Stenosis*

When commissural fusion of a semilunar valve and/or leaflet thickening are present, the rapidly rising ventricular pressure in early systole drives the abnormal valve leaflets upward. At the precise moment of maximum ascent, the taut valve cusps bulge or dome into their respective great vessel, producing a high-frequency sound (Fig. 1.19A). Flow across the stenotic valve occurs only after maximal valve opening has been reached, and the resultant systolic ejection murmur immediately follows the ejection click. When the valve stenosis is extremely severe and the valve cusps are relatively immobile or heavily calcified, both the ES and the respective valve component of $S_2$ are diminished or even absent.

*Aortic Stenosis.* An ejection click is almost always present in congenital abnormalities of the aortic valve (see Chapter 8) (Figs. 1.18

and 1.19). Most often an aortic ES indicates a bicuspid aortic valve. An isolated ejection click may be heard in the absence of an ejection murmur. In these situations, echocardiography is mandatory to assess the possibility of a bicuspid or otherwise thickened aortic valve. In *acquired* aortic valve stenosis, usually of rheumatic or degenerative origin, ejection clicks are much less common.

*Pulmonary Stenosis.* ES are common in valvular pulmonary stenosis. As with the aortic valve, the presence of ES localizes the obstruction to the valve level. Infundibular pulmonary stenosis does not produce an ejection click. In very mild or very severe pulmonary stenosis, the pulmonic ejection click may not be heard. *Practical Point: The most characteristic attribute of the pulmonic valve ES is its marked variability with respiration.* In contradistinction to almost all other right-sided acoustic phenomena, which become louder with inspiration, the pulmonic valve ejection click typically *softens* or *disappears* with inspiration.

### Nonvalvular Ejection Sounds

An ES with a normal semilunar valve typically is associated with dilation of the aorta or pulmonary artery, which occurs in conditions of increased stroke volume and/or increased force of ejection (Fig. 1.19B).

*Aortic Root Ejection Sounds.* These sounds are found in subjects with aortic arteriosclerosis, aortic aneurysm, aortic regurgitation, or systemic hypertension.

*Pulmonary Ejection Sounds.* Pulmonary ES may occur in any condition resulting in pulmonary hypertension. In such situations, respiratory variation of the pulmonic ES is not common. Early ejection of blood into a tense, noncompliant pulmonary artery is thought to be the cause of the ES.

### *Clues to Auscultation of Ejection Sounds*

#### *Quality and Timing*

Both aortic and pulmonic ejection clicks typically are high-frequency, sharp, discrete sounds that are at least equal in intensity to $S_1$ (Fig. 1.18). They are best heard with the diaphragm of the stethoscope. The later the ES, the more audible it is. An early ES may merge with $S_1$ or, more likely, is thought by the examiner to be part of the $S_1$ complex (split $S_1$). In pulmonary stenosis, the more severe the valve obstruction, the earlier the click. In these cases, the ES is easily confused with $S_1$.

#### *Location*

Aortic ES are audible at the cardiac base and the aortic area. They usually are well heard at the apex, and often the sound is heard only at the apex. This is particularly true in the elderly or in patients with chronic lung disease. The systolic murmur of both aortic and pulmonary stenosis begins with the click, and this may obscure separate identification of the click at the base.

Pulmonic ES are best heard at the second and third left interspace and are poorly heard or inaudible at the apex. An *inspiratory decrease* in ES amplitude is of valvular pulmonary stenosis. A pulmonic click at the pulmonic area may be mistaken for $S_1$, which usually is quite soft at the left second or third interspace. In patients suspected of having pulmonary stenosis, listen with the subject in the upright position. The resultant decrease in RV venous return often results in the click becoming more audible both in inspiration and expiration.

### Heart Murmurs

Physicians should be able to assess heart murmurs accurately to properly evaluate patients with congenital or valvular heart disease. In the general population, systolic murmurs are widespread but reflect abnormal cardiac structure in only a small percentage of persons. The presence of a heart murmur raises questions regarding prophylaxis for endocarditis, restriction from athletics, eligibility for life insurance or employment, risk of pregnancy to the mother or fetus, and safety of noncardiac surgery. In the practice of medicine, physicians confront these issues daily and must be able to distinguish heart murmurs in subjects who have no intrinsic cardiac abnormalities from those that indicate organic disease.

### Significance of a Murmur

When someone is found to have a murmur, several issues require resolution. The first question to ask is whether the murmur is organic or pathologic or a normal variant. Based on the information derived from the cardiac physical examination, one then can determine the likeliest hemodynamic cause of the murmur. Once the anatomic origin of an organic murmur is characterized, the possible etiologies of the heart disease should be investigated, and the severity of the underlying condition can be assessed.

Usually, a capable clinician can resolve these questions after a careful physical examination. Although ancillary diagnostic testing (ECG, chest roentgenogram, M-mode or two-dimensional echocardiogram, cardiac catheterization) often is important, typically these studies provide additional data about the severity of a problem that already has been identified and roughly quantitated by the physical examination.

When a heart murmur is believed to be "innocent" (see Table 1.5), the diagnosis of *non-disease* should be made firmly and without equivocation. *Practical Point: Heart murmurs with no intrinsic cardiac abnormality are far more common than those with organic cardiovascular disease. Thus, "ruling out" significant heart disease is an important aspect of everyday clinical practice.*

### Physiology

Turbulence is the primary factor in the genesis of heart murmurs. Turbulent blood flow produces both physiologic murmurs and organic murmurs. An important determinant of turbulence is the velocity of blood flow. Increases in velocity result in marked increases in turbulence, often producing audible sound. Obstruction to blood flow, such as stenosis, produces abnormal turbulence, which is related both to the velocity of blood flow and to alterations in accelerating forces. Turbulence increases as the gradient across the valve becomes larger.

### Normal Ejection

During the first part of systole, there is a small pressure or "impulse" gradient between each ventricle and its respective great vessel (Fig. 1.20) that may account for sufficient turbulence to produce cardiac sound.

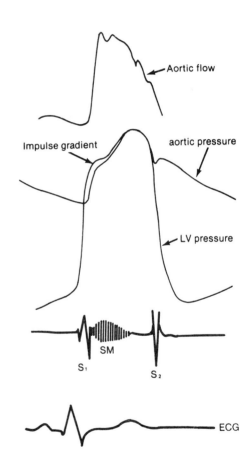

**FIG. 1.20.** Pressure flow relationships of the systolic ejection or flow murmur. During early systole, peak blood flow and velocity are maximal, producing sufficient turbulence for the production of audible sound. A typical systolic ejection murmur ends within the first two thirds of systole. Note the small "impulse gradient" in early systole. (Auscultation of Heart Murmurs. PC 1981;7:21–43.)

## Sound Frequency

In general, turbulent flow produces random sound that has many frequencies and results in mixed frequency murmurs. High flow rates or large gradients produce more high-pitched sound; low flow rates and/or small gradients result in low-pitched sound.

## Transmission

Transmission or radiation of cardiac sound results from vibration of cardiac structures and blood vessels set up by turbulence or eddy formation. High-frequency sound does not transmit well downstream. Low-frequency vibrations are better heard downstream and thus transmit more widely.

### General Principles of Cardiac Auscultation

#### Use of the Stethoscope

The bell of the stethoscope is ideal for low-frequency murmurs (25 to 125 cps). When the bell is used, light skin contact is desirable to maximize detection of low-pitched sound (Fig. 1.3). The diaphragm is best for high-frequency or mixed-frequency murmurs. Increasing pressure on the diaphragm will attenuate lower-pitched sounds and accentuate the higher frequencies. One should routinely alter stethoscope pressure during auscultation to optimally assess the frequency characteristics of heart sounds and murmurs.

#### Grading Murmurs

The familiar 1 through 6 grading protocol provides a systematic and consistent method of evaluating the intensity of heart murmurs.

*Grade 1:* Faintest murmur that can be heard under optimal conditions (quiet room, relaxed patient and physician)

*Grade 2:* Soft but readily audible murmur

*Grade 3:* Prominent murmur that should always stimulate a careful search for cardiac disease

*Grade 4:* Very loud murmur that is palpable (thrill)

*Grade 5:* Louder still (thrill)

*Grade 6:* Murmur audible with the stethoscope held off the chest wall (thrill)

Most innocent or functional murmurs will be grade 1/6 to 2/6; some will be grade 3/6. Murmur grades of 5/6 or 6/6 are rare.

#### Valve Areas

Customarily, specific locations on the chest have been designated as relating to a particular cardiac valve. This practice stems from observations regarding the site where a specific murmur (e.g., aortic stenosis) usually is best heard. Thus, the second right interspace is known as the "aortic area"; the second to third left interspace is the "pulmonary area"; the lower left sternal border is the "tricuspid area"; and the apex is the "mitral area." However, there are many exceptions to this oversimplified approach.

### Classification of Heart Murmurs

The general classification of murmurs proposed by Aubrey Leatham in 1958 has been widely adopted (Table 1.5). Leatham divided systolic murmurs into two major types: *midsystolic ejection* and *pansystolic* or *regurgitant. Diastolic* and *continuous* murmurs are the other two major types of heart murmurs. *Ejection murmurs* not caused by valvular narrowing are known as *flow, functional,* or *innocent* murmurs. When defining or classifying a murmur, it is desirable to use a physiologic descriptor as well as an indication of the timing of the murmur (e.g., late systolic regurgitant murmur or early systolic ejection murmur).

#### Systolic Murmurs

*Ejection Murmurs.* The most common murmur heard in everyday practice is the ejection or flow murmur produced by rapid ejection of blood during the first part of systole. Peak acceleration of blood flow occurs in early systole just after aortic valve opening. During the last third of systole, very little for-

**TABLE 1.5.**  *Classification of heart murmurs*

Systolic
  Ejection murmurs
    Flow or functional murmurs
      Innocent murmur
      Physiologic murmur (related to increased cardiac output), e.g., anemia, thyrotoxicosis, postexercise
    Pathologic or significant murmurs
      Abnormal but nonstenotic aortic or pulmonary valve
      Aortic or pulmonary valve stenosis
      Dilation of aorta or pulmonary artery
      Left or right ventricular outflow tract obstruction (nonvalvular)
  Regurgitant murmurs
    Mitral regurgitation
    Tricuspid regurgitation
    Ventricular septal defect
Diastolic
  Semilunar valve incompetence
    Aortic or pulmonary regurgitation
  Ventricular filling murmurs
    Mitral or tricuspid stenosis
    Augmented atrioventricular valve flow (e.g., mitral regurgitation, ventricular septal defect, atrial septal
      defect)
    Presystolic murmur due to atrial contraction (e.g., mitral or tricuspid stenosis)
Continuous
  Communication between high-pressure chamber or artery with low-pressure chamber or vein (e.g., patent
    ductus arteriosus, coronary arteriovenous fistula, sinus of Valsalva to right atrial communication)

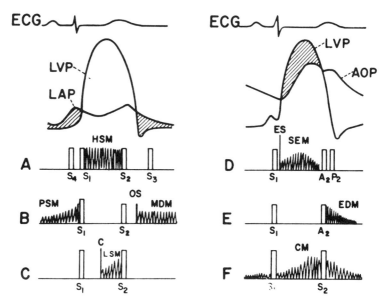

**FIG. 1.21.**  Intracardiac pressures and heart murmurs in the major cardiac valve abnormalities. See text for discussion of specific murmurs. AOP, aortic pressure; C, mid-systolic click; CM, continuous murmur; EDM, early diastolic murmur; ES, ejection sound; HSM, holosystolic murmur; LAP, left atrial pressure; LSM, late systolic murmur; LVP, left ventricular pressure; MDM, mid-diastolic murmur; OS, opening snap; PSM, presystolic murmur; SEM, systolic ejection murmur. (From Crawford MH, O'Rourke RA. A systematic approach to the bedside differentiation of cardiac murmurs and abnormal sounds. Curr Probl Cardiol 1979;1:1, with permission.)

ward flow occurs across the semilunar valves (Fig. 1.20). *Early systolic murmurs are common, even in the presence of normal valves and a basal cardiac output.* Irregular, thickened, or stenotic semilunar valves leaflets result in greater turbulence and increased murmur intensity.

The typical systolic or flow ejection murmur begins after $S_1$ at the completion of isovolumic contraction (Figs. 1.20, 1.21D, and 1.22A), peaks early (crescendo), and then falls away (decrescendo). *The systolic ejection murmur usually ends before $S_2$.* However, with severe semilunar valve stenosis, prolonged ventricular emptying may produce a late peaking murmur that can extend to or beyond $A_2$ or $P_2$. The intensity of the ejection murmur is related to the velocity of blood flow, valve orifice area, and accelerating forces. A large stroke volume results in a louder and longer murmur.

*Systolic Regurgitant Murmurs.* Systolic regurgitant murmurs are generated by a continuous systolic pressure gradient produced by an abnormal structural or functional communication between two chambers of the heart. A typical regurgitant murmur begins during the development of ventricular pressure (isovolumic contraction) and continues up to $S_2$ (Figs. 1.21A and 1.22B). If a large pressure gradient between two cardiac chambers persists into late systole, blood flow and cardiac sound will continue until the onset of diastole. The classic regurgitant murmur is holosystolic or pansystolic with a constant amplitude and shape throughout systole (Figs. 1.21A and 1.22B). Systolic regurgitant murmurs are present in mitral and tricuspid regurgitation and ventricular septal defects. Late systolic murmurs, beginning after $S_1$ and extending to $S_2$, typically reflect mild degrees of mitral regurgitation (Figs. 1.21C and 1.22C).

### Diastolic Murmurs

*Semilunar Valve Regurgitation.* Semilunar valve regurgitation murmurs begin with semilunar valve closure ($S_2$) and usually are decrescendo in configuration (Figs. 1.21E and 1.22D). The shape and length of the murmur reflect the diastolic pressure gradient between aorta or pulmonary artery and the respective ventricle. Because of the high velocity of regurgitant blood flow from the great vessels, murmurs of semilunar valve incompetence typically are of high frequency.

*Ventricular Filling Murmurs. Atrioventricular valve stenosis.* These murmurs are caused by obstruction to inflow of blood to the LV or RV in patients with mitral or tricuspid valve stenosis (Figs. 1.21B and 1.22E). The onset of the murmur follows complete opening of the AV valve, and the murmur is mid-diastolic in timing. Typically, these murmurs are low pitched because of the relatively small pressure gradients between the atrium and ventricles, which result in low flow velocity even with severe stenosis.

*Increased atrioventricular valve flow without valvular stenosis.* Under conditions of exces-

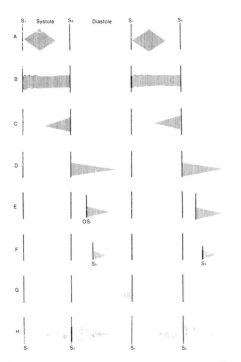

**FIG. 1.22.** Major types of cardiac murmurs. See text for description. (Auscultation of Heart Murmurs. PC 1981;7:21–43.)

sive atrial blood volume and augmented flow across the mitral or tricuspid valve, a short, mid-diastolic "filling murmur" often can be heard. Such a murmur may begin with a ventricular filling sound ($S_3$) (Fig. 1.22F). Mid-diastolic flow murmurs are common when there is increased flow across an AV valve due to a left to right shunt (atrial septal defect, ventricular septal defect, or patent ductus arteriosus). The Austin Flint murmur of aortic regurgitation is another variant of the "functional" diastolic filling murmur (see Chapter 9).

*Presystolic murmurs.* Late diastolic or presystolic murmurs may be heard in patients with mild to moderate mitral or tricuspid stenosis who are in sinus rhythm. This results from augmentation of AV flow following atrial contraction.

### Continuous Murmurs

Continuous murmurs result from a persistent gradient between a high-pressure site (arterial or ventricular) and a low-pressure site (vein or right heart chamber). These murmurs typically begin in systole and "spill over" into early diastole, peaking in mid to late systole. Rarely, they are audible in late diastole (Figs. 1.21F and 1.22H).

### Diagnosis of Organic Murmurs

Because nonpathologic or innocent flow murmurs are so common in normal persons, the clinician has a great responsibility to determine whether or not a heart murmur is pathologic. There are few criteria that absolutely identify the organic or pathologic cardiac murmur.

1. *All diastolic murmurs are pathologic.* There should be no cardiac sound during diastole.
2. *All pansystolic and late systolic murmurs are pathologic.* Cardiac sound typically is absent during the last third of ejection. Murmurs that extend to $S_2$ are organic and indicate continuing turbulent blood flow at a time when silence is expected.

**TABLE 1.6.** *Factors affecting the loudness of heart murmurs*

Increased intensity
  High cardiac output (hyperdynamic) states
  Thin chest wall
  Narrow thoracic diameter, e.g., "straight back," pectus excavatum
  Anemia (decreased blood viscosity)
  Tortuous aorta (close to chest wall)
Decreased intensity
  Obesity
  Muscular or thick chest wall
  Obstructive lung disease
  Barrel chest (increased anteroposterior diameter)
  Pericardial thickening or fluid
  Decreased cardiac output (congestive heart failure, low ejection fraction)

3. *Continuous murmurs always indicate organic heart disease.* A murmur that continues up to $S_2$ and spills over into diastole must reflect a continuing pressure differential between two cardiovascular structures and, therefore, is abnormal.
4. *Very loud murmurs usually are pathologic.* Any murmur associated with a thrill (grade 4 or greater) has a pathologic basis. Table 1.6 lists common noncardiac conditions associated with an increase or decrease in murmur intensity. These factors should always be kept in mind during auscultation of the patient.
5. *Associated cardiac abnormalities* raise the likelihood that a given heart murmur is organic.
6. *Frequency, shape* or *contour,* and *radiation* characteristics of heart murmurs are too nonspecific to establish definitively the organic etiology of a murmur.

### Evaluation of Heart Murmurs

The clinician should take a systematic approach to the accurate assessment of heart murmurs. The following features of murmurs should be consciously analyzed in each patient:

- Whether the murmur is *systolic* or *diastolic*
- *Timing* of the murmur within systole or diastole—early, mid, or late

- *Duration* of the murmur
- *Intensity* or *loudness* of the murmur, i.e., its grade
- *Transmission* of the murmur
- *Frequency* and *shape* of the murmur
- *Other cardiac abnormalities* present on examination that may relate to the etiology of the murmur

Once it is clear that a given murmur is systolic or diastolic, it is necessary to clarify whether the murmur is early, mid, or late in systole or diastole. This will help identify the probable cause of the murmur.

### Systole

Ejection murmurs, whether or not pathologic, are all early to mid-systolic in timing. When there is a severe degree of obstruction to outflow, ejection murmurs will lengthen and peak later in systole. Not all early systolic murmurs are ejection murmurs. In some patients, the murmur of a ventricular septal defect or AV valve regurgitation tapers off in late systole, ending before $A_2$.

A late systolic murmur should not be confused with an ejection murmur. Late systolic murmurs usually represent mitral regurgitation (Figs. 1.21C and 1.22C) (see Chapter 6). These murmurs begin in mid systole, with sound vibrations heard up to $A_2$.

### Diastole

Early diastolic murmurs result from semilunar valve incompetence (aortic or pulmonary regurgitation). Mid-diastolic murmurs are produced by flow across either the mitral or tricuspid valve during passive filling of the ventricles or with stenosis of either AV valve. Diastolic murmurs are caused by narrowed and obstructive orifices. Such murmurs lengthen in proportion to the severity of valvular obstruction, and cardiac sound may persist up to $S_1$. Mid-diastolic murmurs also can occur without narrowing of the AV valve if there is markedly augmented blood flow with rapid ventricular filling. Here, the mur-

mur is brief and usually follows an $S_3$. Late diastolic and presystolic murmurs are produced by atrial contraction in the presence of mitral or tricuspid stenosis.

*Continuous murmurs* represent cardiac sound that spills over into diastole. Care must be taken to differentiate these murmurs from the combination of a long systolic and early diastolic murmur that can be heard in mixed semilunar valve stenosis and regurgitation.

### Duration

*Systole.* The most important characteristic of systolic murmurs relates to their length. *Practical Point: Whether a systolic murmur extends to $S_2$ and, therefore, is holosystolic is the most valuable part of murmur analysis.*

The presence of a long systolic murmur should stimulate a careful evaluation of late systole through the use of selective listening. Careful focus on the last 25% of systole is important (Fig. 1.23) If sound vibrations end before $S_2$, the murmur is usually an ejection murmur. If the murmur truly extends to $S_2$ (pansystolic), the differential diagnosis should include regurgitant lesions as well as severe, semilunar valvular stenosis.

*Diastole.* The duration of diastolic murmurs is important, particularly in assessment of LV filling murmurs. Flow across a nonobstructive or mildly stenotic AV valve produces a short mid-diastolic murmur. A long diastolic murmur following an opening snap is indicative of a persistent AV gradient and significant mitral stenosis.

Murmurs of semilunar valve regurgitation usually are quite long and may be pandiastolic, continuing to $S_1$. Usually, these high-frequency murmurs are of low intensity and may be very faint in late diastole. With severe aortic regurgitation, particularly in acute valvular incompetence, the murmur may be surprisingly short.

### Intensity

The intensity or loudness of a murmur is directly related to the degree of turbulence.

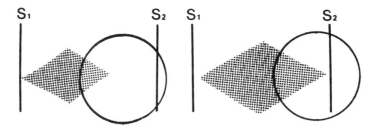

**FIG. 1.23.** Importance of late systole in evaluation of systolic murmurs. It is essential to assess the last part of systole to determine whether a murmur is ejection in nature or is holosystolic. **Left:** Early peaking murmur ends before the last third of systole. This is the rule in functional murmurs or with mild semilunar valve stenosis. **Right:** Long ejection murmur that peaks later in systole. Sound vibrations extend to $S_2$, suggesting severe obstruction to ventricular outflow. In severe semilunar valve stenosis, the vibrations may extend beyond $S_2$. (Auscultation of Heart Murmurs. PC 1981;7:21–43.)

Increased volume and/or velocity of flow results in enhanced turbulence and louder murmurs.

Often, it is assumed that the intensity of a murmur is directly related to the severity of the underlying condition. Although this is frequently true, there are many exceptions. The careful auscultator should be aware of the various factors that may modify the intensity of murmurs (Table 1.6).

*Transmission*

Radiation and transmission patterns of murmurs are directly related to the intensity or loudness of the murmur. Loud murmurs transmit widely; soft murmurs do not.

*Shape*

Assessing the contour or shape of heart murmurs may help the clinician to distinguish systolic ejection murmurs (crescendo-decrescendo) from regurgitant (holosystolic) murmurs.

There are important exceptions to the classic descriptions of murmur contour. For example, the pansystolic murmur of mitral regurgitation may have late systolic accentuation or can taper off in late systole. It is useful to diagram the shape of the murmur in the clinical record.

*Frequency*

The pitch or frequency of a heart murmur has some diagnostic value. Because of a large proportion of dominant higher frequencies, higher-pitched murmurs are more musical or pure in tone than lower frequencies. These often are called "blowing" murmurs. Very harsh murmurs (e.g., aortic valve stenosis) are mixtures of medium and high frequencies; the ear best perceives the lower tones, which tend to mask the higher frequencies. Murmurs with a preponderance of a particular frequency often have a certain resonance that is called "musical" or "vibratory." Murmurs with a relatively clear pitch and pure fundamental tone often are called "cooing" or "seagull" murmurs.

**Systolic Ejection Murmur**

A variety of normal and abnormal conditions can produce the relatively nonspecific "ejection" murmur. Most systolic murmurs heard in everyday practice are related to physiologic blood flow and are of no clinical importance. It is imperative for the physician to be able to properly identify these murmurs, thus avoiding the need for referral to a cardiologist, additional diagnostic tests, prophylaxis against acute rheumatic fever and bacterial endocarditis, and restriction of activities or employment.

*Innocent or Functional Murmurs*

The innocent murmur, by far the most common murmur heard in clinical practice, has certain characteristics that should enable the careful examiner to identify it accurately more than 90% of the time. *The sine qua non is that the underlying cardiovascular system is entirely normal and that the murmur is audible at rest.*

The use of such descriptive terms as "flow," "innocent," "functional," or "physiologic" murmur is important, as it clearly implies that a systolic ejection murmur is not the result of an organic valve lesion or an abnormal communication within the heart or great vessels.

*Etiology.* Innocent or physiologic murmurs are due to rapid early ejection of blood into the aorta, producing sufficient turbulence to yield audible sound.

*Age and Incidence.* Under optimal acoustic conditions, experienced clinicians hear sound vibrations in systole in as many as 80% to 90% of children and young adults. With increasing age, the innocent murmur tends to attenuate or disappear; nevertheless, it is common (30% to 40% of individuals) to hear a soft systolic ejection murmur in normal adults.

*Systolic Murmur of Aging.* Many older subjects in their 60s through 90s have an audible systolic ejection murmur that may have a different etiology than the innocent murmur of youth. These murmurs typically radiate well to the aortic area (second right interspace) and neck and may also be well heard at the apex. They often have a rougher quality than the typical innocent murmur of childhood and are particularly common in patients with hypertension. These systolic murmurs reflect underlying aortic valve sclerosis. They can simulate valvular aortic stenosis and, on occasion, may present a difficult differential problem. When there are accompanying ECG changes or cardiovascular symptoms, it is easy to confuse these murmurs with those reflecting organic heart disease. Particular attention should be paid to the carotid pulse for signs of aortic stenosis, although this can be misleading because of age-related compliance changes in the peripheral vessels (see Fig. 1.5). The length of the systolic murmur also is useful in assessing whether the murmur is significant (Fig. 1.23). If the murmur ends well before S$_2$, important aortic valve stenosis is unlikely. *Practical Point: Echocardiography should be used in doubtful cases to assess the thickness and excursion of the aortic valve cusps.*

*Location, Loudness, and Radiation.* The innocent murmur is best heard along the left sternal border at the second to fourth interspace, most often between the apex and lower sternal border. Innocent murmurs are uncommonly loudest at the apex. As a rule, they do not radiate well into the neck, although loud flow murmurs may be easily heard throughout the precordium. Normal flow murmurs typically are of low or moderate intensity (usually 1/6 to 2/6) and are never grade 4/6 intensity.

*Length, Shape, and Quality.* The typical innocent murmur occupies less than two thirds of systole and is crescendo-decrescendo in configuration (Fig. 1.20). The murmur is usually of low to medium frequency (60 to 180 Hz) and often has a preponderance of relatively pure frequencies. It may appear to be vibratory to the ear; terms such as "whirring," "buzzing," and "humming" are not uncommon descriptors. The intensity or loudness of an innocent or flow murmur will be enhanced by anything that increases the velocity of blood flow, such as exertion, anxiety, or excitement. The typical functional murmur may become much softer or even disappear when the patient is in the upright position.

*Associated Findings.* The presence of an accompanying cardiovascular abnormality makes the diagnosis of an innocent murmur more problematic. For example, a coexisting systolic ejection or nonejection click, diastolic murmur, opening snap, or LV heave indicates that there is a probable cardiac abnormality. Nevertheless, such a finding may exist in association with an unrelated innocent murmur. The characteristics of S$_2$ may be useful. Completely normal splitting of S$_2$ makes an atrial septal defect or pulmonary stenosis most unlikely. In uncertain cases, a full cardiac evaluation is necessary, including an ECG and echocardiogram.

### Physiologic Murmurs

The distinction between an innocent murmur and a physiologic flow murmur is that the latter is caused by a *transient increase* in blood volume and/or velocity of ejection. When the causative factor for the augmented blood flow is removed (e.g., correction of anemia, lysis of fever, childbirth), the murmur no longer is audible or there is only a faint (grade 1/6 to 2/6) innocent murmur.

# 2

# The Normal Color Doppler Echocardiogram

Carlos A. Roldan

*Department of Internal Medicine, University of New Mexico School of Medicine; and Department of
Internal Medicine, Veterans Affairs Medical Center, Albuquerque, New Mexico*

## INTRODUCTION

Color Doppler echocardiography is a highly accurate imaging modality frequently used for assessment of the structure and function of the heart. This technique is noninvasive, is less expensive and free of risk compared with other imaging techniques, is easily available, allows immediate availability of results, requires minimal personnel involvement, and does not require the presence of a physician during performance of the most commonly used transthoracic echocardiography (TTE).

Use of echocardiography as a screening tool is not cost effective and may lead to misdiagnoses by an inexperienced observer unaware of normal variants of heart structure and function. Color Doppler echocardiography frequently can detect a trivial to mild degree of regurgitation of normal valves, detect valve excrescences, misclassify increased leaflet reflectance or thickness, and misdiagnose mitral leaflet prolapse. Misinterpretation of the study can lead to unnecessary patient anxiety and expenses. The diagnostic accuracy of echocardiography depends not only on the experience of interpreters, but also on the experience of technical personnel, adequacy of equipment, and standardization of methods.

Heart murmurs, ejection clicks, and third and fourth heart sounds are common manifestations of valvular, congenital, and myocardial disease; therefore, they are indicators of the need for echocardiography. However, heart murmurs are common (30% to 40%) in healthy subjects, including pregnant females. Also, third heart sounds are a normal variant in young athletes, and fourth heart sounds are highly prevalent in healthy subjects >65 years old. Therefore, the physical examination alone may not always accurately separate subjects with or without heart disease.

Color Doppler echocardiography should be considered only after a careful and complete history and physical examination, electrocardiogram (ECG), or chest radiography has been performed and assessed. These clinical data should determine the need for TTE, transesophageal echocardiography (TEE), stress echocardiography, or contrast echocardiography (1).

Complete TTE or TEE study includes M-mode and two-dimensional (2-D) images, as well as pulse, continuous, and color Doppler analysis. These imaging techniques allow complete assessment of cardiac chamber size; left ventricular (LV) and right ventricular (RV) wall thickness and wall motion; LV and RV systolic and diastolic function; left atrial (LA) and right atrial (RA) pressures; structure and function of the heart valves; presence or absence of intracardiac shunts; assessment of aortic root and pericardium; and estimate of atrial and pulmonary artery pressures. Surrounding noncardiac structures (lung, liver, and mediastinum) incidentally seen on routine cardiac imaging planes should be assessed during interpretation of studies. A complete echocardiogram, independent of its indication, should provide all that information.

The purpose of this chapter is to provide a guide to normal echocardiographic parameters and variants, with a brief description of appropriate imaging techniques and imaging planes.

## LEFT VENTRICLE

### Size and Volume

LV anteroposterior and mediolateral end-diastolic and end-systolic diameters are measured by TTE from the parasternal long- and short-axis views and apical four- and two-chamber views at the level of the papillary muscle tips (by M-mode or 2-D) (Fig. 2.1). By TTE, the anteroposterior LV diameters are measured from the leading edge of the interventricular septum to the leading edge of the posterior wall.

By TEE, LV diameters also are measured using the transgastric short- and long-axis views at the papillary muscle tips. When using the mid-esophageal TEE four- and two-chamber views, the transducer should be in a neutral or slightly retroflexed position to pre-

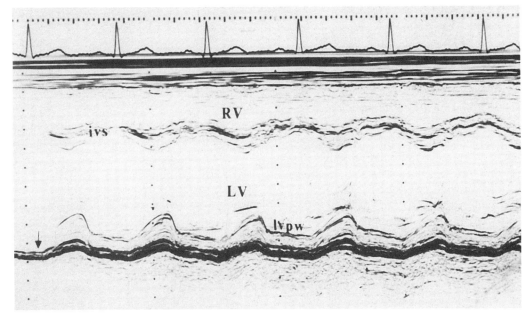

**FIG. 2.1.** M-mode echocardiogram of the right ventricle (RV) and left ventricle (LV) just above the papillary muscle level illustrates normal ventricular cavities, ≥30% systolic thickening of the interventricular septum (ivs) and posterior (lvpw) walls, and pericardial layers, especially after decreasing the gain transmit *(arrow)*

vent LV foreshortening, underestimation of LV volume, and overestimation of LV ejection fraction.

By TTE, LV end-diastolic anteroposterior and mediolateral diameter ranges from 3.4 to 5.6 cm and 3.3 to 5.6 cm, respectively (2–5). By TEE, these diameters measured from inner edge to inner edge range from 3.3 to 5.5 cm and 2.3 to 5.4 cm, respectively (6,7). By either technique, LV end-systolic diameters range from 2.3 to 4.3 cm and 2.4 to 4.8 cm, respectively. LV dilation is present when LV end-diastolic diameter is >5.6 cm.

Applying Simpson's rule using 2-D images for calculation of LV volumes by planimetry from the TTE or TEE four- and two-chamber views probably is the most accurate method to assess LV size, especially when LV geometry is abnormal (8). LV end-diastolic volume is proportional to body surface area and ranges from 59 to 157 mL. The upper limit of normal LV volume index is 65 mL/m$^2$. LV volumes are lower in women than in men.

**Wall Thickness and Mass**

LV end-diastolic wall thickness is reliably assessed by M-mode images of the septal and posterior walls from the TTE parasternal or TEE transgastric long- and short-axis views (Fig. 2.1). The upper limit of normal thickness is 1.1 cm for the septum and 1.0 cm for the posterior wall. LV posterior wall thickness and mass increase with age from about 0.9 cm and 125 g in subjects 20 years old to 1.1 cm and 150 g in subjects >50 years old (4,9).

LV mass can be calculated as 1.05 (total LV volume − LV cavity volume) using the 2-D short-axis view to obtain the myocardial volume and the area–length geometric formula to obtain the LV volume. LV mass also can be calculated from TTE M-mode images obtained from the long parasternal or short-axis views of the LV using the following formula: $0.80 \times 1.04[(\text{septal thickness} + \text{posterior wall thickness} + \text{LV internal diameter})^3 - \text{LV inter-}$

nal diameter[3]] (10). The upper limit of normal is <294 g (<143 g/m$^2$) for men and <198g (<102 g/m$^2$) for women.

## Wall Motion

The LV normally is divided into 16 myocardial segments for which a specific arterial supply has been determined. The basal, mid, and apical anterior; basal, mid, and apical anterior septum; and apical lateral wall blood supply corresponds to the left anterior descending artery (LAD). The basal and mid-anterolateral walls are supplied by the LAD or circumflex arteries. The basal and mid-inferior wall and the basal and mid-inferior septum are supplied by the right coronary artery (RCA). The apical inferior wall arterial supply corresponds to either the RCA or LAD. Finally, the basal and mid-inferolateral walls are supplied by the circumflex artery (Fig. 3.4).

TTE parasternal long- and short-axis and apical views and TEE transgastric short- and long-axis as well as mid-esophageal four- and two-chamber views are used to assess LV wall motion.

Normal resting LV wall motion is best defined by ≥30% endocardial thickening from baseline and less specifically by inward wall motion. Similarly, a normal wall-motion response to exercise or dobutamine echocardiography demonstrates hyperdynamic and symmetric ≥30% endocardial thickening. Each LV segment is scored as 1 = normal, 2 = hypokinetic, 3 = akinetic, or 4 = dyskinetic. Therefore, a normal global wall-motion score is 16 and a normal wall-motion score index is 1 (11).

## Systolic Function

The most commonly used parameters of LV systolic function include ejection fraction, fractional shortening, E point-septal separation, systolic descent of the LV annulus, and aortic root motion. Less commonly used parameters include calculation of stroke volume

and cardiac output and the ratio of preejection period to ejection period.

LV ejection fraction can be assessed by using the Simpson's rule (diastolic volume − systolic volume/diastolic volume). A normal ejection fraction by this method is ≥55%. However, visual estimation of ejection fraction using all TTE or TEE 2-D imaging planes has been demonstrated to be a practical, accurate, and reproducible method (8).

LV fractional shortening using TTE or TEE M-mode images is defined as the diastolic dimension minus the systolic dimension/diastolic dimension. A normal fractional shortening is ≥35%. LV ejection fraction is estimated by multiplying the fractional shortening by a constant of 1.7 (12).

"E point-septal separation," the distance between the most posterior septal endocardium (systole) and the most anterior motion of the anterior mitral valve during early (E) LV filling, generally is ≤5 mm. E point-septal separation is influenced by LV size and stroke volume or transmitral volume flow. These factors are important determinants of LV ejection fraction. As the LV dilates and mitral inflow decreases, E point-septal separation increases. Therefore, an E point-septal separation <7 mm reliably predicts preserved LV systolic function (13).

Systolic descent of the mitral annulus toward the LV apex of >1 cm predicts normal LV systolic function. Descent of the base of <8 mm has 98% sensitivity and 82% specificity for detection of an ejection fraction <50% (14).

The anteroposterior motion of the aortic root is determined by LA filling and emptying (preload or stroke volume) and LV contractility. In patients with normal LV systolic function, the aortic root moves >1 cm or 30- to 45-degree angle from end-diastole to its maximal anterior systolic excursion.

Stroke volume is calculated using the following formula: 0.785(LV outflow tract diameter)$^2$ or $\pi r^2$ × LV outflow velocity time integral (15). LV outflow tract diameter is measured from TTE long parasternal 2-D im-

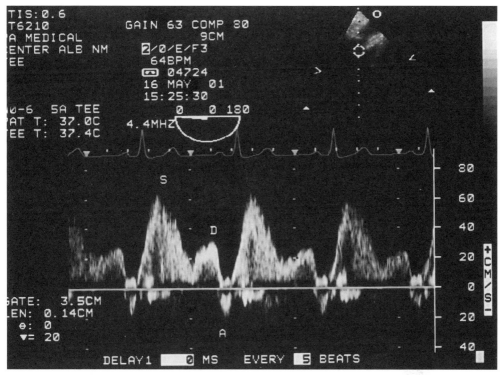

**FIG. 2.2.** *Continued.* **C:** Transesophageal echocardiographic tracing of the left upper pulmonary vein in another middle-aged healthy subject demonstrates systolic (S) predominance, systolic filling fraction >50%, and atrial reversal (A) of small amplitude and duration.

## LEFT ATRIA

### Size and Volume

LA size or volume is largest at end-systole; therefore, the LA anteroposterior diameter is measured at end-systole (end of T wave in the ECG) from the parasternal long- or short-axis views using TTE M-mode or 2-D images. It is measured from the trailing edge of the anterior atrial wall to the leading edge of the posterior wall. By TEE, the anteroposterior and mediolateral diameters are measured from the mid-esophageal four-chamber view from the walls inner edge to inner edge. By TTE, the maximal anteroposterior, mediolateral, and superoinferior diameters of the LA range from 2.2 to 4.1 cm, 2.5 to 4.5 cm, and 3.1 to 6.8 cm, respectively. LA anteroposterior diameter is generally the best defined and, therefore, the most commonly used to assess LA size. Similar values for the anteroposterior and mediolateral LA diameters using 2-D TEE images have been reported. Thus, LA enlargement is considered present when LA measures ≥4.2 cm. Another visual or quantitative parameter of normal LA size is an LA to aortic root ratio of 1.1:1.

LA volumes can be measured by Simpson's rule using TTE four- and two-chamber views from which the entire atria can be delineated. Normal LA volume ranges from 20 to 60 mL (20). Men, nonathletes, and subjects >50 years old have larger volumes than women, athletes, and younger subjects. LA area obtained from TTE parasternal long- and short-axis or apical views ranges from 9 to 23 cm².

Because of the proximity of the TEE transducer to the LA superoposterior portion, complete delineation of the LA is commonly not possible. Therefore, assessment of LA volume and area is difficult and less reliable by TEE. By TEE, the maximum length (anteroposterior) and mediolateral diameter of the LA appendage ranges from 1.5 to 4.3 cm and 1.0 to 2.8 cm, respectively.

## Function

The LA is a reservoir of blood during LV systole, a conduit for blood during early LV filling, and a contractile chamber. During LV systole, LA volume is the highest and pressure is high. During atrial contraction, LA pressure is the highest. After atrial contraction, LA volume and pressure are the lowest. LA contractility and ejection fraction are dependent on atrial preload (Frank Starling mechanism) and afterload (determined by LV compliance or diastolic pressure before atrial contraction). Normal atrial stroke volume is 20% to 40% of LV stroke volume, and LA fractional emptying is about 60%.

## Left Atrial Pressure and Pulmonary Veins

Flow from LA to LV occurs during early and late filling (E and A waves, respectively). E wave velocity is driven by the pressure gradient between LA and LV at the time of mitral valve opening. In young people, this gradient is high because a rapidly relaxing LV causes an abrupt fall in LV diastolic pressure. This transient high gradient produces a high E wave velocity (Fig. 2.2A). With aging, LV relaxation slows, E wave velocity decreases, and A wave velocity becomes predominant. However, with significant LV diastolic dysfunction, mean LA pressure rises, the LA–LV pressure gradient is high at the time of mitral opening, and a high E wave velocity is seen. Because LV end-diastolic pressure is so high at the time of atrial contraction, a small A wave velocity occurs. This mitral inflow pattern may be misinterpreted as the normal pattern seen in normal young adults. Therefore, in older persons or patients with heart disease, an E/A ratio >2:1 is a reliable indication of elevated mean LA pressure (pulmonary capillary wedge pressure ≥18 mm Hg) (17–19).

Four pulmonary veins drain into the LA. The upper and lower pulmonary veins from the right lung drain into the superior and medial areas of the LA and the respective veins from the left lung insert into the superior and lateral portions of the LA.

By TTE, the right pulmonary veins occasionally may be seen in the long parasternal view and the left pulmonary veins in the basilar short-axis view. From the suprasternal short-axis view, the four pulmonary veins can be visualized posterior to the aorta and right pulmonary artery. However, the most appropriate TTE view for assessment of pulmonary vein flow is the apical four-chamber view. From this view, two lateral and one medial (right lower) pulmonary veins generally are identified (Fig. 2.2B).

By multiplane TEE, from the midesophageal short-axis view and at 0 to 30 degrees of rotation, the four pulmonary veins, especially the upper veins, can be identified and their flow patterns assessed. Clockwise and counterclockwise rotations from the short-axis view of the aortic valve allow visualization of the left and right upper pulmonary veins, respectively. From those views, a slight advancement of the TEE probe allows visualization of the lower pulmonary veins.

The best signal and higher pulmonary veins velocities are obtained by placing the sample volume 0.5 to 1 cm into the pulmonary vein. A normal pulmonary vein flow pattern consists of four phases (Fig. 2.2B–C). The first antegrade systolic flow (S1) occurs during atrial relaxation (after the P wave of the ECG). The second antegrade systolic flow (S2) occurs due to a fall in LA pressure during the annular displacement associated with LV contraction (believed to produce a suction effect). The third antegrade diastolic flow (D) occurs soon after mitral valve opening (which causes LA pressure to fall), and its flow and peak velocity are dependent on the LV-pulmonary vein pressure gradients. Pulmonary vein peak diastolic velocity and deceleration time should be similar to those of the mitral E wave. The final and retrograde flow occurs during atrial contraction (A) and generally is of smaller amplitude and duration than the mitral A wave, but its peak velocity and duration increase proportional to LV end-diastolic pressure. In young normal subjects (<30 years old), because of the low LA pressure and LA–LV pressure gradient, systolic velocities normally are lower than diastolic velocities. With increasing age (>40 years old), LV relaxation and compliance decrease; consequently, increases in systolic flow velocities and ratio of systolic to diastolic velocities are observed. In addition, flow reversal after atrial contraction increases.

In normal subjects, the velocity time integral of antegrade systolic flows of the pulmonary veins constitutes 60% to 70% of the sum of the velocity time integrals of the systolic and diastolic velocities (termed "systolic fraction") and normally is >50%. Therefore, a systolic fraction <50% indicates LA hypertension or high pulmonary capillary wedge pressure (≥18 mm Hg) (17–19).

## MITRAL VALVE

The mitral valve apparatus consists of the mitral leaflets, chordae tendineae, fibromuscular mitral annulus, papillary muscles, and LV walls where the papillary muscles attach. The normal mitral valve area is 4 to 6 cm$^2$.

### Leaflets

The mitral valve has two major leaflets, the anterior and posterior leaflet. Mitral leaflet thickness, echo-reflectance, mobility, and length are best assessed by M-mode or 2-D images obtained from TTE parasternal long- and short-axis views and TEE mid-

esophageal four- and two-chamber views at 0 degrees (excludes the LV outflow tract).

### *Thickness*

By TTE, limited data are available regarding normal valve thickness values. By TEE M-mode and 2-D images obtained from the mid-esophageal four- and two-chamber views during systole (using a narrow sector scan and at a depth of 6 to 8 cm), normal mitral leaflet thickness at any portion ranges from 0.7 to 3 mm (Fig. 2.3) (21). The leaflet base and tip portions are thicker than the mid portions, and the thickness of the anterior leaflet is similar to that of the posterior leaflet.

Because measurement of leaflet thickness is time consuming, leaflet thickness usually is assessed visually. Using quantitative measurements of leaflet thickness as the standard, the specificity of visual assessment for mitral valve thickness is 87% by TEE and 83% by TTE.

### *Echo-reflectance*

Normally, the echo-reflectance of the mitral leaflets is homogeneous and of soft tissue, but it is slightly higher than that of the myocardium.

### *Mobility*

Mobility of the mitral leaflets is dependent on LV preload, LA–LV pressure gradient, LV compliance, and LV contractility. Mitral leaflet mobility is best assessed during rapid filling of the LV. By M-mode images obtained using 2-D recordings and from the TTE parasternal long-axis view, the normal motion of the anterior leaflet appears as an M shape and that of the posterior leaflet as a blunted W. Initial opening of the anterior leaflet generally forms an angle ≥70 degrees from the point of closure (D to E slope). Similarly, immediately after cessation of LV filling and as result of increased LV volume and diastolic pressure, the anterior mitral leaflet partially closes and forms the E to F slope of ≥70 degrees. By 2-D images, both an-

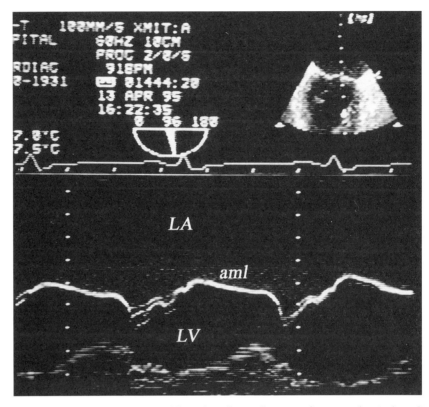

**FIG. 2.3.** Normal mitral valve thickness. M-mode echocardiogram of a normal anterior mitral leaflet (aml) obtained from the mid-esophageal two-chamber view. Note the perpendicular alignment between the ultrasound beam and the mitral leaflet during systole. Note the uniformly thin (<2 mm) leaflet. From the same view, a similar tracing was obtained for the posterior leaflet. Similar M-mode tracings can be obtained from the four-chamber view. LA, left atrium; LV, left ventricle.

terior and posterior leaflets show a parallel motion in relation to the interventricular septum (anterior leaflet) and posterior wall (posterior leaflet). The distance between the leaflets and respective LV wall is <5 mm during their maximum excursion. Because the posterior leaflet is shorter and has a larger area of attachment to the mitral annulus, its mobility is less than that of the anterior leaflet.

### Length

The anterior leaflet is longer than the posterior leaflet and constitutes about two thirds of the mitral annulus diameter during systole. However, the posterior leaflet has a larger area of attachment to the mitral annulus.

### Annulus

Mitral valve annulus diameter generally is measured during early diastole when mitral leaflets are at their most open and nearest position to their respective LV walls. It is measured from the base of the anterior to the base of the posterior leaflet and from the apical TTE or TEE four-chamber views. By either technique, mitral annulus diameter ranges from 2.0 to 3.8 cm.

### Subvalvular Apparatus

The mitral leaflets are anchored by a network of chordae tendineae that insert at or near the free edges and less commonly into the body of the leaflets and commissural portions. Chordae tendineae arising from the postero-medial papillary muscle insert into the medial half of the anterior and posterior leaflets and those arising from the anterolateral papillary muscle insert into the lateral half of both leaflets. They appear as thin, linear, and ho-mogeneously echo-reflectant structures that extend from the papillary muscles to the mitral leaflet tips. Use of harmonic imaging im-proves visualization and definition of inser-tion points of the chordae tendineae.

The papillary muscles are extensions of the LV muscular trabeculae, are located in the posterior half of the LV, and are oriented par-allel to the mitral leaflets' closure line. By TTE, the posterolateral papillary muscle mus-cle is best seen from the parasternal long- and short-axis, apical, and subcostal views. The anterolateral papillary muscle is best seen in the parasternal short-axis view. By TEE, pap-illary muscles are best seen in the transgastric short- and long-axis and mid-esophageal four- and two-chamber views. The posterome-dial papillary muscle is thicker than the an-terolateral papillary muscle. They are of conic shape and their maximum thickness is about 1 to 1.5 cm.

## Regurgitation

The overall prevalence of mitral regurgita-tion in healthy subjects by color Doppler ranges from 38% to 45%. Most (70% to 80%) of these subjects have a trivial degree of re-gurgitation characterized by early systolic, central, narrow, and small jets (<2 cm long and <1 cm$^2$ jet area). The prevalence of mitral regurgitation does not change among healthy subjects aged 10 to 50 years (22).

## AORTIC VALVE AND OUTFLOW TRACT

The aortic valve consists of the right, left, and noncoronary cusps. Normal aortic valve area is 3 to 5 cm$^2$. Components of the aortic valve apparatus include the cusps, annulus, LV outflow tract, and aorta. By TTE, the aor-tic valve apparatus is best seen from the parasternal long- and short-axis and apical three- or five-chamber views. By multiplane TEE, it is best assessed from the mid-esophageal short-axis view with the multi-plane at an angle between 30 and 60 degrees. This view allows assessment of commissures, cusps margins, and coronary sinuses. The valve should be scanned from the outflow tract to the sinus portion of the aortic root by slowly withdrawing or advancing the TEE probe. From the short-axis view, the plane ro-tated to a longitudinal view (80 to 120 de-grees) allows assessment of the LV outflow tract, noncoronary (sometimes the left) and right coronary cusps, aortic annulus, and aor-tic root.

## Cusps

### Thickness

Normal thickness of the aortic cusps ranges from 0.5 to 2 mm by TEE M-mode and 2-D recordings obtained during systole from the mid-esophageal long- and short-axis views (Fig. 2.4). The thickness of the three cusps is similar. Using quantitative aortic cusp mea-surements as the standard, visual assessment of aortic cusp thickness has a specificity of 92% by TEE and 87% by TTE (21).

### Location

The right coronary cusp is located antero-medially and the noncoronary cusp posteriorly and in close proximity to the most distal por-tion of the interatrial septum. These two cusps are seen in most TTE or TEE views. The left coronary cusp is located laterally and is seen in TTE parasternal and subcostal short-axis and TEE mid-esophageal short-axis views.

### Reflectance

As for the mitral valve leaflets, the aortic cusps are homogeneously echo-reflectant and of slightly higher echo-reflectance than that of the myocardium.

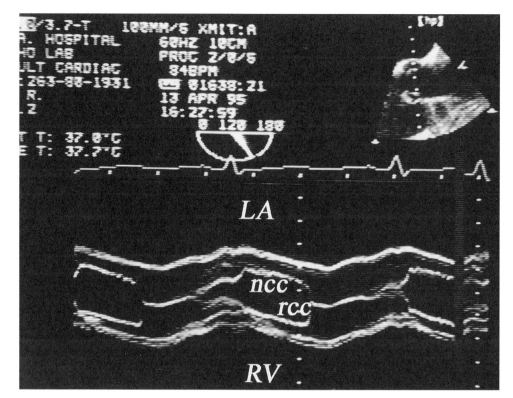

**FIG. 2.4.** Normal aortic valve thickness. M-mode echocardiogram of normal aortic noncoronary cusp (ncc) and right coronary cusp (rcc) obtained from the mid-esophageal longitudinal view of the aortic valve. Note the perpendicular alignment between the ultrasound beam and the cusps during systole. Also note that the cusps have similar and uniform thickness (<2 mm). Similar tracings can be obtained from the short-axis view of the aortic valve (about 30 degrees). LA, left atrium; RV, right ventricle.

### Mobility

Mobility of the aortic cusps is determined by LV stroke volume and contractility. Normally the aortic cusps have a 90-degree excursion from the aortic annulus. During systole, the cusps lie parallel and within a few millimeters of the aortic root walls. Normal cusp separation is ≥2 cm.

### Length

The normal length of the aortic cusps is approximately 1.5 to 2 cm.

### Annulus

The aortic annulus is best delineated from TTE or TEE views longitudinal to the outflow tract or aortic root. Its landmarks are the junction of the aortic root anterior wall with the interventricular septum and the junction of the aortic posterior wall with the base of the anterior mitral leaflet (intervalvular fibrosa). Annulus diameter at end-diastole ranges from 1.4 to 2.6 cm by TTE and 1.8 to 2.7 cm by TEE.

### Outflow Tract

As for the aortic annulus, the LV outflow tract is assessed during systole by TTE or TEE views longitudinal to the aortic root. The inner portion of the proximal interventricular septum and the intervalvular fibrosa delineate it. LV outflow tract diameter measured within 1 cm of the aortic annulus ranges from 1.8 to 2.4 cm.

## Valve and Outflow Tract Flow Velocities

The normal aortic valve flow is laminar with an acceleration time shorter than the deceleration time. Normal aortic valve and outflow tract velocities range from 1.0 to 1.7 m/s and 0.7 to 1.1 m/s, respectively (23). Two preejection velocities normally can be seen in the LV outflow tract (Fig. 2.5).The first and predominant velocity or A wave is the result of atrial contraction causing extension of flow into the LV apex and then into the aortic valve. The second component corresponds to flow produced by LV isovolumetric contraction and mitral valve closure. This last velocity is of lower amplitude than that of the A wave.

## Regurgitation

The prevalence of aortic regurgitation in normal subjects 10 to 50 years old ranges from 0% to 2% and is almost always of trivial degree. Recent studies in healthy but obese subjects reported prevalence rates up to 7% (24). The prevalence of aortic regurgitation increases as healthy subjects age beyond 50 years; by age ≥70 years it is the most commonly regurgitant valve.

## AORTA

The aorta consists of the ascending aorta, aortic arch, and descending aorta.

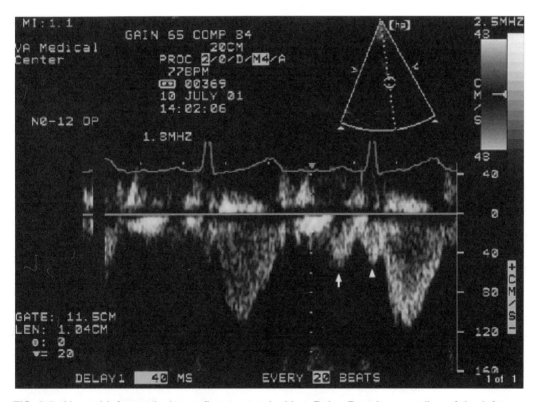

**FIG. 2.5.** Normal left ventricular outflow tract velocities. Pulse Doppler recording of the left ventricular outflow tract in a young healthy subject demonstrates normal laminar flow velocity during the ejection period of about 1 m/s with a short acceleration, but longer deceleration time. Two preejection velocities also are noted. The first and predominant velocity or A wave *(arrow)* is the result of atrial contraction causing extension of flow into the left ventricular apex and then into the aortic valve. The second velocity *(arrowhead)* results from flow produced by left ventricular isovolumetric contraction and mitral valve closure. This last velocity is of lower amplitude than that of the A wave.

## Ascending Aorta

The ascending aorta extends for about 5 cm from the annulus level to its junction with the aortic arch. It is subdivided into the sinuses and tubular portions. It is best assessed by TTE parasternal long-axis and TEE mid-esophageal long-axis views (at about 80 to 120 degrees).

### *Aortic Sinuses*

The sinuses of Valsalva and named right, left, and noncoronary sinuses are outpouchings of the aortic root located just above the aortic cusps with a diameter 3 to 5 mm larger than the annulus and tubular portion. At this level, the end-diastolic aortic diameter ranges from 2.1 to 3.5 cm. The right and left coronary sinuses give rise to their respective coronary arteries, provide a reservoir for diastolic coronary flow, and allow a separation during systole of the aortic cusps and the coronary ostia. At this level, the thickness of the anterior and posterior aortic root walls assessed by TEE M-mode or 2-D images normally is <2.2 mm (25).

### *Tubular Aorta*

The tubular aorta extends for about 3 cm from the sinotubular junction (located about 2 cm from the aortic annulus). It has a smaller diameter than the sinus portion but is slightly larger than the annulus. Its diameter measured from the inner edge of the anterior wall to the leading edge of the posterior wall ranges from 1.7 to 3.4 cm. The thickness of the aortic walls at this level is similar to that at the sinus level (<2.2 mm).

Aortic root motion is dependent on LV contractility and stroke volume and normally is >1 cm or of a 30- to 45-degree angle from end-diastole to its maximal systolic anterior excursion.

## Aortic Arch

From the suprasternal notch view, the aortic arch and its three major branches (left subclavian, left common carotid, and innominate arteries) are commonly visualized. By TEE, the distal portion and especially its anterior wall are best visualized. By TEE, about 2 cm of the arch in front of the trachea is not visualized (the "blind spot").

## Descending Aorta

The descending aorta is seen posterior to the atrioventricular groove and distal portion of the LA on TTE parasternal long-axis view. Its normal diameter ranges from 2 to 2.5 cm. The proximal descending aorta is slightly larger than the distal portion. From the TTE long parasternal short-axis view of the LV at the papillary muscle level, the descending aorta is located posteromedially and at the aortic valve level is located posterolaterally.

## RIGHT VENTRICLE

### Size

RV size cannot be quantitated accurately by routine echocardiography due to its crescentic shape and its anterosuperior position in relation to the LV. The parasternal long-axis and subcostal four-chamber views frequently transect the RV at its anterosuperior and posterolateral horn, respectively. Therefore, RV size frequently is underestimated from these views. The TTE apical four-chamber view may transect the RV oblique to its long axis and overestimate its size. Thus, visual assessment of the RV size should integrate all echocardiographic planes.

RV maximal anteroposterior dimension from the TTE parasternal or TEE transgastric long-axis or mid-esophageal four-chamber view (by M-mode or 2D) should not exceed 3.5 cm. End-diastolic mediolateral diameter of the RV mid-cavity from the apical four-chamber view ranges from 2.1 to 4.2 cm. LV size provides a valuable comparison in the four-chamber views for assessing RV size. With mild dilation, RV area remains less than LV area. The apex of the RV should fall short of the LV apex by approximately one third of the distance from the base to the apex. Any alteration suggests RV enlargement.

For all those reasons and lack of a standard, data on normal RV volumes by echocardiography are limited.

### Wall Thickness

Normal RV wall thickness ranges from 2 to 5 mm and is best assessed from TTE parasternal long- and short-axis views using M-mode images. In these views, the ultrasound beam generally is perpendicular to the RV anterolateral wall. Therefore, RV hypertrophy is present when RV wall thickness measures >5 mm. Assessment of RV wall thickness from other views is less accurate. Due to decreased ultrasound lateral resolution, the RV lateral wall endocardium frequently is not well defined from the apical four-chamber view. In addition, the RV walls are lined with multiple trabeculae carneae (small muscle bands). Therefore, visual assessment of normal RV wall thickness lacks specificity.

### Wall Motion

Assessment of RV wall motion is limited due to difficulties in defining systolic thickening of its thin endocardium and lack of a standard. Therefore, RV wall motion is subjectively defined and based on its inward motion rather than its endocardial thickening. It is best assessed from TTE parasternal and subcostal long- and short-axis views.

### Systolic Function

As for RV size and wall thickness, RV systolic function is visually assessed. TTE parasternal long- and short-axis views, parasternal long-axis view of RV inflow, apical and subcostal four-chamber views, and TEE transgastric short- and long-axis views of the RV as well as mid-esophageal four-chamber views offer the best images for assessment of RV systolic function. A systolic excursion of the tricuspid annulus toward the cardiac apex of ≥2 cm denotes normal RV systolic function. This parameter has demonstrated a good correlation with nuclear methods ($R = 0.92$) (26). A

systolic excursion <0.5 cm indicates severe RV systolic dysfunction. Although not standardized, normal values currently are available. The inward motion of the RV free wall highly correlates with RV systolic function. Difficulties measuring RV volumes have made methods for measuring RV ejection fraction difficult and often inaccurate. Using nuclear techniques, normal RV ejection fraction is ≥40%.

Tissue Doppler imaging of the tricuspid annulus recently was shown to be a valuable parameter for assessment of RV systolic function. A peak systolic annular velocity ≥11.5 cm/s (normal range 11.6 to 21.1 cm/s) is predictive of an RV ejection fraction >45%. Time from onset of the ECG QRS complex to the peak systolic annular velocity of >200 ms also is predictive of RV ejection fraction >45% (27).

### Diastolic Function

Diastolic function of the RV has not been studied as extensively as that of the LV. It can be assessed by RV IVRT and tricuspid inflow and inferior vena cava (IVC) or hepatic vein Doppler flow velocities. These parameters follow a similar pattern to those of LV relaxation time and mitral and pulmonary vein inflow Doppler variables (28,29).

### RIGHT ATRIA

#### Size

The size and volumes of the RA are best evaluated from the apical four-chamber view. The parasternal long-axis view of RV inflow, the subcostal four-chamber view, and less optimally the parasternal short-axis view can complement the four-chamber views. By TEE, the transgastric long-axis view of the RV is adequate.

In normal subjects, the end-systolic superoinferior and mediolateral dimensions of the RA range from 3.4 to 4.9 cm and 2.9 to 4.6 cm, respectively. Normal RA area ranges from 8.3 to 19.5 cm$^2$. As a rule, RA area should not exceed LA area.

**Venous Vessels and Right Atrial Pressure**

Three principal venous vessels drain into the RA. The IVC drains into its right inferior portion, the superior vena cava into the right anterosuperior wall, and the coronary sinus into its posterior portion above the tricuspid annulus and distal to the inferior portion of the interatrial septum.

Echocardiographic evaluation of the size of the IVC and its response to respiration in the supine position provides a rough estimate of mean RA pressure. The negative intrathoracic pressure generated by inspiration normally is 5 to 10 mm Hg and normally causes the IVC to collapse. Therefore, normal RA pressure is 5 to 10 mm Hg.

RA pressure is low (<5 mm Hg) if the IVC is small (<1.5 cm) and collapses with inspiration; normal (5 to 10 mm Hg) if the IVC mea-

sures 1.5 to 2.5 cm and collapses >50%; mildly elevated (10 to 15 mm Hg) if the IVC is of normal size and collapses <50%; moderately elevated (15 to 20 mm Hg) if the IVC is >2.5 cm and collapses <50%; and severely elevated (>20 mm Hg) if the hepatic veins are dilated and the IVC does not collapse with inspiration (30). Also, failure of the IVC to collapse with a sniff indicates RA pressure >20 mm Hg.

Flow from the hepatic veins is determined by the pressure gradient between these vessels and the RA. From the subcostal view, flow from these vessels is parallel to the Doppler sample volume and, therefore, ideal for assessing RA pressure. The sample volume placed near the junction of the hepatic veins and IVC allows for the best Doppler velocity recordings.

The first predominant forward flow of the hepatic veins in systole is due to a fall in RA pressure after atrial relaxation (after the P wave

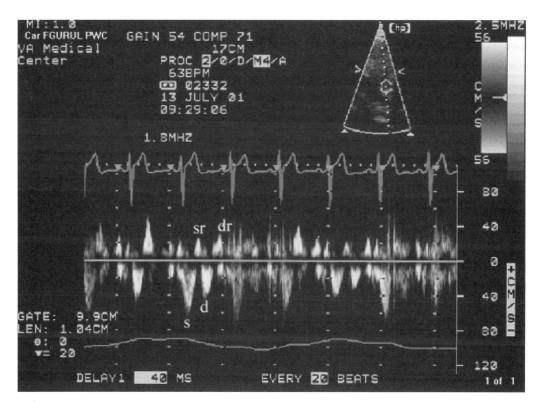

**FIG. 2.6.** Normal flow pattern of hepatic veins. Hepatic vein pulse Doppler flow pattern obtained from the subcostal view and recorded at 25 cm/s paper speed demonstrates the normal predominance of the systolic (s) over the diastolic (d) component, more noticeable in this tracing at the end of inspiration. Also note the respective systolic flow reversal (sr) as well as diastolic reversal (dr) following atrial contraction.

of the QRS) and downward displacement of the tricuspid annulus during RV contraction. The second forward diastolic flow is related to a fall in RA pressure during RV filling. Minimal retrograde flows (toward the transducer) are seen at the end of atrial and ventricular systole (Fig. 2.6). During inspiration, systolic and diastolic forward flow velocities increase and the reversal velocities decrease. Opposite changes occur during expiration and apnea. With decreased RV compliance, atrial reversal increases, systolic flow decreases, and the diastolic velocity becomes predominant.

In normal subjects, the time velocity integral of the antegrade systolic flow of the hepatic veins constitutes >50% of the sum of the systolic and diastolic velocity time integrals (termed "systolic fraction," normally >50%). Therefore, a systolic proportion of total forward flow of <50% and <20% are sensitive and specific for RA pressure >8 mm Hg and >15 mm Hg, respectively (28,30,31).

## TRICUSPID VALVE

The tricuspid valve apparatus includes the anterior, septal, and posterior leaflets; annulus; chordae tendineae; papillary muscles corresponding to each leaflet; and RV myocardium. The tricuspid valve is larger and more complex than the mitral valve. The best TTE views to assess the anterior and posterior tricuspid leaflets are the parasternal long-axis view of the RV inflow, parasternal short-axis view, and apical and subcostal four-chamber views. Rarely, the papillary muscles are visualized from these views. By TEE, the transgastric long-axis view of the RV allows detailed visualization of the anterior and posterior leaflets, chordae, and corresponding papillary muscles

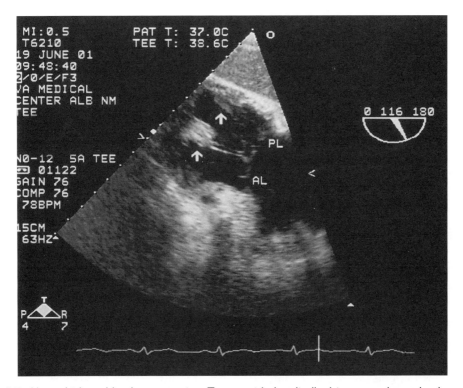

**FIG. 2.7.** Normal tricuspid valve apparatus. Transgastric longitudinal transesophageal echocardiographic view of the right ventricle demonstrates normal appearance of the posterior (PL) and anterior (AL) tricuspid leaflets, thin chordae tendineae, and corresponding small posterior and large anterior papillary muscles *(arrows).*

(Fig. 2.7). The transgastric short-axis view allows assessment of the three tricuspid leaflets. The TEE mid-esophageal four-chamber and short-axis views allow assessment of the anterior and septal leaflets. From all these TTE or TEE views, the tricuspid valve can be interrogated by Doppler techniques to determine the presence, severity, and peak velocity of tricuspid regurgitation (TR). The TTE four-chamber view is the most appropriate for assessment of the severity and peak velocity of TR and tricuspid valve inflow Doppler velocities.

## Leaflets

### *Thickness*

By TTE, no data currently are available about normal thickness values of the tricuspid leaflets. By multiplane 2-D TEE images, the thickness of the basal, mid, and tip portions of the anterior and septal TV leaflets can be measured from the mid-esophageal four-chamber view in most subjects. The posterior TV leaflet can be measured from the transgastric RV long-axis view. By TEE, the normal thickness of the tricuspid leaflets ranges from 0.7 to 3 mm and is similar among the three leaflets (21). As for the mitral valve, the basilar and tip portions are the thickest. Using quantitative tricuspid leaflet measurements as the standard, visual assessment of tricuspid valve thickness has a specificity of 99% by TEE and 97% by TTE.

### *Mobility*

As for the mitral valve, no standards have been defined regarding normal mobility of the tricuspid leaflets. However, the anterior and posterior leaflets follow a mobility pattern similar to that of the mitral leaflets. The septal leaflet is the least mobile.

### *Length*

The anterior tricuspid leaflet is the largest and extends from the anterior to the inferolateral portion of the tricuspid annulus. The septal leaflet is the shortest, extends from the muscular to the membranous interventricular septum,

and inserts more apically than the anterior mitral leaflet. The posterior leaflet extends from the inferior septum to the inferolateral wall and is of similar length to that of the anterior leaflet.

## Annulus

Tricuspid valve annulus diameter is measured during early diastole (when leaflets are in their most open and nearest position to their respective RV walls). It is measured from the base of the anterior leaflet to the base of the septal leaflet from the TTE or TEE four-chamber views. Similar values ranging from 2 to 4 cm have been reported by both techniques. The tricuspid and mitral annulus diameters are similar.

## Subvalvular Apparatus

The anterior papillary muscle is the largest, is located behind the commissures of the anterior and posterior leaflets, and is attached to free RV anterolateral wall and partly to the moderator band. The posterior papillary muscle is small and lies behind the commissure of the posterior and septal leaflets. The small septal papillary muscle tethers the anterior and septal leaflets against the infundibular wall.

From the TTE parasternal long-axis view of the RV inflow and from the subcostal four-chamber view, the anterior and posterior papillary muscles are partially visualized. From the TEE transgastric long-axis view of the RV, the posterior and anterior papillary muscles and their chordal attachments are generally well defined (Fig. 2.7).

## Regurgitation

The prevalence of TR as determined by color Doppler ranges from 15% to 78%. Its prevalence is highest (60% to 65%) in younger subjects 10 to 30 years old and lowest (15% to 35%) in those 30 to 50 years old. In highly trained athletes, the prevalence is up to 90% in contrast to <25% in those with sedentary lifestyles. The degree of TR in healthy subjects is predominantly (>80%) of trivial degree, with centrally located small jets having areas <1.5 cm² (22). The decrease of TR with aging may be related to decreased ultrasound penetration and image resolution.

## PULMONIC VALVE

The pulmonic valve is located left, anterior, and superior to the aortic valve and consists of the anterior, right posterior, and left posterior cusps. From TTE parasternal and subcostal views and TEE transgastric and mid-esophageal short-axis views, with the imaging plane parallel to the RV outflow tract, the anterior and right posterior cusps, RV outflow tract, annulus, and main pulmonary artery can be assessed. All three cusps can be seen with a mid-esophageal short-axis multiplane TEE view (at 0 to 30 degrees) slightly above the aortic valve cups. All these views allow evaluation of pulmonic valve flow, RV stroke volume, and regurgitation.

### Cusps

Although M-mode recordings have been used to assess the structural characteristics of the pulmonic cusps, adequate tracings in normal subjects are rarely obtained. As for other heart valves, no TTE data on normal leaflets thickness values have been reported. By TEE 2-D images, leaflet thickness measured at the mid portion from the mid-esophageal short-axis and longitudinal views ranges from 0.7 to 2 mm (values similar to those of the aortic valve cups) (21). Using quantitative pulmonic leaflet measurements as the standard, visual assessment of pulmonic valve thickness has a specificity of 97% by TEE and 94% by TTE. The reflectance, mobility, and length of the pulmonic cusps are similar to those of the aortic cusps. Laminar flow velocities across the pulmonary valve in normal adults range from 0.6 to 0.9 m/s. RV outflow tract diameter (measured within 1 cm from the annulus) and the pulmonic valve annulus by TTE 2-D images measure 1.8 to 3.4 cm and 1.0 to 2.2 cm, respectively. By TEE, normal RV outflow tract diameter ranges from 1.6 to 3.6 cm.

### Regurgitation

The prevalence and distribution of pulmonic regurgitation (PR) in healthy subjects is similar to that of TR, ranging from 28% to 88%. Prevalence rates are highest in subjects <30 years old and lowest among those 30 to 50 years old. The degree of PR in healthy subjects usually is trivial, with centrally located jets having areas ≤1 cm² (22). As for TR, the decrease in the prevalence of PR with aging may be related to decreased ultrasound penetration and image resolution.

## PULMONARY ARTERY AND PRESSURE

### Anatomy

The main pulmonary artery is best imaged by TTE from the parasternal and subcostal short-axis views and by multiplane TEE from the mid-esophageal short-axis view of the pulmonic valve with the imaging plane parallel to the RV outflow tract (about 30 to 45 degrees). The right and left pulmonary arteries can be imaged from the suprasternal or supraclavicular views. Flow in the pulmonary artery gradually accelerates and decelerates, and increases by 15% during inspiration. Pulmonary artery peak velocities in normal adults are similar to those of the pulmonic valve and range from 0.6 to 0.9 m/s. A normal pulmonary artery acceleration time (from onset of flow to peak velocity) is >110 ms. Normal diameters of the main, right, and left pulmonary arteries by TTE range from 0.9 to 2.9 cm, 0.7 to 1.7 cm, and 0.6 to 1.4 cm, respectively. By TEE, the right pulmonary artery diameter ranges from 1.2 to 2.2 cm.

### Systolic Pressure

TR peak velocity measured by continuous wave Doppler is used to estimate the gradient between RV and RA systolic pressure. RV and pulmonary artery systolic pressures are equal in the absence of pulmonic stenosis. Estimated RA pressure from clinical or echocardiographic data then is added to the transtricuspid gradient to provide an estimate of the pulmonary artery systolic pressure using the modified Bernoulli equation as $4V^2$ (where V = peak TR velocity) plus the estimated RA pressure. A normal pulmonary artery systolic pressure is <30 mm Hg. Due to the variability of TR velocities with respiration and heart rate, it is recommended that three to five beats be averaged to estimate this pressure. The correlation between Doppler-derived and catheter-measured pressure gradients is 0.96, with interobserver and intraobserver observer variability in peak gradients of <2 mm Hg (32).

### Diastolic Pressure

In the presence of PR, pulmonary artery diastolic pressure can be estimated by applying the Bernoulli equation ($4V^2$) to the PR end-diastolic velocity obtained by continuous wave Doppler and adding to this value an estimated RA pressure (33).

## PERICARDIUM

The pericardium is a fibrous membrane that separates the heart from other intrathoracic structures and is formed by the visceral and parietal pericardium. A space between the visceral and parietal pericardium constitutes the pericardial cavity, which contains about 20 to 30 mL of fluid that originates from the subepicardial lymphatics. The pericardial space extends superiorly just above the origin of the great vessels and posteriorly to the insertion of the pulmonary veins and vena cava. The pericardial fluid allows the pericardial layers to slide over each other smoothly during cardiac motion. The pericardial layers and their sliding motion are better appreciated by TTE long parasternal and subcostal four-chamber views and TEE transgastric short- and long-axis views of the LV and RV.

Normally and during diastole, the pericardium appears as a single highly reflective linear structure better noted posterior to the LV. During systole, a few millimeters of separation can be noted among the pericardial layers. To improve visualization of the peri-

cardium, the transmitted pulse or gain can be decreased to attenuate the echo-reflectance of endocardial and myocardial surfaces and allow visualization of a more reflective pericardium (Fig. 2.1). Normal pericardial thickness as determined by TEE is $1.2 \pm 0.8$ mm. Normal intrapericardial pressure is subatmospheric or negative (−1 to −3 mm Hg) and allows a positive transmural pressure gradient and, therefore, filling of the heart chambers. Pericardial pressure is more negative during inspiration, which leads to a higher filling and stroke volume, especially of the right heart.

## NORMAL VARIANTS OF THE LEFT HEART

### Bridging Trabeculations or False Tendons

Bridging trabeculations are fibromuscular structures that appear echocardiographically as linear or bandlike structures that traverse the LV cavity in variable directions and are characteristically slightly more echo-reflectant than the myocardium (34). They frequently are seen in the distal third of the LV and extend from the apical lateral wall to the interventricular septum or from the basal to the mid and distal septum. Rarely, false tendons are seen connecting a papillary muscle(s) to the septum or free wall. They may be single or multiple. With the current use of harmonic imaging, bridging trabeculations are now detected in at least 25% to 30% of studies. The importance of their recognition is their potential misinterpretation as LV thrombi. The underlying normal inward wall motion, endocardial thickening, and their separation from the endocardium, especially during systole (forming a systolic slack), should help to differentiate them from thrombi.

### Pectinate Muscles

Pectinate muscles are muscle ridges of the LA appendage and are located in its lateral wall. On the TEE mid-esophageal short-axis view, they appear as nonmobile linear projections or indentations of the appendage wall,

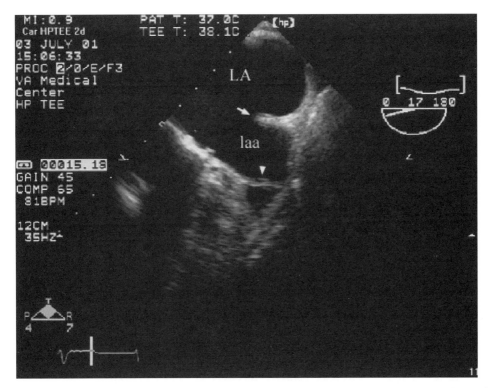

**FIG. 2.8.** Left atrial appendage pectinate muscle and ridge. Transesophageal echocardiographic view of the left atrial appendage (laa) demonstrates a prominent pectinate muscle *(arrowhead)* traversing the appendage from its lateral to medial wall. Note that this muscle echo-reflectance is similar to that of the atrial wall and myocardium. Also note the prominent ridge *(arrow)* at the most superior aspect of the appendage. This ridge is formed by the junction of the inferior wall of the left upper pulmonary vein and the lateral wall of the left atrial appendage.

have echo-reflectance similar to that of the appendage wall, and can commonly be seen traversing the entire appendage (Fig. 2.8). Occasionally, similar muscle ridges are seen on the lateral wall of the RA appendage. The importance of their recognition is their differentiation from thrombi.

### Left Upper Pulmonary Vein Ridge

The junction of the inferior wall of the left upper pulmonary vein and the lateral wall of the LA appendage forms a prominent ridge that is more noticeable in its most medial and superior portion (Fig. 2.8). This ridge frequently appears prolapsing into the LA cavity and can mimic an LA mass. It usually is seen in the TEE mid-esophageal short-axis view of the LA appendage and infrequently in the TTE apical four-chamber view.

### Valve Excrescences

Valve excrescences are thin (0.6 to 2 mm wide), elongated (4 to 16 mm long), and hypermobile structures seen at the coaptation point of the aortic or mitral valve leaflets and rarely on the right-sided valves (35). They are seen on the aortic valve prolapsing into the LV outflow tract during diastole (Fig. 2.9). Valve excrescences on the mitral valve prolapse into the LA during systole. They are detected almost exclusively by TEE in up to 35% to 40% of apparently healthy subjects. They persist unchanged over time and probably are not associated with increased cardioembolic risk. They result from the constant bending and buckling of the leaflets, which lead to tearing of the subendocardial collagen and elastic fibers that subsequently endothelialize.

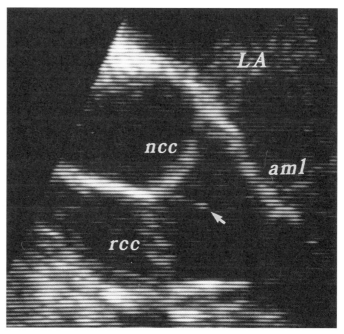

**FIG. 2.9.** Aortic valve excrescence. Longitudinal close-up transesophageal echocardiographic view of the aortic valve in a healthy young subject demonstrates a thin and elongated valve excrescence located at the coaptation point of the noncoronary cusp (ncc) and right coronary cusp (rcc) and prolapsing into the left ventricle during diastole.

### Nodes of Arantius

The nodes of Arantius are tiny and localized or nodular thickening at the tip of each of the aortic cusps. They become more noticeable with aging and are seen almost exclusively by TEE. The proportion of subjects in whom these nodes are seen is unknown.

## NORMAL VARIANTS OF THE RIGHT HEART

### Moderator Band

The moderator band is a large muscle bundle that extends from the distal third of the interventricular septum to the apical anterolateral RV wall and base of the anterior papillary muscle (Fig. 2.10). The moderator band is seen by TTE or TEE in at least two thirds of normal subjects.

### Eustachian Valve

The eustachian valve is a fold or ridge of atrial endocardium that originates from the in-

ferior portion of the crista terminalis and extends from the IVC to the interatrial septum above the fossa ovale. It appears echocardiographically as a linear, nonmobile echo-density that originates from the inferior aspect of the IVC junction with the RA (behind the tricuspid annulus), runs through the most posterior aspect of the atrial wall, and extends to the proximal portion of the fossa ovale (Fig. 2.11). It is best visualized by the TTE parasternal long-axis view of the RV inflow tract and the apical and subcostal four-chamber views.

### Chiari Network

The Chiari network is a remnant of the embryonic sinus venosus and is a variant of the eustachian valve. As for the eustachian valve, it extends from the inferior inlet of the IVC through the posterior atrial wall into the fossa ovale. In contrast to the eustachian valve, this network is a thin, filamentous, and undulating hypermobile struc-

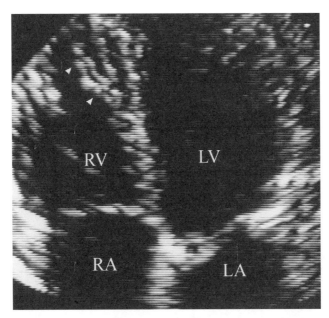

**FIG. 2.10.** Transthoracic echocardiographic four-chamber view demonstrates a prominent moderator band *(arrowheads)* traversing from the distal third of the interventricular septum to the apical right ventricular lateral wall. Note that this muscle band has similar echo-reflectance to that of the myocardium. LV, left ventricle; RA, right atrium; RV, right ventricle.

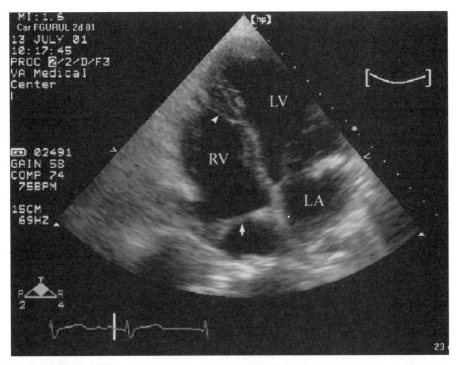

**FIG. 2.11.** Transthoracic four-chamber view demonstrates a prominent eustachian valve *(arrow)* appearing as a bandlike structure that extends from the inferolateral aspect of the right atrial wall (area of junction with the inferior vena cava) to the fossa ovale area. Also note the prominent moderator band *(arrowhead)* in the right ventricle.

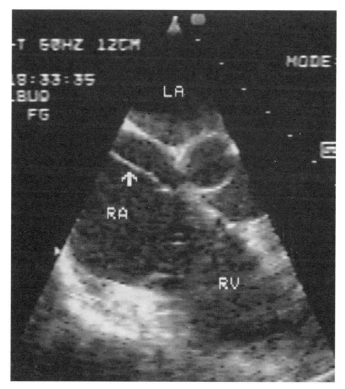

**FIG. 2.12.** Transesophageal echocardiographic four-chamber view in a healthy subject demonstrates a Chiari network *(arrow)* appearing as a homogeneously echo-reflectant and thin or linear structure extending parallel to the interatrial septum from the superior to the inferior aspect of the right atrium.

ture (Fig. 2.12). Its prevalence is <2% by TTE and 5% to 10% by TEE. This network is seen in the same views as described for the eustachian valve. As for the eustachian valve, the importance of its recognition is its distinction from tricuspid valve vegetations or atrial thrombi.

## NORMAL VARIANTS COMMON TO THE LEFT AND RIGHT HEART

### Interatrial Septal Aneurysm

This structure is defined as an outpouching of the interatrial septum that moves 11 to 15 mm in either direction (toward either atrium) and has a base or mouth of >15mm. More commonly it involves the fossa ovale area and rarely the entire interatrial septum. Its prevalence in normal subjects is <1% by TTE and 3% to 8% by TEE. It frequently is associated with a patent foramen ovale (up to 77%). Its prevalence in patients with suspected cardioembolism increases to 15%, but a causal relationship has not been established.

### Patent Foramen Ovale

A patent foramen ovale is a small gap in the foramen ovale resulting from failure of the secundum and primum septum to fuse. It forms a one-way valve allowing flow from RA to LA. It is highly prevalent in normal subjects, up to 10% by TTE and up to 30% by TEE. It also is highly (40%) associated with atrial septal aneurysm. Higher prevalence rates have been reported in patients undergoing TEE for suspected cardioembolism, but a causal relationship has not been established.

The diagnosis is confirmed by the demonstration during a saline contrast study of a small amount of bubbles entering the LA within the first three cardiac cycles. Valsalva maneuver performed during a saline contrast study increases the detection of shunting of bubbles. The appearance of bubbles in the LA after four cycles suggests the presence of a pulmonary arteriovenous fistula.

### Negative Saline Contrast Effect

During saline contrast echocardiography, a negative contrast effect on the RA side of the fossa ovale is induced by IVC inflow. This phenomenon is observed in TTE apical and subcostal four-chamber views and TEE midesophageal four-chamber view. The absence of LA bubbles or of a color Doppler jet entering the RA from the LA through the interatrial septum, and color Doppler flow from the IVC into the RA (area of negative contrast effect) exclude an interatrial septal defect causing a negative contrast effect due to left to right shunting.

### Epicardial Fat

Subepicardial fat is more common in the elderly, the obese, diabetics, and women. It is predominantly located anterior to the heart,

especially anteroapical to the RV; has a characteristic speckled or granular echo-reflectance; and is best seen in the TTE long parasternal and subcostal views. Posteriorly located subepicardial fat is rare (up to 6.5%) in a general population (<1% in subjects <30 years old and up to 15% in those >80 years old).

### SUMMARY

### Diagnostic Value of Echocardiography

Although normal echocardiographic values of the heart chambers and great vessels do not increase linearly with an increase in body surface area, they do with an increase in age, conditioning, and heredity. However, the effect of these factors on normal values is minimal and mostly of no clinical relevance. Therefore, indexing normal values for body surface area is clinically nonimportant and impractical. Also, normal mean values by TTE or TEE are of limited value when applied to an individual subject. Therefore, in this chapter we present ranges of normal values reported by series using TTE and some data using TEE (Tables 2.1–2.6).

**TABLE 2.1.** *Normal values of the left heart chambers by TTE and TEE*

| Measurement | TTE | TEE |
|---|---|---|
| LV anteroposterior, diastole (cm) | 3.5–5.7 | 3.3–5.5 |
| LV anteroposterior, systole (cm) | 2.5–4.3 | 1.8–4.0 |
| LV mediolateral, diastole (cm) | 3.7–5.6 | 2.3–5.4 |
| LV mediolateral, systole (cm) | 2.5–4.8 | 1.8–4.2 |
| LV volume, diastole (mL) | 59–157 | — |
| LV volume, systole (mL) | 18–68 | — |
| LV area, diastole (cm$^2$) | 18–47 | — |
| LV area, systole (cm$^2$) | 8–32 | — |
| LV fractional shortening (%) | 30–35 | 30–35 |
| LV ejection fraction (%) | ≥55 | ≥55 |
| LV interventricular septal thickness, diastole (cm) | 0.6–1.1 | 0.6–1.1 |
| LV posterior wall thickness, diastole (cm) | 0.6–1.0 | 0.6–1.0 |
| LV mass (g) | <294 in men, <198 in women | — |
| LV outflow tract, systole (cm) | 1.8–3.4 | — |
| LA anteroposterior, systole (cm) | 2.2–4.1 | 2.0–5.2 |
| LA mediolateral, systole (cm) | 2.5–4.5 | 2.4–5.2 |
| LA volume (mL) | 20–77 in men, 15–59 in women | — |
| LA area (cm$^2$) | 9–23 | — |
| LA appendage length (cm) | — | 1.5–4.3 |
| LA appendage diameter (cm) | — | 1.0–2.8 |

LA, left atrial; LV, left ventricular; TEE, transesophageal echocardiography; TTE, transthoracic echocardiography.

**TABLE 2.2.** *Normal values of the right heart chambers by TTE and TEE*

| Measurement | TTE | TEE |
| --- | --- | --- |
| RV anteroposterior, diastole (cm) | 2.5–3.8 | — |
| RV anteroposterior, systole (cm) | 2.0–3.4 | — |
| RV mediolateral, diastole (cm) | 2.1–4.2 | — |
| RV mediolateral, systole (cm) | 1.9–3.1 | — |
| RV area, diastole (cm$^2$) | 11–36 | — |
| RV area, systole (cm$^2$) | 5–20 | — |
| RV ejection fraction (%) | ≥40 | — |
| RV free-wall thickness (mm) | 2–5 | — |
| RV outflow tract, systole (cm) | 1.8–3.4 | 1.6–3.6 |
| RA anteroposterior, systole (cm) | — | 2.8–5.2 |
| RA mediolateral, systole (cm) | 2.9–4.6 | 2.9–5.3 |
| RA volume (mL) | 15–58 in men, 14–44 in women | — |
| RA area (cm$^2$) | 8.3–19.5 | — |

RA, right atrial; RV, right ventricular; TEE, transesophageal echocardiography; TTE, transthoracic echocardiography.

**TABLE 2.3.** *Normal measurements of the left heart valves and great vessels*

| Measurement | TTE | TEE |
| --- | --- | --- |
| Mitral valve area (cm$^2$) | 4–6 | 4–6 |
| Mitral annulus, diastole (cm) | 2.0–3.4 | 2.0–3.8 |
| Mitral leaflets thickness (mm) | ≤4 | 0.7–3 |
| Mitral regurgitation (overall %) | 38–45 | 70–80 |
| Pulmonary veins (mm) | 8–15 | 7–16 |
| Aortic valve area (cm$^2$) | 3–5 | 3–5 |
| Aortic annulus, systole (cm) | 1.4–2.6 | 1.8–2.7 |
| Aortic regurgitation (overall %) | 0–2 | 3–4 |
| Aortic root sinuses, diastole (cm) | 2.1–3.5 | — |
| Aortic root tubule, diastole (cm) | 1.7–3.4 | — |
| Aortic arch (cm) | 2.0–3.6 | — |
| Descending aorta (cm) | 2.0–2.5 | 1.4–3 |

TEE, transesophageal echocardiography; TTE, transthoracic echocardiography.

**TABLE 2.4.** *Normal measurements of the right heart valves and great vessels*

| Measurement | TTE | TEE |
| --- | --- | --- |
| Tricuspid valve area (cm$^2$) | 4–6 | 4–6 |
| Tricuspid annulus, diastole (cm) | 2.0–4.0 | 2.0–4.0 |
| Tricuspid leaflet thickness (cm) | ≤4 | 0.7–3 |
| Tricuspid regurgitation (overall %) | 15–78 | 20–50 |
| Superior vena cava (cm) | — | 0.8–2.0 |
| Proximal inferior vena cava (cm) | 1.2–2.3 | — |
| Hepatic vein (cm) | 0.5–1.1 | — |
| Coronary sinus (cm) | — | 0.4–1.0 |
| Pulmonic valve area (cm$^2$) | 3–5 | — |
| Pulmonic valve annulus (cm) | 1.0–2.2 | — |
| Pulmonic regurgitation (overall %) | 28–88 | 20–50 |
| Right ventricular outflow tract, systole | 1.8–3.4 | 1.6–3.6 |
| Main pulmonary artery | 1.0–2.9 | — |
| Right or left pulmonary artery | 0.7–1.7 | 1.2–2.2 |

TEE, transesophageal echocardiography; TTE, transthoracic echocardiography.

**TABLE 2.5.** *Normal left and right ventricular Doppler filling parameters*

| Parameter | Left ventricle | | Right ventricle | |
|---|---|---|---|---|
| | <50 yr | >50 yr | <50 yr | >50 yr |
| Peak E[a] (cm/s) | 72 ± 14 | 62 ± 14 | 51 ± 7 | 41 ± 8 |
| Peak A[b] (cm/s) | 40 ± 10 | 59 ± 14 | 27 ± 8 | 33 ± 8 |
| E/A ratio[c] | 1.9 ± 0.6 | 1.1 ± 0.3 | 2.0 ± 0.5 | 1.34 ± 0.4 |
| Decelaration time (ms) | 179 ± 20 | 210 ± 36 | 188 ± 22 | 198 ± 23 |
| Isovolumetric relaxation time (ms) | 76 ± 11 | 90 ± 17 | 76 ± 11 | 90 ± 17 |
| PV/SVC peak S (cm/s) | 48 ± 9 | 71 ± 9 | 41 ± 9 | 42 ± 12 |
| PV/SVC peak D (cm/s) | 50 ± 10 | 38 ± 9 | 22 ± 5 | 22 ± 5 |
| PV/SVC actual reversal (cm/s) | 19 ± 4 | 23 ± 14 | 13 ± 3 | 16 ± 3 |
| Left atrial filling fraction (%) | 0.25 ± 0.05 | 0.35 ± 0.06 | — | — |

[a]After age 20, E peak velocity decreases by 2–6 cm/s per decade of life.
[b]After age 20, A peak velocity increases by 2–9 cm/s per decade of life.
[c]After age 20, E/A ratio decreases by 0.15–0.30 per decade of life.
PV, pulmonary vein; SVC, superior vena cava.
Klein AL, Cohen GI. Doppler echocardiographic assessment of constrictive pericarditis, cardiac amyloidosis and cardiac tamponade. Cleve Clin J Med. 1992;59:278–290.

By TTE or TEE, LA and RA anteroposterior and mediolateral dimensions, volumes, and areas; mitral and tricuspid annulus diameters; and aortic root and RV outflow tract dimensions are similar.

By TEE, the thicknesses of the mitral and tricuspid leaflets are similar; the mitral and tricuspid leaflets are thicker than the aortic and pulmonic valves; and aortic valve cusps are slightly thicker than those of the pulmonic valve. For each valve, there is no difference in thickness between genders and among the different age decades. LA size and the diameters of the aortic root, descending aorta, and pulmonary artery increase proportionally with age. In contrast, gender does not appear to have an effect on heart chamber dimensions.

### Limitations of Echocardiography

1. Measurement of LV diameters is subject to error due to variations in cardiac position and shape.

2. From the TEE mid-esophageal four-chamber view, foreshortening of the LV is common and leads to underestimation of LV volume, overestimation of LV ejection fraction, and misinterpretation of normal motion of apical segments.

3. Use of Simpson's rule for calculation of LV ejection fraction is time consuming, and errors due to underestimation of volumes, especially in end-systole, lead to overestimation of LV ejection fraction.

4. Fractional shortening can be altered by an abnormal preload or afterload.

5. IVRT is not a true reflection of LV relaxation in the presence of a high or low aortic diastolic pressure and/or the presence of mitral or aortic regurgitation.

6. Mitral inflow parameters lose specificity during tachycardia because A velocity increases and the E/A ratio decreases.

7. In the assessment of pulmonary vein Doppler patterns, the early forward systolic and atrial reversal velocities are seen in only about 30% to 40% of nor-

**TABLE 2.6.** *Normal aortic and pulmonic valve velocities in adults <50 years old*

| Parameter | Aortic valve | Pulmonic valve |
|---|---|---|
| Peak velocity (cm/s) | 72–120 | 44–78 |
| Ejection time (ms) | 265–325 | 280–380 |
| Acceleration time (ms) | 83–118 | 130–185 |

mal subjects by TTE and 75% to 100% by TEE.

8. In the assessment of RV size, false-positive results can occur if the transducer probe is not located over the LV apex. False-negative results can occur when the LV is concurrently enlarged.

9. Assessment of RV wall thickness from the subcostal four-chamber view may be overestimated because the ultrasound beam may be tangential to the posterolateral RV wall.

10. Difficulties in measuring RV volumes have made methods for measuring RV ejection fraction difficult and inaccurate.

11. A markedly negative intrathoracic pressure with inspiration may cause IVC collapse despite an elevated RA pressure. These conditions include obstructive airway disease, pleural effusions, and respiratory distress of other causes. Also, patients on positive-pressure ventilation may not have IVC collapse despite normal RA pressure.

12. Underestimation or overestimation errors in calculating pulmonary artery systolic pressure by Doppler echocardiography are generally related to errors in estimating RA pressure.

13. Pulmonary artery pressure cannot be estimated in most normal subjects because the prevalence of TR is low and predominantly of trivial degree. In subjects with normal pulmonary artery pressure, the proportion of measurable TR jet velocities is <75%.

14. By TEE, pulse and continuous Doppler interrogation of the aortic and pulmonic valves is generally inadequate. Occasionally, a parallel alignment of the ultrasound and the aortic valve can be obtained from the transgastric view at about 60 to 90 degrees.

15. By 2-D or M-mode TEE images, measurements of mitral and aortic valve thickness can be obtained in 80% to 90% of subjects. By 2-D TEE images, tricuspid and pulmonic leaflet measurements can be obtained in 80% and 60% of sub-

jects, respectively. By TTE, adequate measurements of leaflet thickness of any heart valve are accomplished less frequently and commonly are inaccurate.

## REFERENCES

1. Cheitlin MD, Alpert JS, Armstrong WF, et al. ACC/AHA guidelines for the application of echocardiography. Circulation 1997;95:1686–1744.
2. Triulzi M, Gillam L, Gentile F, et al. Normal adult cross-sectional echocardiographic values: linear dimensions and chamber areas. Echocardiography 1994;1:403–426.
3. Knutsen K, Stugaard M, Michelsen S, et al. M-mode echocardiographic findings in apparently healthy, non-athletic Norwegians aged 20–70 years: influence of age, sex and body surface area. J Intern Med 1989;225:111–115.
4. Gardin J, Henry W, Savage D, et al. Echocardiographic measurements in normal subjects from infancy to old age. Circulation 1980;62:1054–1061.
5. Schnittgher I, Gordon E, Fitzgerald P, et al. Standardized intracardiac measurements of two-dimensional echocardiography. J Am Coll Cardiol 1983;2:934–938.
6. Cohen G, White M, Sochowski R, et al. Reference values for normal adult transesophageal echocardiographic measurements. J Am Soc Echocardiogr 1995;8:221–230.
7. Drexler M, Erbel R, Muller U, et al. Measurement of intracardiac dimensions and structures in normal young adult subjects by transesophageal echocardiography. Am J Cardiol 1990;65:1491–1496.
8. Schiller NB, Shah PM, Crawford MH, et al. Recommendations for quantitation of the left ventricle by two-dimensional echocardiography: American Society of Echocardiography Committee on Standards, subcommittee on quantitation of two-dimensional echocardiograms. J Am Soc Echocardiogr 1989;2:358–367.
9. Kitzman D, Scholz D, Hagan P, et al. Age-related changes in normal human hearts during the first 10 decades of life, part II (maturity): a quantitative anatomic study of 765 specimens from subjects 20 to 99 years old. Mayo Clin Proc 1988;63:137–146.
10. Devereux RB, Reichek N. Echocardiographic determination of left ventricular mass in man. Anatomic validation of the method. Circulation 1977;55:613–618.
11. Armstrong WF, Pellikka PA, Ryan T, et al. Stress echocardiography: recommendations for performance and interpretation of stress echocardiography. J Am Soc Echocardiogr 1998;11:97–104.
12. Quinones MA, Pickering E, Alexander JK. Percentage of shortening of the echocardiographic left ventricular dimension. Its use in determining ejection fraction and stroke volume. Chest 1978;74:59–65.
13. Massie BM, Schiller NB, Ratshin RA, et al. Mitral-septal separation: a new echocardiographic index of left ventricular function. Am J Cardiol 1997;39:1008–1016.
14. Simonson JS, Schiller NB. Descent of the base of the left ventricle: an echocardiographic index of left ventricular function. J Am Soc Echocardiogr 1989;2:25–35.
15. Lewis JF, Kuo LC, Nelson JG, et al. Pulsed Doppler echocardiographic determination of stroke volume and

cardiac output: clinical validation of two new methods using the apical window. Circulation 1984;70:425–431.

16. Pinamonti B, DiLenarda A, Sinagra G, et al. Restrictive left ventricular filling pattern in dilated cardiomyopathy assessed by Doppler echocardiography: clinical, echocardiographic and hemodynamic correlations and prognostic implications. Heart Muscle Disease Study Group. J Am Coll Cardiol 1993;22:808–815.

17. Appleton CP, Galloway JM, Gonzalez MS, et al. Estimation of left ventricular filling pressures using two-dimensional and doppler echocardiography in adult patients with cardiac disease: additional value of analyzing left atrial size, left atrial ejection fraction and the difference in duration of pulmonary venous and mitral flow velocity at atrial contraction. J Am Coll Cardiol 1993;22:1972–1982.

18. Brunaszzi MC, Chirillo F, Pasqualini M, et al. Estimation of left ventricular diastolic pressures from precordial pulsed-Doppler analysis of pulmonary venous and mitral flow. Am Heart J 1994;128:293–300.

19. Yamamoto K, Nishimura RA, Burnett JC, et al. Assessment of left ventricular end-diastolic pressure by Doppler echocardiography: contribution of duration of pulmonary venous versus mitral flow velocity curves at atrial contraction. J Am Soc Echocardiogr 1997;10:52–59.

20. Wang Y, Gutman YM, Heilbron D, et al. Atrial volume in a normal adult population by two-dimensional echocardiography. Chest 1984;86:595–601.

21. Crawford MH, Roldan CA. Quantitative assessment of valve thickness in normal subjects by transesophageal echocardiography. Am J Cardiol 2001;87:1419–23.

22. Yoshida K, Yoshikawa J, Shakudo M, et al. Color Doppler evaluation of valvular regurgitation in normal subjects. Circulation 1988;78;840–847.

23. Gossler K, Goldberg S. Velocity gradients across normal cardiac valves. Am J Cardiol 1991;67:99–102.

24. Shively BK, Roldan CA, Gill EA, et al. Prevalence and determinants of valvulopathy in patients treated with dexfenfluramine. Circulation 1999;100:2161–2167.

25. Roldan CA, Chavez J, Weist P, et al. Aortic root disease and valve disease associated with ankylosing spondylitis. J Am Coll Cardiol 1998;32:1397–1404.

26. Jian L, Siu SC, Handschumacher MD, et al. Three-dimensional echocardiography: in vivo validation for right ventricular volume and function. Circulation 1994;89:2342–2350.

27. Meluzin J, Spinarova L, Bakala J, et al. Pulse Doppler tissue imaging of the velocity of tricuspid annular systolic motion. Eur Heart J 2001;22:340–348.

28. Spencer KT, Weinert L, Lang RM. Effect of age, heart rate and tricuspid regurgitation on the Doppler echocardiographic evaluation of right ventricular diastolic function. Cardiology 1999;92:59–64.

29. Ozer N, Tokgozoglu L, Coplu L, et al. Echocardiographic evaluation of left and right ventricular diastolic function in patients with chronic obstructive pulmonary disease. J Am Soc Echocardiogr 2001;14:557–561.

30. Kircher BJ, Himelman RB, Schiller NB. Noninvasive estimation of right atrial pressure from the inspiratory collapse of the inferior vena cava. Am J Cardiol 1990; 66:493–496.

31. Nagueh SF, Kopelen H, Zoghbi W. Relation of mean right atrial pressure to echocardiographic and Doppler parameters of right atrial and right ventricular function. Circulation 1997;95:537–538.

32. Berger M, Haimowitz A, Van Tosh A, et al. Quantitative assessment of pulmonary hypertension in patients with tricuspid regurgitation using continuous wave doppler ultrasound. J Am Coll Cardiol 1985;6:359–365.

33. Lee RT, Lord CP, Plappert T, et al. Prospective Doppler echocardiographic evaluation of pulmonary artery diastolic pressure in the medical intensive care unit. Am J Cardiol 1989;64:1366–1370.

34. Stoddard M, Liddell N, Longaker R, et al. Transesophageal echocardiography: normal variants and mimickers. Am Heart J 1992;124:1587–1598.

35. Roldan CA, Shively BK, Crawford MH. Valve excrescences: prevalence, evolution and risk for cardioembolism. J Am Coll Cardiol 1998;30:1308–1314.

# 3

# The Patient with Coronary Artery Disease

Michael A. Chizner and *Carlos A. Roldan

*Department of Medicine, University of Miami School of Medicine, Miami, Florida; Department of Medicine, University of Florida College of Medicine, Gainesville, Florida; and The Heart Center of Excellence, North Broward Hospital, Fort Lauderdale, Florida; *Department of Internal Medicine, University of New Mexico School of Medicine; and Department of Internal Medicine, Veterans Affairs Medical Center, Albuquerque, New Mexico*

## INTRODUCTION

Coronary artery disease (CAD) represents the most common clinical problem in adult cardiology. In this modern era of catheter-based interventions and aggressive new pharmacologic management strategies for ischemic syndromes, a rapid, accurate, and cost-effective evaluation of the patient who presents with chest pain suggestive of acute or chronic CAD remains an important and continuing diagnostic challenge. A meticulous and thoughtful clinical history and physical examination remain the cornerstone in the initial and ongoing assessment and treatment of the patient with known or suspected myocardial ischemia or infarction. When skillfully performed, a careful detailed history and physical examination helps guide physicians in the appropriate utilization of additional diagnostic techniques, when needed, for further documentation of the presence and severity of ischemic heart disease.

Echocardiography is an important complementary diagnostic tool to the history, physical examination, and electrocardiography (ECG) in patients with known or suspected CAD. Resting, exercise, pharmacologic (dobutamine, adenosine, or dipyridamole), contrast, and transesophageal echocardiography (TEE) are proven to be of diagnostic and prognostic value in these patients. In addition, echocardiography is highly accurate in detecting mechanical complications after myocardial infarction (MI). Finally, echocardiography has an important role in the differentiation of an acute MI (AMI) or ischemia from other serious conditions, such as pericarditis, pulmonary embolism, and aortic dissection.

### Prevalence and Incidence

CAD affects >12 million Americans and remains the single leading cause of death in the United States. Annually, there are more than five million emergency department visits for evaluation of chest discomfort suggestive of acute cardiac ischemia. More than one million Americans experience a new or recurrent AMI each year. Many more are hospitalized for unstable angina or evaluated and treated for stable coronary syndromes (1–6).

### Clinical Spectrum and Pathogenesis

The clinical manifestations of CAD comprise a spectrum, ranging from chronic stable angina pectoris to unstable angina, non–Q-wave MI (non–ST-segment elevation), Q-wave MI (ST-segment elevation), and sudden cardiac death. The most common clinical presentation is stable (exertional) angina caused by "fixed" obstructive atheromatous plaques that limit myocardial oxygen delivery during periods of increased myocardial oxygen demand ("demand ischemia").

The acute coronary syndromes are initiated by the spontaneous rupture of a "vulnerable" atherosclerotic plaque (characterized by a lipid-rich core, surrounding inflammation, and a thin overlying fibrous cap) with superimposed thrombus formation. Endothelial dysfunction and increased coronary vasomotor tone also may play an active role in the acute ischemic event. Plaques prone to rupture often are only mild to moderately stenotic (i.e., not flow limiting) and, therefore, do not cause clinical angina. In patients with unstable angina, a partial but nonocclusive platelet-rich thrombus forms at the site of a ruptured atheromatous plaque and limits coronary blood flow. Most patients with non–Q-wave MI have transient thrombotic occlusion with early spontaneous reperfusion or sustained thrombotic occlusion in the presence of well-developed collaterals. Acute Q-wave MI occurs when persistent and complete fibrin-rich thrombotic occlusion (without early recanalization, rapid relief of spasm, or adequate distal collateralization) leads to irreversible ischemic cell damage and usually transmural myocardial necrosis (Table 3.1) (7–12).

### Natural History and Prognosis

The clinical course of patients with CAD may wax and wane over long periods of time, i.e., asymptomatic phase ("silent ischemia") alternating with symptomatic phase (chronic stable angina), or it may be interrupted abruptly by an acute ischemic event. The prognosis of CAD is determined by the location, extent, and severity of obstructive CAD, and, importantly, the status of left ventricular (LV) function. Advancing age and diabetes mellitus are powerful independent adverse predictors of patient outcome.

Significant CAD is defined as ≥70% narrowing of one or more major epicardial coronary arteries. Patients with severe CAD (left main, triple-vessel, or double-vessel disease involving the proximal left anterior descending coronary artery [LAD]) are at high risk for an adverse cardiac event. The mortality risk is even greater when there is associated

**TABLE 3.1.** *Clinical spectrum of coronary artery disease*

| Asymptomatic (subclinical) phase | |
|---|---|
| Symptomatic phase | Silent myocardial ischemia |
| Stable subsets<br>(stable "fixed" atherosclerotic plaque) | Chronic coronary artery disease<br>• Stable (exertional) angina pectoris<br>  "Fixed threshold" angina secondary to flow-limiting coronary<br>  stenoses (demand ischemia)<br>• Variant or Prinzmetal angina<br>  "Spontaneous" angina at rest secondary to dynamic coronary<br>  narrowing (vasospasm) superimposed on obstructive coronary artery<br>  disease or normal coronary arteries (supply ischemia)<br>• Mixed angina<br>  "Variable threshold" angina secondary to vasoconstriction<br>  superimposed on fixed atherosclerotic plaque (demand and supply<br>  ischemia) |
| Unstable subsets<br>(unstable "vulnerable" plaque rupture<br>  with superimposed thrombus) | Acute coronary syndromes<br>• Unstable angina pectoris<br>  *New-onset angina* (severe and <2 mo duration)<br>  *Increasing (crescendo) angina* (more severe, prolonged, or frequent)<br>  *Angina pectoris at rest* (usually prolonged >20 min and within 1 wk<br>    of presentation)<br>  *Postinfarction angina* (within 2 wk of acute MI)<br>• Acute MI (with or without complications)<br>  *Non–Q wave MI* (transient thrombotic occlusion with early<br>    spontaneous reperfusion)<br>  Smaller infarct size with high risk for recurrent ischemia, reinfarction,<br>    and sudden death<br>  *Q wave MI* (total thrombotic occlusion)<br>  Larger infarct size with higher in-hospital mortality and complication<br>    rate<br>• Sudden ischemic cardiac death<br>  Secondary to malignant ventricular tachyarrhythmias (ventricular<br>    tachycardia/ventricular fibrillation) |

MI, myocardial infarction.

LV systolic dysfunction. Patients with moderate to severe LV systolic dysfunction have almost three times the mortality rate than those with normal LV function, even in the presence of a similar extent of CAD (4,8,13).

The prognosis in many individuals may be more dependent on the biologic activity of coronary lesions ("stable" vs. "unstable") than on the extent of stenosis. However, severe chronic symptoms (especially with low levels of physiologic stress or at rest) are generally associated with severe angiographic CAD and a poorer prognosis. Patients with unstable angina who have prolonged ongoing pain at rest, particularly when accompanied by signs of new or worsening LV systolic dysfunction and hemodynamic instability, usually have severe underlying CAD with ex-

tensive areas of jeopardized ischemic myocardium. These patients are at high risk for nonfatal MI and death and thus require more aggressive management strategies than those with chronic stable angina (5,10,11,13).

Patients with AMI represent a heterogeneous population. At one end of the spectrum are younger patients with a first, small, uncomplicated MI; preserved LV function; no residual ischemic pain; and no ventricular tachyarrhythmias. These patients have a low prevalence of multivessel CAD and have a very good prognosis. At the other end of the spectrum are older patients, often female, with a previous history of MI, angina pectoris, hypertension, or diabetes mellitus, whose AMI is large, complicated by severe LV dysfunction or shock, post-MI angina, heart block, atrial fib-

**TABLE 3.2.** *Clinical risk stratification in acute coronary syndromes*

|  | Unstable angina | Acute myocardial infarction |
|---|---|---|
| Low risk | • New-onset Canadian Cardiovascular Society class III or IV angina in the past 2 wk to 2 mo *without* prolonged, rest, or nocturnal episodes, ECG changes, or serum cardiac marker elevation<br>• No signs of LV dysfunction or hemodynamic instability | • First, small, uncomplicated MI<br>• No post-MI angina<br>• No signs of LV dysfunction or hemodynamic compromise<br>• No complex ventricular arrhythmias |
| High risk | • Accelerating tempo of ischemic symptoms (within 48 hr)<br>• Prolonged, ongoing (>20 min) rest pain with dynamic ECG changes and serum cardiac marker elevation (e.g., troponins, C-reactive protein)<br>• Post-MI angina<br>• Signs of new or worsening LV dysfunction and/or hemodynamic instability (e.g., $S_3$, rales, pulmonary edema, MR murmur, hypotension, tachycardia)<br>• Older age (≥70 yr)<br>• Diabetes mellitus | • Prior MI, diabetes mellitus<br>• Older age (≥70 yr)<br>• Female gender<br>• Post-MI angina<br>• Large (particularly anterior) transmural MI complicated by signs of severe LV dysfunction or shock, mechanical defects (ventricular septal defect, acute MR, LV aneurysm with thrombus), right ventricular infarction with inferior MI, atrial fibrillation, heart block, sustained ventricular tachycardia |

ECG, electrocardiographic; LV, left ventricular; MI, myocardial infarction; MR, mitral regurgitation.

rillation, and complex ventricular arrhythmia or mechanical complications. In general, patients with anterior MI have a higher mortality than patients with inferior MI. A patient with a Q-wave MI carries a higher in-hospital mortality and complication rate than a patient with a non–Q-wave MI. The early survival advantage for non–Q-wave MI may soon be lost, however, because these patients are at particularly high risk for recurrent ischemia, reinfarction, and sudden death (Table 3.2) (10,12,14).

## HISTORY

The clinical history plays an essential role in the diagnosis and management of the patient with suspected myocardial ischemia or infarction. In general, the typical history is relatively straightforward and diagnostic (10,15–17).

### Clinical Characteristics of Ischemic Symptoms: an Overview

Chest pain or discomfort is the most frequent presenting symptom of myocardial ischemia or infarction. In the patient with uncomplicated CAD, the chest pain history typically is far more helpful than the physical examination (which usually is entirely normal). In eliciting the history of chest pain, the physician should ask the patient to describe the character, location, radiation, and duration of the pain; the factors that precipitate and relieve the pain; the frequency, pattern, and setting of the pain occurrence; and whether or not there are any associated symptoms. Ischemic discomfort typically is described as tightness, pressure, heaviness, a weight ("as if someone were sitting on my chest"), aching, squeezing, viselike or bandlike constriction, a feeling of fullness, gas ("I need to belch"), burning, or even "indigestion." The pain is deep seated rather than superficial, comes on gradually, and lasts minutes (rather than seconds) or longer (>30 minutes) if due to evolving AMI. It generally is felt beneath the breastbone (retrosternal), spreads across the precordium with predilection for the left side, and commonly radiates to (but on occasion may originate in) the neck, throat ("choking" sensation), lower jaw, teeth ("toothache"), upper back, interscapular area, epigastrium ("heartburn"), chest ("the flu"), shoulders ("arthritis" or "bursitis"), and down the inner (ulnar) aspect of one or both arms (usually the left) to the elbows, wrists, and fingers, where it often is described as a numbness and tingling ("pins and needles") sensation rather than actual pain (Fig. 3.1) (4,7,8,10,14).

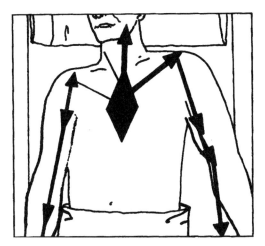

**FIG. 3.1.** Radiation of chest pain of myocardial ischemia or infarction. (From Harvey WP. Cardiac pearls. Cedar Grove, NJ: Laennec Publishing, 1993, with permission.)

Many patients have difficulty describing the feeling of myocardial ischemia and deny that their discomfort is truly "pain." Some make a clenched fist over the sternum (so-called "Levine sign"), a type of "language of the hands," as they grope for the words to describe the sensation. Associated or primary symptoms of myocardial ischemia or infarction include shortness of breath, sweating, nausea, vomiting, lightheadedness, weakness, fatigue, apprehension, and fear of impending doom. Thus, although chest pain is the classic symptom in the majority of patients, it is by no means present in all. Dyspnea (secondary to an elevated LV filling pressure [diastolic dysfunction] and/or transient ischemic mitral regurgitation [MR]), or extreme fatigue, weakness, and dizziness, may be the cardinal manifestations of myocardial ischemia (anginal "equivalent"). Chest pain may be truly absent (so-called "silent ischemia") in as many as 25% or more of patients, especially in those with diabetes mellitus, in whom pain perception may be altered by neuropathy ("defective warning system"); in the elderly, in whom atypical symptoms, such as confusion, lightheadedness, syncope, breathlessness, or gastrointestinal upset, may be the presenting complaint; or in those in the postoperative state recovering from anesthesia and/or receiving analgesics. Women have a higher incidence of atypical symptoms, such as jaw pain, sharp chest pain, abdominal pain, shortness of breath, nausea, and fatigue, which often result in significant delay in receiving medical attention. On the other hand, women have more non-CAD chest pain than men.

## Stable Angina Pectoris

Pain brought on by exertion, physical effort, mental or emotional stress, sexual activity, exposure to cold and/or hot, humid weather, or after eating a heavy meal, which is relieved promptly (within a period of 30 seconds to several minutes) by rest or sublingual nitroglycerin, suggests classic stable angina pectoris. Characteristically, the patient stops activity and prefers to remain in the sitting or standing position to obtain relief. Redistribution of intravascular volume (increase in venous return) in the recumbent position may increase oxygen demand and thus aggravate ischemic chest discomfort ("angina decubitus"). Carotid sinus massage, by increasing vagal tone and decreasing heart rate and blood pressure (BP), can bring about relief of angina in some patients; if effective, it is a useful diagnostic maneuver. It should be applied cautiously, especially in older patients.

Chronic stable angina usually comes on gradually and reaches its maximum intensity over 2 to 5 minutes. Reproducibility of discomfort with a predictable and fairly constant level of physical activity is a helpful clue ("fixed threshold" angina). Many patients, however, have a "variable threshold" for angina, with "good days" and "bad days." Pain may occur unpredictably during an effort usually well tolerated, while the patient is inactive ("rest angina"), or even while the patient is asleep ("nocturnal angina"). Transient increases in coronary vascular tone (vasospasm) superimposed on fixed atherosclerotic CAD is believed to play a role in such patients. Angina tends to be more readily provoked by early morning activities. It may occur early in the course of a given activity (e.g., during the first hole of golf, while walking to the bus stop on the way to work ["first-effort" or "warm-up" angina]) and then subside as the individual continues on and

**TABLE 3.3.** *Canadian Cardiovascular Society classification of angina pectoris*

| | |
|---|---|
| Class I | Ordinary physical activity, e.g., walking or climbing stairs, does not cause angina. Angina may occur with strenuous, rapid, or prolonged exertion at work or recreation. |
| Class II | Slight limitation of ordinary activity. Angina may occur with walking or climbing stairs rapidly; walking uphill; in the cold or into the wind; walking or climbing stairs after meals; while under emotional stress; or only during the first few hours after awakening. Walking more than two blocks on a level surface and climbing more than one flight of ordinary stairs at a normal pace and in normal conditions may bring on angina. |
| Class III | Marked limitation of ordinary physical activity. Angina may occur when walking one or two blocks on the level or climbing one flight of stairs in normal conditions and at a normal pace. |
| Class IV | Inability to carry out any physical activity without discomfort. Angina may be present at rest. |

Adapted from Campeau L. Grading of angina pectoris [Letter]. Circulation 1976;54:522–523.

"walks through" the discomfort. Some patients may be able to tolerate the same or even more strenuous activity after a period of rest ("second-wind" phenomenon). These phenomena have been attributed to the opening of collateral blood vessels during the initial episode of ischemia. A useful and widely accepted classification system for grading the functional severity of angina pectoris has been developed by the Canadian Cardiovascular Society (CCS). (Table 3.3) (8,10,13,17).

### Unstable Angina

Unstable angina is a transitory clinical syndrome associated with a change in the pattern (increased tempo or intensity) of ischemic chest pain. It may occur de novo (new-onset angina) in previously asymptomatic individuals, in patients with a history of chronic stable angina, or in those who had a recent MI, percutaneous coronary intervention within the past 6 months (restenosis), or prior coronary bypass surgery. In general, patients with unstable angina have recurring ischemic episodes that are more severe (CCS class III or IV), more frequent, more easily provoked (or occur at rest), more prolonged (>20 minutes), and more difficult to relieve with nitroglycerin than those with stable angina (but without ECG or enzymatic evidence of MI).

### Acute Myocardial Infarction

The clinical syndrome of AMI can present in a typical manner or with a variety of atypical symptoms and signs that may obscure the correct diagnosis (Table 3.4). In the clas-

**TABLE 3.4.** *Clinical presentation of acute myocardial infarction*

Typical
* Middle-aged, older male; older postmenopausal female
* Severe, prolonged chest pain (discomfort): pressure tightness, heaviness, squeezing, crushing, viselike, burning
* Location: retrosternal, radiating to precordium, neck, jaw, epigastrium, interscapular area, shoulders, arms (left side common)
* Associated symptoms: nausea, vomiting, diaphoresis, shortness of breath, weakness, anxiety, feeling of impending doom

Atypical
* Pain localized to extrathoracic sites: arms, shoulders, back, jaw, teeth, epigastrium ("arthritis," "bursitis," "toothache," "indigestion")
* "Gastrointestinal" symptoms alone: nausea, vomiting, heartburn, gas
* Profound fatigue, weakness, anxiety, nervousness
* Palpitations, dizziness, syncope
* Sudden onset of congestive heart failure, pulmonary edema, or shock
* Cerebral or peripheral embolism (stroke, cold extremity)
* Acute confusional state, psychosis
* "Silent," especially in elderly, diabetic, female, perioperative state

Modified from Chizner MA. Acute myocardial infarction and its complications: clinical spectrum, diagnosis and management. In: Chizner MA, ed. Classic teachings in clinical cardiology: a tribute to W. Proctor Harvey, M.D. Cedar Grove, NJ: Laennec Publishing Inc., 1996:843.

sic clinical presentation, the pain of AMI, although similar to stable angina in character, location, and radiation, is usually (but not always) more intense, longer lasting, and as likely to occur unexpectedly during inactivity as during effort, not infrequently in the early morning hours. It typically builds in intensity; often becomes severe and unrelenting (although it can be deceptively mild); may be associated with nausea, vomiting, and diaphoresis; and lasts for up to several hours if not relieved by narcotic analgesics or aggressive intervention. Inasmuch as the extent of myocardial necrosis plays a crucial role in the prognosis, it is important for the clinician to determine, as quickly as possible, the presence and time of onset of AMI symptoms in order to establish eligibility for reperfusion therapy and thus maximize the likelihood of myocardial salvage ("time is muscle") (Table 3.5). Chest pain associated with AMI generally subsides within 12 to 24 hours. Recurrent or persistent pain beyond 24 hours is an adverse prognostic sign. Patients with non–Q-wave MI are at particularly high risk for recurrent ischemia and reinfarction, as this represents an incomplete thrombotic occlusion of the infarct-related coronary artery (10,12,14).

## Past Medical History and Risk Factors

Evaluation of the patient with chest pain suggestive of myocardial ischemia includes a detailed history of prior ischemic events (angina pectoris, MI) and/or cardiac procedures (coronary angioplasty/stenting, bypass surgery). A history of cerebrovascular or peripheral vascular disease should heighten the suspicion that the chest pain is ischemic. A careful search should be made for the presence of traditional CAD risk factors, such as cigarette smoking, hypertension, hyperlipidemia, diabetes mellitus, and a family history of premature CAD. If present, these features increase the likelihood of underlying CAD and serve as potential targets for intervention. Although CAD manifests about 10 years later in women than in men, it is the most common cause of mortality in women, accounting for twice as many deaths as all forms of cancer. Inquiry into the use of cocaine or "over-the-counter" sympathomimetic agents and other stimulant drugs, such as sumatriptan (Imitrex), which is prescribed for migraine and cluster headaches, should be made in a patient who presents with chest pain.

## PHYSICAL EXAMINATION

A properly conducted physical examination often can provide useful information in the

**TABLE 3.5.** *Clinical characteristics predictive of acute myocardial infarction in patients with chest pain in the emergency room*

|  | Probability of acute myocardial infarction (%) |
| --- | --- |
| Description of pain | |
| • Pressure, tightness, crushing | 24 |
| • Burning, indigestion | 23 |
| • Ache | 13 |
| • Sharp, stabbing | 5 |
| • Partially pleuritic or positional | 7 |
| • Fully pleuritic or positional | 1 |
| Radiation of the pain to the jaw, neck, left arm, or left shoulder | 19 |
| Reproducibility | |
| • Pain partially reproducible by chest wall palpation | 6 |
| • Pain fully reproducible by chest wall palpation | 5 |
| Combination of variables | |
| • Sharp or stabbing pain; no prior angina or myocardial infarction; pain pleuritic, positional, or reproducible by palpation | 0 |

From Gaspoz JM, Lee TH, Goldman L. Emergency room evaluation and triage strategies for patients with acute chest pain: lessons from the pre-thrombolytic era. In: Califf RM, Mark DB, Wagner GS, eds. Acute coronary care, 2nd ed. Philadelphia: Mosby-Year Book, 1995:256, with permission.

**TABLE 3.6.** *Physical examination in acute myocardial ischemia and infarction*

General: Anxious, agitated, anguished faces, clenched fist ("Levine sign")—classic hand gesture
Skin: Cool, clammy, pale, ashen
Low-grade fever: Nonspecific response to myocardial necrosis
Hypertension, tachycardia: High sympathetic tone (anterior MI)
Hypotension, bradycardia: High vagal tone (inferior-posterior MI)
Small-volume pulses: Low cardiac output
Fast, slow, or irregular pulse: Atrial or ventricular arrhythmias, heart block
Paradoxical "ectopic" systolic impulse: LV dyskinesis, ventricular aneurysm (anterior MI)
Soft $S_1$: Decreased LV contractility; first-degree atrioventricular block (inferior MI)
$S_4$ gallop: Decreased LV compliance
Paradoxically split $S_2$ (rare): Severe LV dysfunction, left bundle branch block
$S_3$ gallop, pulmonary rales, pulsus alternans: LV systolic dysfunction (signs of congestive heart failure: >25%
  of myocardium infarcted)
Hypotension: Skin—cold, clammy, cyanotic; central nervous system—altered mental status; kidneys—oliguria
  (signs of cardiogenic shock—>40% of myocardium infarcted)
Jugular venous distention: Kussmaul's sign, hypotension, RV $S_4$ and $S_3$ gallops, clear lungs—RV infarction
Systolic murmur of mitral regurgitation: Papillary muscle dysfunction or rupture (apex; palpable thrill rare)
Systolic murmur of ventricular septal defect: Ventricular septal rupture (left sternal border; palpable thrill
  common)
Pericardial friction rub: Early contiguous pericarditis (accompanies transmural MI)—late postmyocardial
  infarction (Dressler) syndrome
Signs of cardiac tamponade, electromechanical dissociation: Cardiac rupture

Modified from Chizner MA. Acute myocardial infarction and its complications: clinical spectrum, diagnosis and management. In: Chizner MA, ed. Classic teachings in clinical cardiology: a tribute to W. Proctor Harvey, M.D. Cedar Grove, NJ: Laennec Publishing Inc., 1996:852.

evaluation of the patient with known or suspected CAD. The spectrum of clinical findings varies greatly, ranging from none to a myriad of signs, depending on the temporal relation of the examination to an acute ischemic event; the presence (or absence) of MI; the state of LV function; and whether there are associated mechanical complications. Although the physical examination usually is entirely normal between episodes of angina, close evaluation during an ischemic attack can be helpful. Furthermore, because the clinical features of AMI may change dramatically during the first few hours and days following the acute event, careful repeated examination can provide important clues to the clinical course and prognosis (Table 3.6) (10,15,16,18–21).

**General Appearance**

The classic stereotypical appearance of the "coronary-prone" individual is that of a short, balding, overweight, sedentary, chain-smoking, middle-aged or older male (or postmenopausal female), with stigmata of underlying risk factors for CAD, such as nicotine-stained fingers or teeth (cigarette smoking); cutaneous and tendon xanthomas, xanthelasmas, or corneal arcus senilis (hyperlipidemia); a diagonal earlobe crease; and perhaps an aggressive, highly competitive and/or hostile (so-called "type A") personality. Obviously, such characteristics occur uncommonly in a general population. While chest pain is still present, the patient with AMI may appear restless, anxious, and agitated, often thrashing about in bed in an effort to find a more comfortable position. In contrast, those with exertion-related angina pectoris tend to remain quiet, and sit or stand still in an effort to obtain relief, recognizing that movement may enhance the pain. The patient may have an anguished facial expression, clenching his or her fist against the sternum while complaining of discomfort ("Levine sign"). During an AMI, the subject may exhibit evidence of marked sympathetic discharge, appearing ashen, pale, and profusely diaphoretic, with cool and clammy skin, even in the absence of shock, due to vasoconstriction.

Respiratory distress, characterized by dyspnea, orthopnea, dry nonproductive cough, and wheezing ("cardiac asthma"), may dominate the clinical picture when ischemic LV dysfunction and/or significant MR is present. The patient may be tachypneic, sitting upright in bed, gasping and struggling for breath, and coughing frothy pink sputum if acute ("flash") pulmonary edema ensues. Some patients with heart failure and a poor cardiac output, especially those who are older with underlying cerebrovascular disease (particularly during sleep and/or sedation), may manifest a cyclic breathing pattern (hyperpnea) alternating with apnea, referred to as Cheyne-Stokes respiration.

If cardiogenic shock is the predominant feature, due to extensive impairment of LV function and/or one of the mechanical complications of AMI, signs of peripheral circulatory collapse, such as cold and clammy skin, marked facial pallor, cyanosis of the lips and nail beds, and bluish-red mottling of the extremities, may become evident. The individual may be confused or mentally obtunded, reflecting an altered sensorium resulting from cerebral hypoperfusion. In the patient receiving thrombolytic therapy, especially those who are older, female, hypertensive, of low body weight, and who are receiving aggressive adjunctive anticoagulation therapy, the sudden onset of lethargy, stupor, or coma should alert the clinician to the possibility of intracranial bleeding. It should be realized, however, that acute confusion and altered mental status is a common atypical presentation of AMI (especially in the elderly) that, by itself, may deter the physician from administering fibrinolytic therapy.

Fortunately, these dramatic clinical manifestations of AMI usually are not present. Many affected individuals appear to be in good health, with no visible abnormality in appearance or behavior, and show no signs of circulatory impairment, even as an MI of substantial size evolves. It may, in fact, be difficult to convince these patients they are seriously ill. At times, patients may present with alterations in emotional state (e.g., denial, anger, fear, anxiety, and depression), particularly those with their first clinical experience with CAD, which can have a major negative psychological impact. Occasionally, a low-grade temperature elevation may be present for several days following an AMI. This is a nonspecific response to tissue necrosis, usually occurring after the first 24 hours and reaching its peak on the second or third day post-MI.

**Blood Pressure and Arterial Pulse**

Even in the absence of preexisting hypertension, the systemic BP may be elevated during an anginal episode or the early stages of AMI (particularly anterior) due to marked endogenous catecholamine release resulting from pain, agitation, and apprehension. The majority of such patients demonstrate a gradual decline in BP following the acute event. Severe uncontrolled hypertension (BP >180/110 mm Hg), however, remains a relative contraindication to thrombolytic therapy. If persistent, it can increase myocardial oxygen demand and predispose the patient to mechanical complications, such as infarct expansion and rupture. Hypotension may result from many factors, including the venodilating effects of nitrate and morphine administration; reduced cardiac output due to impaired LV function; right ventricular (RV) infarction; or hypovolemia secondary to vomiting, excessive diaphoresis, inadequate fluid intake, or overzealous use of diuretics, beta blockers, angiotensin-converting enzyme inhibitors, calcium channel blockers, and certain thrombolytic agents (e.g., streptokinase). Marked and persistent hypotension, when accompanied by signs of vital organ hypoperfusion, is one of the diagnostic hallmarks of cardiogenic shock. Many patients with inferior wall MI are hypotensive (even in the absence of cardiogenic shock) due to intense parasympathetic discharge. This vagally mediated (Bezold-Jarisch) reflex induces bradycardia, peripheral vasodilation, and hypotension. It is seen most frequently when inferior wall MI is associated with RV infarction, commonly appears following nitroglycerin therapy, and occurs in response to sudden reperfusion of the occluded MI-related artery.

Careful palpation of the arterial pulse can reveal useful information about heart rate and rhythm. During an anginal attack or the early phase of AMI (especially in young patients with anterior wall MI), sinus tachycardia often is present (±25% of patients) due to sympathetic nervous system overactivity related to fever, pain, fear, or anxiety. If persistent, it may represent an unfavorable prognostic sign reflecting a compensatory response to diminished stroke volume in the setting of significant LV dysfunction. Tachycardia also may result from hypovolemia and concurrent occult complications, including infection, pericarditis, pulmonary embolism, and borderline cardiogenic shock. Bradycardia is associated with inferoposterior wall MI (up to 50% of patients) due to excess vagal tone and/or ischemia of the sinus and atrioventricular (AV) nodes. Iatrogenic causes, such as use of morphine sulfate, beta blockers, or rate-slowing calcium antagonists, also may be responsible.

Information about LV function may be derived from a detailed assessment of the character, rate of rise, and amplitude of the arterial pulse. A small, weak (hypokinetic) pulse suggests the presence of diminished stroke volume and decreased LV contractility. A brisk, "quick rise" (hyperkinetic) pulse may be present in patients with hemodynamically significant MR due to papillary muscle dysfunction and/or rupture, or an acute ventricular septal defect (VSD). Gentle palpation of the peripheral arterial pulse (radial or femoral) may detect pulsus alternans, a valuable sign of LV systolic dysfunction. In pulsus alternans, there is a variation in the amplitude and/or rate of rise of the arterial pulse with alternate beats (stronger alternating with weaker arterial pulse). Pulsus alternans often is palpable transiently after premature ventricular contractions (PVCs), but may be sustained when severe LV systolic dysfunction is present. It often is brought out or accentuated in the sitting or upright position (due to a decrease in venous return). Pulsus alternans should alert the examiner to search carefully for alteration in the intensity of heart sounds (particularly the second heart sound [$S_2$]), murmurs, and a ventricular diastolic (third heart sound [$S_3$]) gallop. Examination of the peripheral arteries for diminished or absent pulses (peripheral vascular disease), carotid arteries for bruits (carotid artery disease), and abdominal aorta for expansive and pulsatile masses (aortic aneurysm) are important clinical findings that, if found, increase the likelihood that significant CAD also will be present.

## Venous Pulse

When the right atrium contracts against a closed tricuspid valve, large "cannon" A waves will be visualized in the jugular venous pulse (JVP). These waves these can be seen in complete heart block, during ventricular tachycardia, and with PVCs (due to the presence of AV dissociation). When effective atrial activity is no longer present, jugular venous A waves will be absent and only V waves will remain. If the arterial pulse is "irregularly irregular," atrial fibrillation is present. In the setting of AMI, this may result from an acute increase in left atrial (LA) pressure secondary to LV dysfunction and/or MR or pericarditis and as such may have adverse prognostic implications.

The height of the JVP usually is normal (or only slightly elevated) in patients with AMI, even in the presence of mild to moderate LV failure. Marked elevation of the JVP occurs in the presence of pulmonary hypertension or associated RV infarction. In a patient with acute inferoposterior wall MI, the presence of the classic triad of hypotension, clear lungs, and elevated JVP (increasing with inspiration [Kussmaul sign]) provides valuable clues to the clinical diagnosis of an RV infarction. Large or "giant" A waves may be seen in the JVP when there is vigorous right atrial contraction due to increased resistance to emptying, resulting from RV infarction, pulmonary hypertension associated with LV failure, or pulmonary emboli complicating an AMI. The jugular V wave, normally smaller than the A wave, may become accentuated with tricuspid regurgitation (TR) resulting from RV papillary muscle necrosis or in the presence of an RV infarction.

## Precordial Examination

Careful palpation of the precordium, with the patient lying in the supine position, allows the physician to estimate heart size at the bedside. The normal apical impulse will be palpated at the fifth left intercostal space within the mid-clavicular line as a brief outward movement in early systole. Abnormal precordial impulses may be palpated during an acute ischemic event. Palpable presystolic distinstion of the LV (the tactile counterpart of the fourth heart sound [$S_4$] gallop) occurs as the result of vigorous atrial contraction into a ventricle reduced in compliance from the stiffened area of ischemic or infarcted myocardium (diastolic dysfunction). It is best assessed by palpation using the pulps of the fingertips while the patient is turned to the left lateral decubitus position. If LV systolic dysfunction occurs, a palpable outward movement of the LV may develop in early diastole (corresponding to the $S_3$ gallop). An $S_3$ also may be palpable when early diastolic filling of the LV is accentuated, as may occur with VSD or MR due to papillary muscle rupture. In such situations, a markedly increased volume of blood flows into the LV immediately after mitral valve opening in early diastole. At times, evidence of a gallop rhythm can be seen and felt, even when not well heard.

An "ectopic" systolic impulse (bulge) may be palpated in the third and fourth intercostal spaces between the lower left sternal border and cardiac apex (Fig. 3.2). This represents the infarcted, dyskinetic segment of myocardium expanding paradoxically during systole, and, if persistent (along with ST-segment elevation on the ECG), may be a clue to the presence of a ventricular aneurysm. An LV aneurysm results most commonly from a Q-wave anterior wall infarction and may present with signs of congestive heart failure, systemic embolism (due to mural thrombus formation), or recurrent ventricular tachycardia. They usually begin to develop within hours of the acute event and may enlarge and become more prominent over the ensuing weeks or months as a result of infarct expansion and dilation (so-called LV "remodeling"). In some patients, the "ectopic" impulse is palpable medial and superior to the cardiac apex, clearly separable from the apical LV impulse. Careful simultaneous palpation of the apex and "ectopic" area with two hands will help reveal the asynchrony between the two impulses. In other patients, the abnormal outward movement may be diffuse. It may

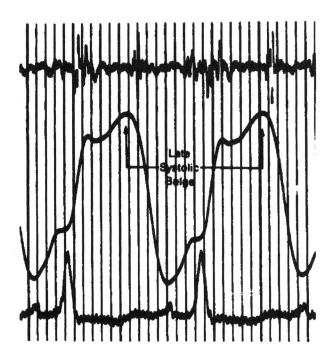

**FIG. 3.2.** Apexcardiogram in left ventricular aneurysm. A prominent late systolic bulge, or outward movement, is palpable at the cardiac apex. (From Delman AJ, Stein E. Dynamic cardiac auscultation and phonocardiography: a graphic guide. Philadelphia: WB Saunders, 1979, with permission.)

merge with the LV apical impulse and produce a systolic lifting of the entire precordium with palpable and audible presystolic ($S_4$) and diastolic ($S_3$) filling sounds, along with the systolic murmur of MR. Rarely, generalized heaves or bulges (dyskinesia) also can be transiently palpable during an episode of angina pectoris or in the acute phase of AMI prior to anatomical thinning of the myocardium. These may be considered "physiologic" aneurysms because they are present when the heart is ischemic or in its early stages of infarction (10,18,19).

If a grade 4/6 or more systolic murmur of acute VSD or MR is present, the vibrations may be transmitted to the surface of the chest and be perceived as a palpable thrill. A diligent search for the location of the maximal systolic thrill, although less frequent with acute MR (at the apex) than VSD (at the left sternal border), occasionally is rewarding and of great importance if detected.

## Auscultation

### *First and Second Heart Sounds*

During AMI or an episode of angina, the first heart sound ($S_1$) may be faint due to diminished myocardial contractility. $S_1$ increases in intensity as healing commences and/or ischemia subsides. A soft $S_1$ also may reflect the presence of a prolonged PR interval, as occurs in first-degree AV block associated with inferior wall MI. Variation in the intensity of $S_1$ can be appreciated when the PR interval varies, as occurs in complete heart block, ventricular tachycardia, or changes in cycle length during atrial fibrillation.

Attentive auscultation may reveal reversed or paradoxic respiratory splitting of $S_2$ ($P_2$-$A_2$) in AMI patients with marked LV dysfunction or left bundle branch block (LBBB) due to delayed activation and/or contraction of the LV. Patients who present with ischemic chest discomfort and new (or presumably new) LBBB, caused by occlusion of the LAD, should be screened quickly and considered for reperfusion therapy. Uncommonly, transient paradoxic splitting of $S_2$ also may be heard during an acute anginal episode. Is-

chemic LV dysfunction with prolongation of ventricular systole is responsible for the delay in aortic valve closure ($A_2$).

Abnormally wide or exaggerated "physiologic" respiratory splitting of $S_2$ ($A_2$-$P_2$) may occur in patients with right bundle branch block due to delayed activation of the RV or an acute VSD due to increased RV stroke volume and delayed pulmonic valve closure ($P_2$). Severe MR and a ruptured VSD also may cause wide "physiologic" splitting of $S_2$. This is due to earlier closure of the aortic valve, caused by rapid LV emptying as blood flows from the LV into both the aorta and LA (MR), and into the aorta and RV (VSD). If pulmonary hypertension is present, resulting from LV failure or pulmonary emboli complicating an AMI, $P_2$ may be accentuated in intensity.

### *Third and Fourth Heart Sounds*

Careful auscultation of the cardiac apex may reveal atrial ($S_4$) or ventricular ($S_3$) gallop sounds. The $S_4$ gallop is an expected finding heard in virtually all patients with AMI (who are in sinus rhythm), reflecting a reduction in LV compliance due to stiffening of the infarcted myocardium. It may be faint, but often is louder during the early phase of AMI (or during an episode of acute ischemia). The absence of an $S_4$ gallop, therefore, should raise serious doubts as to the diagnosis of an AMI.

Patients with systolic or diastolic dysfunction may present with moist rales over the lung fields, which do not clear on coughing. The appearance of an $S_3$ gallop, however, signals the presence of (and is an auscultatory hallmark for) LV systolic dysfunction. It denotes more severe impairment of LV function associated with abnormally elevated LV filling pressure and, when louder and persistent, carries a poor prognosis. $S_3$ gallops frequently are detected in AMI (but not nearly as often as the $S_4$ gallop). They are heard more commonly in patients with larger Q-wave anterior MI than in those with smaller inferior or non–Q-wave MI. Prompt subsidence of an $S_3$ gallop suggests that LV function has improved with recovery of reversibly dysfunctional but viable ("stunned" or "hibernating") myocardium, indicating a favorable response to therapy and thus an improved outlook.

Four subgroups of AMI patients have been classified (classes I to IV) from low to high mortality risk based on the degree and severity of LV dysfunction by clinical examination (so-called Killip classification). Patients in class I have an uncomplicated MI without any evidence of heart failure, i.e., no $S_3$ gallop or pulmonary rales. Class II patients have mild to moderate heart failure with an $S_3$ gallop and bibasilar rales. Class III patients have clear-cut pulmonary edema with rales extending up to the apices of the lungs. Class IV patients have signs of cardiogenic shock. Pulmonary edema usually is indicative of moderate to severe LV systolic dysfunction and/or significant ischemic MR. Although an $S_3$ gallop is an expected finding, it may not be readily detected due to the difficulty of cardiac auscultation in the presence of loud respiratory noise (or if diastolic dysfunction alone is the main culprit).

Cardiogenic shock represents the leading cause of death from AMI and results from extensive damage to the LV (or RV) myocardium, or from a potentially remediable mechanical defect (e.g., VSD or papillary muscle rupture). LV systolic dysfunction accounts for most of the cases and can occur early, within 6 to 24 hours of the onset of the acute event. Although correlation of the physical examination with hemodynamic measurements may not be precise (in part related to "phase lags" as pulmonary congestion develops or resolves), meticulous clinical evaluation, when coupled with information derived from color flow Doppler echocardiography, usually will enable accurate assessment of the patient's status in the majority of cases (10,12,14).

It should be noted that a "pathologic" $S_3$ does not always indicate LV failure. It also may be heard when MR or VSD is present, and it may be accompanied by a mid-diastolic rumble related to increased blood flow across the mitral valve into the LV. $S_3$ and $S_4$ gallop sounds also can originate in the RV. Right-sided gallops are heard best at the lower left sternal border, increase in intensity with inspiration, and often are associated with other features of RV involvement, e.g., parasternal lift, accentuated $P_2$, or elevated JVP with large A or V waves. These findings suggest pulmonary hypertension caused by LV failure, pulmonary emboli, or RV infarction.

### Heart Murmurs

Systolic murmurs, transient or persistent, are commonly audible in patients with acute myocardial ischemia or infarction. A new systolic murmur may represent MR resulting from papillary muscle dysfunction (due to ischemia, geometric distortion of the mitral apparatus with LV dilatation, or ventricular aneurysm formation) or rupture (Fig. 3.3). The murmur of papillary muscle dysfunction (present in 30% to 50% of patients) may be persistent or intermittent, appearing only during the ischemic episode, disappearing once ischemia has subsided or following prompt restoration of coronary blood flow and mitral valve competence. The systolic murmur can be early, mid, late, or holosystolic in timing. It is best heard at the cardiac apex and may radiate to the base (posteromedial papillary muscle) or axilla (anterolateral papillary muscle). Papillary muscle rupture is a rare (<1% of patients) but catastrophic complication, usually of an acute inferior or posterolateral Q-wave or non–Q-wave MI resulting in acute severe MR, sudden overwhelming pulmonary edema, and cardiogenic shock. The regurgitant murmur typically is loudest at the cardiac apex and may be accompanied by a palpable systolic thrill. It is holosystolic but decrescendo in the latter part of systole (tapers off well before $S_2$) due to the abrupt rise in pressure in the noncompliant LA, which results in rapid equilibration of LA and LV pressures and decreases regurgitant flow. Little correlation exists, however, between the intensity of the murmur and the degree of MR. If cardiogenic shock or severe LV systolic function is present, the systolic murmur may be deceptively soft or completely absent, even in the presence of hemodynamically severe MR.

Rupture of the interventricular septum is a rare (1% to 3% of patients) but devastating

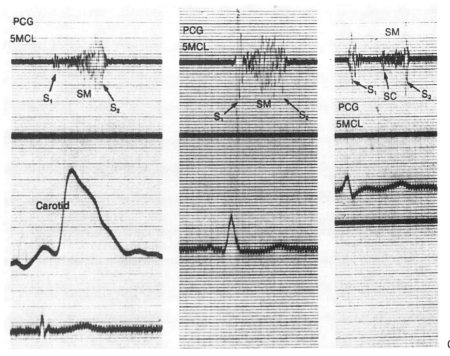

**FIG. 3.3.** Spectrum of the systolic murmur (SM) of papillary muscle dysfunction. **A:** Classic late systolic murmur that begins in early to mid systole and crescendos to $S_2$. **B:** Louder and longer systolic murmur that is crescendo-decrescendo in configuration. Note the increased $S_1$. **C:** Late systolic murmur with a mid-systolic click. (From Delman AJ, Stein E. Dynamic cardiac auscultation and phonocardiography: a graphic guide. Philadelphia: WB Saunders, 1979, with permission.)

complication of acute anteroseptal or inferoseptal MI, producing a harsh holosystolic crescendo-decrescendo murmur loudest at the lower left sternal border, which radiates across the chest from left to right and frequently is accompanied by a palpable systolic thrill. Risk factors for acute VSD include age >65 years old, first infarction, no angina preceding MI, history of hypertension, and female gender. The clinical presentation usually is catastrophic, characterized by the rapid onset of right heart failure (elevated JVP), signs of LV failure, and increasing cardiogenic shock. Wide splitting of $S_2$ also is heard and, in the presence of LV systolic dysfunction, pulsus alternans, alternation of heart sounds and the systolic murmur, along with an $S_3$ gallop can all be appreciated. Although differentiation between VSD and acute MR may be difficult at times, a careful search for the lo-

cation of the maximal systolic murmur and thrill (left sternal border for VSD, apex for acute MR) provides the clues that help establish the correct diagnosis. (10,12,14,15,18, 19,21).

TR may result from acute RV failure complicating LV failure, RV papillary muscle dysfunction, or RV infarction. It may be recognized by a holosystolic murmur, also heard best at the lower left sternal border, but, unlike the murmur of acute VSD, characteristically becomes louder during inspiration due to the increase in blood return to the right side of the heart. This murmur is often deceptively short, soft, or absent during expiration.

### Pericardial Friction Rub

Pericardial friction rubs, resulting from inflammation of the adjacent pericardium, usually occur several days into the course of a Q-wave MI. Rubs usually are absent within the first 24 hours, but they may be present when the patient is first seen, especially if there has been a delay in receiving medical attention. Friction rubs are audible in up to 20% of patients, but are notorious for their evanescence. Frequent repeated cardiac auscultation, therefore, is necessary for their identification. Pericarditis occurs more frequently in patients with a large anterior wall MI and after RV infarction. In patients who receive reperfusion therapy, however, the incidence of pericardial friction rubs has diminished dramatically (≤5%), presumably as a result of limiting transmural extension of infarction. A loud, persistent rub, therefore, suggests the presence of a large transmural MI with a higher incidence of associated heart failure and thus represents a poor prognostic sign. Pericardial friction rubs occurring later than 1 week after onset of AMI suggest post-MI (Dressler) syndrome, an autoimmune phenomenon very rarely seen in the reperfusion era. A pericardial friction rub also may accompany free-wall rupture. Cardiac rupture classically is heralded by prolonged chest pain, restlessness, agitation, repetitive vomiting, dyspnea, hypotension, neck vein distention (signs of cardiac tamponade), and ECG evidence of electromechanical dissociation. Death usually occurs within minutes.

Rubs often are best heard over the left sternal border or occasionally at the cardiac apex by applying firm pressure on the diaphragm of the stethoscope. They are to-and-fro scratchy sounds, which often increase in intensity with inspiration.

## ISCHEMIC CARDIOMYOPATHY

Acute or chronic CAD often results in significant LV damage, with impaired regional or global LV systolic function. Furthermore, many patients with preserved LV systolic function will manifest diastolic dysfunction. The latter group will have little in the way of an abnormal examination, although such patients may experience dyspnea on exertion and have a prominent LV impulse and a palpable $S_4$ heart sound on the physical examination.

Significant systolic LV dysfunction due to overt MI, chronic myocardial ischemia, or LV fibrosis without an established infarct on ECG or by patient history is common. LV dysfunction may be mild or severe. In a minority of cases, an actual apical LV aneurysm may be present. When sufficient loss of LV muscle results in congestive heart failure, the cardiac physical examination becomes abnormal in a predictable fashion. However, in the absence of an ectopic LV impulse or huge LV apical heave suggestive of an aneurysm, the physical findings are similar to those in subjects with heart failure due to other conditions.

### General Appearance

Patients with overt LV systolic dysfunction may appear normal. If they have severe and/or chronic heart failure, orthopnea, tachypnea, rales, jugular venous distention, hepatomegaly, and peripheral edema may be present (not all signs will be found in every patient).

### Jugular Venous Pulse

If there is associated right heart failure (biventricular heart failure), the mean venous pressure will be elevated. The jugular A wave will be dominant unless there is severe associated TR, usually related to pulmonary artery hypertension. If atrial fibrillation is present, the venous pulse will consist of only V waves.

### Arterial Pulse

The arterial pulse may be normal, but often of small volume. Pulsus alternans may be detected.

### Precordial Motion

If the LV apical impulse is palpable, it will characteristically be abnormal. A sustained

LV heave is common, as is a palpable atrial sound. The latter is best and often only felt with the patient in the left lateral position. Ectopic impulses reflect palpable LV activity distant from the normal apical site, typically medial and somewhat caudal to the expected point of maximal impulse or apical impulse. They represent dyskinetic LV segments. In subjects with severe systolic abnormalities, the LV impulse may be felt over a large area, be forceful in nature, and may be associated with a palpable $S_3$ or $S_4$. Furthermore, parasternal RV motion may be noted if the pulmonary artery pressure is high or if there is severe TR.

## Auscultation

The first and second heart sounds are normal to attenuated. An $S_4$ is very common; an $S_3$ should be carefully sought. With an increased pulse rate, there may be a prominent low-frequency diastolic sound known as a summation gallop ($S_3$ and $S_4$ merging together).

The typical heart murmur in ischemic cardiomyopathy is MR. This may be the classic holosystolic apical high-frequency murmur, or the systolic murmur may begin in mid systole (papillary muscle dysfunction) or even taper off before $S_2$. If there is significant TR, a blowing holosystolic murmur at the lower left sternal area may be present that increases with inspiration; in severe cases, a palpable hepatic impulse will be felt.

## Other Findings

Patients with severe ischemic cardiomyopathy can become cachectic, develop hepatomegaly and ascites, and may have severe peripheral edema. Such individuals cannot be differentiated from other causes of end-stage heart disease. Some patients will present initially with overt congestive heart failure and an abnormal cardiac examination without any prior history of angina or MI, and even a nondiagnostic ECG. In these cases, echocardiography is the key to making the diagnosis of CAD.

## ECHOCARDIOGRAPHY

### Introduction

Earlier and accurate diagnosis of myocardial ischemia or MI can lead to an earlier and increased rate of coronary artery patency, preservation of myocardium and LV function, and improved patient survival. The diagnosis of myocardial ischemia or MI can be made in most patients with the integration of history and physical examination, ECG, and measurement of myocardial enzymes. However, independently of limitations in each of these diagnostic techniques, both resting and stress echocardiography have a very important complementary and additive diagnostic and prognostic value in patients with ischemic heart disease. Chest pain frequently is noncharacteristic of myocardial ischemia or infarction; 30% to 35% of patients have ST-T depression (less specific for ischemia than ST elevation); not uncommonly patients have conditions (e.g., hypertension) or are undergoing therapy (digoxin, antiarrhythmics) that can make the ECG ST abnormalities less specific; ECG ST-T segment elevation mimicking acute injury can be seen in acute pericarditis, early repolarization, and LV aneurysm; and, more importantly, 15% to 20% of patients with acute ischemic syndromes have a normal ECG. In addition, myocardial biochemical markers increase are not seen before 6 hours in most patients. On the other hand, of the five million Americans presenting to the emergency rooms with chest pain, 85% will not have AMI, but 3% to 5% will have an unrecognized AMI and are discharged home.

Doppler echocardiography is a rapid, accurate, readily available, versatile, noninvasive technique that can play an important role in the evaluation of the patient with suspected acute or chronic manifestations of CAD. The current use of digital and harmonic imaging, LV myocardial and cavity enhancing contrast agents, and side-by-side (or quad screen) rest and stress images in a cine loop have made resting and stress echocardiography during exercise (treadmill, bicycle) or with pharmacologic stressors or vasodilators (dobutamine, arbutamine, dipyridamole, adenosine) practical and highly accurate for the detection or exclusion of CAD. Resting or stress echocardiography can assist in the initial diagnosis of patients with chest pain or suspected acute coronary syndromes; provide an assessment of myocardial ischemia or infarct size and its location; define the extent of CAD; monitor serial changes in regional and global diastolic and systolic LV function; and facilitate early and accurate diagnosis of post-MI mechanical complications. Therefore, echocardiography not only can help establish the diagnosis of CAD, but also can stratify patients with acute or chronic ischemic heart disease into patients with good versus poor prognosis. Of importance, stress echocardiography provides comparable levels of accuracy (slightly less sensitive but more specific) to nuclear stress imaging (although less expensive, more convenient, and without radiation exposure) and superior levels of accuracy (~85%) to standard ECG stress testing alone (~65%).

## Techniques and Criteria for Echocardiographic Diagnosis of Coronary Artery Disease

The accuracy of resting or stress echocardiography for the diagnosis of CAD is dependent on specific diagnostic criteria.

### Resting Echocardiography

Segmental wall-motion abnormalities are the *sine qua non* of myocardial ischemia or MI. The most commonly used scoring system for defining the location and grading the severity of wall-motion abnormalities is that of the American Society of Echocardiography (22). The LV is divided into 16 myocardial segments for which a specific arterial supply has been determined (Table 3.7 and Fig. 3.4). Each myocardial segment is graded based on wall motion and endocardial thickening on a scale of 1 to 5, where 1 = normal; 2 = hypokinetic; 3 = akinetic; 4 = dyskinetic; and 5 = aneurysmal (Table 3.8).

The extent and severity of wall-motion abnormalities is determined by a wall-motion score and index defined as the sum of each wall segment score divided by the total of segments scored. A patient with normal wall motion should have a global wall-motion score of 16 and an index of 1. The higher the score and index, the worse are the extent and severity of myocardial ischemia or infarction.

### Stress Echocardiography

Comparison of resting with peak stress wall motion and endocardial thickening results in four types of wall-motion response and corresponding clinical assessment (Table 3.9). The diagnostic accuracy of stress echocardiography in the detection of CAD increases as the severity of wall motion and/or number of asynergic segments increase; if the predicted maximal heart rate is achieved or exceeded; and as the severity and extent of CAD increase. If one segment is involved or if wall motion deteriorates by one grade, the positive predictive value is ≤85% compared to ≥95% if four or more segments are involved or if wall

**TABLE 3.7.** *Left ventricular wall segments and corresponding coronary artery supply*

| Echocardiographic segment | Coronary artery |
|---|---|
| Basal, mid, and apical anterior | LAD |
| Basal, mid, and apical anterior septum | LAD |
| Apical lateral | LAD |
| Basal and mid anterolateral | LAD/LCX |
| Basal and mid inferior | RCA |
| Basal and mid inferior septum | RCA |
| Apical inferior | RCA/LAD |
| Basal and mid inferolateral | LCX |

LAD, left anterior descending artery; LCX, left cirfumflex artery; RCA, right coronary artery.

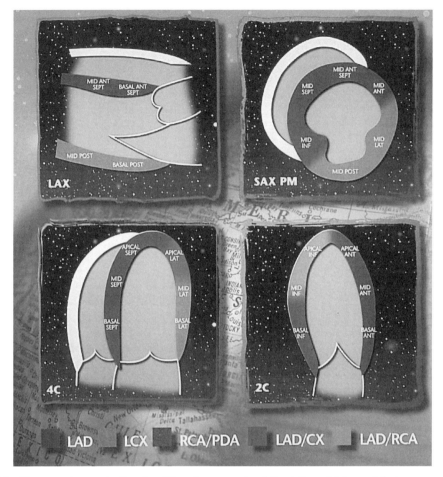

**FIG. 3.4.** Diagram demonstrating the 16 wall segments of the left ventricle and their corresponding coronary artery supply. (Courtesy of Biosound, Inc.) (See Color Figure 3.4.)

motion deteriorates by two or more grades. Similarly, the sensitivity of the test is <70% or >85% if the predictive maximum heart achieved is <75% or >85%, respectively (23). Also, the sensitivity of the test is higher when a major vessel stenosis is >75% or proximally located and with multivessel disease (24). Fi-

nally, the sensitivity of exercise echocardiography is improved when images are obtained at peak rather than postexercise (25).

The overall sensitivity, specificity, and predictive value of the different modalities of stress echocardiography (treadmill or bicycle exercise, dobutamine, adenosine, and high-

**TABLE 3.8.** *Scoring system for grading left ventricular wall motion*

| Score | Wall motion | Systolic wall motion | Endocardial thickening |
|---|---|---|---|
| 1 | Normal | Normal | Normal (>30%) |
| 2 | Hypokinesis | Reduced | Reduced (<30%) |
| 3 | Akinesis | Absent. Reduced if dragged by other normal walls. | Absent. Thinning may be present. |
| 4 | Dyskinesis | Outward | Thinning in most cases |
| 5 | Aneurysmal | Diastolic deformity | Absent and thinning |

**TABLE 3.9.** *Patterns of left ventricular wall motion on stress echo cardiography and their clinical implications*

| Wall motion at rest | Wall motion at peak stress | Clinical implication |
|---|---|---|
| Normal wall excursion and endocardial thickening | Hyperdynamic and symmetric wall thickening | Absent or very low likelihood of CAD |
| Normal wall excursion and endocardial thickening | Hypokinetic, akinetic, uncommonly dyskinetic | CAD (ischemia) without MI |
| Wall hypokinesis or akinesis with partial or full endocardial thickening | Augmented, hypokinetic, akinetic, or dyskinetic | Nontransmural MI with viable stunned (if augmented), ischemic (if worsens), or hybernating myocardium (if a biphasic response noted) |
| Akinetic and thinned wall | Akinetic or dyskinetic | Transmural MI, no viability |

CAD, coronary artery disease; MI, myocardial infarction.

dose dipyridamole) probably are similar (26,27). The sensitivity of dobutamine and atropine is slightly higher than dobutamine alone due to the higher heart rate response achieved. With supine or upright bicycle exercise, the detection and extent of ischemia are slightly higher than with treadmill exercise, mainly because images are obtained at peak exercise and maximum heart rate achieved (28). Also, the diagnostic accuracy of any stress echocardiography modality is improved if second harmonic imaging is utilized (29). Dobutamine or exercise echocardiography may have lower sensitivity in women than in men, especially in patients with single-vessel disease (30,31). Finally, and although not yet widely applied, acoustic quantification, automatic border detection, tissue Doppler imaging, and color kinesis may enhance the diagnostic value of stress echocardiographic techniques for detection of CAD (32,33).

### Assessment of Myocardial Viability

Dobutamine echocardiography currently is a commonly used technique for assessment of myocardial viability. Two patterns of wall-motion response to dobutamine establish the presence of viable myocardium: (i) a resting hypokinetic or akinetic wall that shows improvement in wall motion and endocardial thickening at low dose (≤10 μg/kg/min) but deteriorates at higher dose ("biphasic response") is indicative of viable "ischemic" myocardium with a flow-limiting coronary artery stenosis; and (ii) a rest-

ing hypokinetic or akinetic wall that shows continued (low and high dose) improvement in wall motion and endocardial thickening indicates viable "nonischemic" myocardium with a non–flow-limiting coronary artery stenosis.

### Echocardiography in Patients with Suspected Acute Myocardial Ischemia or Infarction

#### Diagnosis

Segmental wall-motion abnormalities occur within 30 minutes of a coronary artery occlusion and actually before chest pain, ischemic ECG changes, and elevation of myocardial enzyme levels. Therefore, in patients who present to the emergency department with acute chest pain, the presence of any new or worsening (transient or persistent) segmental wall-motion abnormality on resting echocardiography assists in the early detection of acute myocardial ischemia or infarction and helps identify the "culprit" coronary artery (concordance of echocardiography and angiography for predicting infarct related artery in patients with ST elevation is >80%). In general, resting echocardiography detects wall-motion abnormalities in 90% to 100% of patients with ST-segment elevation MI, 75% to 85% of those with non–ST-segment elevation MI, but only 20% of patients with unstable angina. Therefore, wall-motion abnormalities on resting echocardiography have high sensitivity, specificity, and predictive value for AMI (34,35). The combination of findings on resting echocardiography with troponin T levels has improved diagnostic and prognostic value in patients with chest pain (36). *Practical Point: The absence of wall-motion abnormalities during chest pain identifies patients who are highly unlikely to be having an acute coronary event.*

LV diastolic and systolic function can be rapidly assessed, and post-MI mechanical complications can be accurately diagnosed with bedside echocardiography in patients with known or suspected acute myocardial ischemia or AMI. These parameters are of significant prognostic importance.

### Risk Stratification

In patients presenting to the emergency room, a resting echocardiogram can define the extent and severity of wall-motion abnormalities in the infarct- and noninfarct-related coronary artery distributions. In patients with AMI not treated with thrombolytics or primary angioplasty, extensive wall-motion abnormalities (wall-motion score index >1.5 or ≥4 abnormal segments) in the distribution of the infarct-related artery and/or in remote areas are highly predictive of large MI or multivessel CAD, respectively. These patients have higher in-hospital post-MI angina, MI extension or expansion, post-MI mechanical complications, significant ventricular arrhythmias, heart failure, cardiogenic shock, and death (34–38). Patients with LV systolic dysfunction have similar prognosis (39). Therefore, a resting echocardiogram in patients with suspected acute myocardial ischemia or MI can help identify those who should benefit by aggressive antithrombotic or thrombolytic therapy, urgent cardiac catheterization, and percutaneous or surgical coronary revascularization. Such interventions should result in early artery patency, smaller infarct size, preservation of LV function, and improvement in patient short- and long-term survival. In contrast, patients with AMI who have mild or small extent of wall-motion abnormalities tend to

have smaller infarcts and, thus, more favorable short- and long-term prognosis.

A patient with chest pain seen in the emergency room or admitted for further evaluation with suspected CAD despite a normal resting echocardiogram (or no echocardiogram), normal or unremarkable ECG, and at least two negative sets of myocardial isoenzymes can safely undergo an exercise treadmill with or without echocardiography, or dobutamine echocardiography with or without atropine (after at least 12 hours of observation in a chest pain unit). A positive exercise or dobutamine echocardiogram is predictive of increased early and 6-month rates of recurrent nonfatal MI, unstable angina, coronary revascularization, and cardiac death (40–42).

Finally, a bedside echocardiogram performed in the emergency department, intensive care unit, or coronary care unit can detect other potentially life-threatening cardiovascular causes of chest pain, such as valvular aortic stenosis, hypertrophic (obstructive) cardiomyopathy, pericarditis (pericardial effusion), aortic dissection, and pulmonary embolism. If aortic dissection is suspected, TEE, computed tomography, or magnetic resonance imaging is indicated.

### Echocardiography During Hospital Course of Postmyocardial Infarction Patients

### Assessment of Salvaged or Jeopardized Myocardium

Resting echocardiography in post-MI patients can assess the effects of reperfusion therapy. Comparison of initial wall-motion abnormalities with those after reperfusion therapies can determine the extent of myocardial salvage and, therefore, myocardium at risk for subsequent ischemic events. In patients with successful reperfusion therapy, myocardial stunning can resolve within 3 to 5 days. This is of most importance in anterior MI, because the resolution of myocardial stunning and improvement of LV function help identify those patients with no need for anticoagulation therapy. In contrast, patients with persistent significant wall-motion abnormalities, LV aneurysm formation, or LV ejection fraction ≤35% may need long-term anticoagulation for prevention of cardioembolism independently of the presence of LV thrombus.

### Detection of Postmyocardial Infarction Ischemia, Infarct Extension, or Expansion

Patients with resting post-MI angina may, on bedside echocardiogram, have transient or persistent worsening of wall-motion abnormalities in the infarct- or noninfarct-related artery distribution without myocardial enzyme reelevation. Patients with MI extension have reelevation of myocardial enzymes in addition to new or worse wall-motion abnormalities. These two clinical syndromes are suggestive of recurrent thrombosis of the MI-related coronary artery or disease in other vessels. Such patients have poor short- and long-term prognoses. Patients with infarct expansion show an increased area of wall thinning in the infarct zone, especially those with late, unsuccessful, or no reperfusion therapy, and/or large infarcts (most commonly anterior). Infarct expansion is progressive within 7 days post-MI and may lead to aneurysm formation. These patients are at high risk for thrombus formation, heart failure, wall rupture, recurrent ischemia, and ventricular arrhythmias.

### Right Ventricular Infarction

Although ECG is highly sensitive and specific for detection of RV MI, it does not provide information on the extent of infarct and RV function. RV MI occurs in 25% to 30% of patients with posteroinferior MI and implies obstruction of the RCA proximal to the takeoff of the RV and acute marginal branches. The echocardiographic findings are RV dilation and dysfunction, segmental wall-motion abnormalities of the RV free wall, TR of variable severity, paradoxic septal motion, a plethoric inferior vena cava indicative of right atrial hypertension, and rarely shunting from right to left through a patent foramen ovale. Patients with RV MI have an increased incidence of heart failure, mechanical complica-

tions, and mortality independent of the extent of LV dysfunction (43).

### Left Ventricular Diastolic Dysfunction

In post-MI patients with or without clinical heart failure, echocardiography can define the presence of ischemic LV diastolic dysfunction. A decrease in early LV filling leads to a decrease in E wave velocity, prolongation of E deceleration time (>240 ms), decrease in the E/A ratio, and prolongation of the isovolumic relaxation time. All these parameters are indicative of impaired LV relaxation. A decrease in LV compliance can lead to a restrictive LV filling pattern characterized by a high E/A ratio (>1.5), shortened E deceleration time (<140 ms), and shortened isovolumic relaxation time (<110 ms). Mitral inflow with a pseudonormal pattern has a deceleration time between 140 and 240 ms and an E/A ratio <1.5. These last two patterns of LV filling are generally associated with an abnormal inflow pattern of the pulmonary veins. Systolic pulmonary vein inflow is decreased or absent (normally larger than the diastolic inflow), diastolic inflow is predominant (normally smaller than systolic), and atrial reversal velocity is of longer duration than that of mitral A velocity. These three LV filling patterns, but especially the restrictive mitral and pulmonary vein inflows, are predictive of high LV filling pressures (pulmonary capillary wedge >20 mm Hg) and are independent predictors of cardiac death (44).

### Left Ventricular Aneurysm

LV aneurysm is the end result of transmural MI expansion and extensive fibrosis. Its incidence ranges from 8% to 22%, it occurs predominantly (>90%) at the apex after an anterior MI, and it commonly occurs within the first week post-MI. It is defined as an outward diastolic and systolic deformity of the thinned and scarred infarcted area. Transthoracic echocardiography has a sensitivity >95% for detecting LV aneurysm. Patients with LV aneurysm have a high risk for thrombus formation and cardioembolism, and they have increased in-hospital and 1-year mortality.

## *Left Ventricular Thrombus*

LV thrombi occur most commonly (>90%) within the first week after a transmural MI. The incidence is much higher in transmural anterior than in inferior or lateral MI (20% to 50% vs. 1%, respectively). Thrombi are seen most commonly at the LV apex and almost always are associated with an apical aneurysm or apical wall akinesis or dyskinesis. In patients with successful and early reperfusion therapy, the incidence of LV thrombus is <10%. Transthoracic echocardiography has a sensitivity of 90% to 95% and a specificity of 85% to 95% for detection of LV thrombus. The sensitivity is higher with the use of 3.5- and 5-MHz transducers and harmonic imaging. Echocardiographic predictors of LV thrombus formation include a high wall-motion score index (usually apical akinesis or dyskinesis or aneurysm formation), high LV end-systolic and end-diastolic volume indexes, and low ejection fraction (≤40%) (45,46).

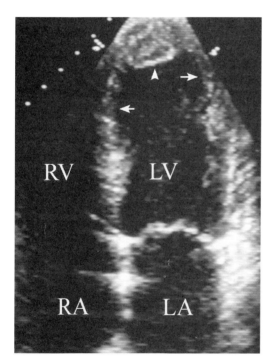

**FIG. 3.5.** Apical four-chamber two-dimensional echocardiogram from a 52-year-old man with a recent anterior myocardial infarction demonstrates an apical aneurysm *(arrows)* with an oval shape apical thrombi *(arrowhead)*. LA, left atrium; LV, left ventricle; RA, right atrium; RV, right ventricle.

LV thrombus is characterized as a distinct mass that usually protrudes into the LV cavity; however, it can be flat and mimic LV endocardium; sessile and oval shaped; or pedunculated and mobile. A recently formed thrombus has similar echo-reflectance to the myocardium. In contrast, old thrombus has heterogeneous increased echo-reflectance (especially in the borders) and may be calcified (Fig. 3.5). A mobile thrombus is associated most commonly with subsequent cardioembolism. The current use of harmonic imaging enhances differentiation and detection of bridging trabeculations (a normal variant), most commonly seen at the LV apex. Bridging trabeculations have a characteristic linear structure with homogeneously increased reflectance and separate from the LV wall during systole. In some cases it may be difficult to differentiate bridging trabeculations from LV thrombus or to exclude an interspersed thrombus. Use of contrast agents for LV cavity opacification can help to differentiate an LV thrombus from an apical bridging trabeculation or artifact.

### *Postmyocardial Infarction Pericarditis*

Pericarditis may occur within 3 to 10 days after a large transmural MI. The incidence of post-MI pericarditis/pericardial effusions (generally small) is up to 25% in transmural infarcts, but it is lower in those treated with thrombolytic therapy or primary angioplasty. Echocardiography is highly sensitive for detection of a pericardial effusion (47). Pericarditis or pericardial effusions occurring 2 weeks or more after MI usually represent Dressler syndrome.

### Echocardiography for Detection of Postmyocardial Infarction Mechanical Complications

Post-MI mechanical complications include partial or complete papillary muscle rupture with severe MR, VSD, and free-wall rupture; incidence rates are 1%, 1%, and 3%, respectively. These catastrophic events occur most commonly within 3 to 5 days post-MI and almost always in patients with transmural MIs. Risk factors include age >65 years, female sex, hypertension, no angina preceding MI, single-vessel disease, and first MI. Free-wall rupture occurs more commonly in patients with a posterolateral infarct (circumflex artery occlusion) and in those with unsuccessful thrombolytic therapy (5.9% vs. 0.5%) (48).

### Ischemic Mitral Regurgitation and Papillary Muscle Rupture

MR in post-MI patients is defined as ischemic when primary valve pathology cannot be identified (49). Its incidence is about 20% and is similar in anterior and inferior MI. In most cases, MR is mild or mild to moderate. The presence of moderate or worse MR is associated with increased short- and long-term mortality. A new systolic murmur (present in only 50% of patients with acute and severe ischemic MR), new-onset heart failure, or pulmonary edema in a patient with a recent posteroinferior MI should raise the suspicion of hemodynamically significant MR. Bedside echocardiography should be performed. The characteristics of ischemic MR vary according to the location of the MI. In patients with inferior MI, the ischemic or infarcted posteromedial papillary muscle causes tethering and decreased mobility, predominantly of the posterior mitral leaflet, leading to leaflet malcoaptation and relative anterior leaflet prolapse or pseudoprolapse (Fig. 3.6). Anterior mitral pseudoprolapse explains the characteristically eccentric and posterolaterally directed MR jet. In patients with anterior MI, LV dilation and dysfunction lead to downward and lateral displacement of the papillary muscles. The mitral leaflets undergo incomplete but symmetric malcoaptation; therefore, the MR jet is central. When papillary muscle rupture is partial, prolapse of one or both mitral leaflets or a flail portion can be demonstrated. When rupture is complete, MR is eccentric and severe, and the involved mitral leaflet with a portion of its papillary muscle becomes flail and prolapses freely into the LA (Fig. 3.7). Because of the associated highly eccentric MR jet, transthoracic echocardiography may underestimate

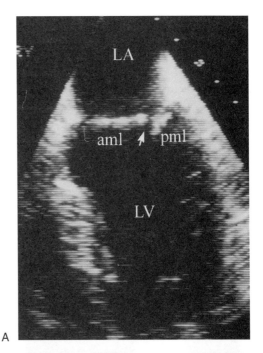

A

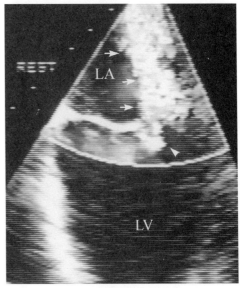

B

FIG. 3.6. A: Four-chamber transesophageal echocardiogram from a 63-year-old male with a recent inferior myocardial infarction, sudden-onset pulmonary edema, and a holosystolic apical murmur demonstrates tethering of the posterior mitral leaflet (pml) and asymmetric and incomplete leaflet malcoaptation (arrow) leading to pseudoprolapse of the anterior mitral leaflet (aml). B: Severe mitral regurgitation demonstrated by color Doppler with a highly eccentric and posterolaterally directed jet extending to the pulmonary veins (arrows). Abbreviations as in previous figures. (See Color Figure 3.6B.)

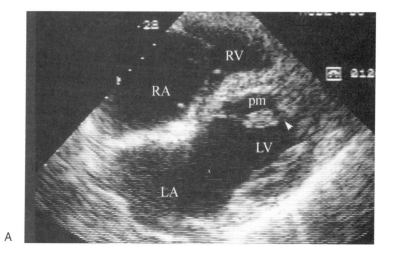

A

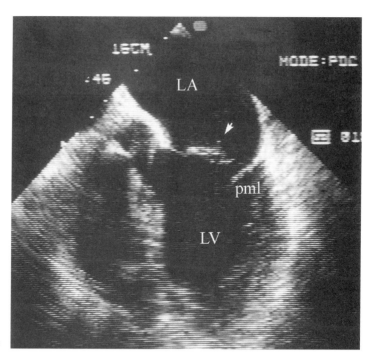

B

**FIG. 3.7. A:** Transthoracic subcostal four-chamber view in a 54-year-old man with a recent posteroinferior myocardial infarction demonstrates complete rupture of the posteromedial papillary muscle (pm) *(arrowhead).* **B,C:** Four-chamber transesophageal echocardiograms demonstrate a flail anterior mitral leaflet with a portion of the posteromedial papillary muscle attached *(arrow)* and
associated severe mitral regurgitation by color Doppler. (See Color Figure 3.7C.)

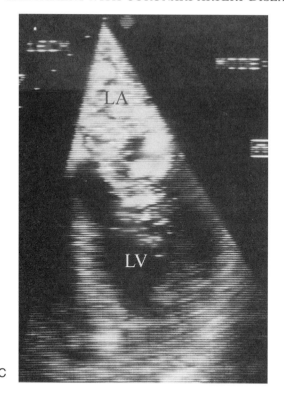

C

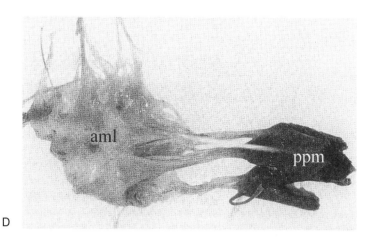

D

**FIG. 3.7.** *Continued.* **D:** Surgical specimen shows the completely transected posteromedial papillary muscle (ppm) with normal morphology of the anterior mitral leaflet (aml). Abbreviations as in previous figures.

the severity and mechanism of MR. There-fore, TEE should be performed promptly in patients suspected of having a ruptured pap-illary muscle.

### Ventricular Septal Defect

Ventricular septal rupture occurs more commonly in the posteroapical septum and distal anterior septum. A septal rupture can be multiple and have a serpiginous course. VSDs are best visualized from the paraster-nal short-axis view below the level of the papillary muscles and from the apical four-chamber view with anterior or posterior an-gulation. Posterior defects also can be visu-alized from the subcostal four-chamber view (Fig. 3.8). The sensitivity of transthoracic color Doppler echocardiography for detec-tion of VSD ranges from 86% to 95%. The sensitivity and specificity of TEE is >95%. The width of the color Doppler jet correlates with the defect size at surgery. Commonly associated acute RV volume overload may lead to RV dilation and dysfunction, para-doxic septal motion, and right atrial hyper-tension and dilation (48).

### Free-Wall Rupture and Pseudoaneurysm

Free-wall rupture manifests on echocardio-graphy predominantly as a pericardial effu-sion (hemopericardium) with or without in-trapericardial densities (clots) and cardiac tamponade, frequently with compression of the left heart chambers. Echocardiography is highly sensitive for detection of free-wall rup-ture (50,51). An LV pseudoaneurysm is a my-ocardial rupture contained by pericardial ad-hesions. The pericardial adhesions form a pouch that communicates with the LV and is characterized on echocardiography by a nar-row neck with a neck to maximum diameter ratio of <0.5. Color Doppler demonstrates flow in and out of the pericardial space at the site of the tear and abnormal swirling flow within the pseudoaneurysm (Fig. 3.9). How-ever, the myocardial tear is infrequently visu-alized.

## Resting and Stress Echocardiography After Treatment of Unstable Angina and Myocardial Infarction

### Diagnosis and Risk Stratification

Resting echocardiography in patients with acute ischemic syndromes and stress echocar-diography (independently of stress modality used) after their stabilization are highly accu-rate for detecting myocardial ischemia in the infarct-related artery or in remote areas (this last implies multivessel CAD), detecting my-ocardial viability and recovery after revascu-larization, and predicting the rate of future cardiac events (Table 3.10).

In patients with medically treated unstable angina or AMI treated with thrombolytics, a wall-motion score index ≥1.5, ejection frac-tion ≤45%, or MR severity >2+ on resting echocardiography are strong predictors of cardiac death, recurrent unstable angina, non-fatal MI, and congestive heart failure over 18 to 24 months of follow-up (52,53).

In patients with medically treated unstable angina, a positive predischarge exercise echocardiogram predicts a 20% risk of car-diac death, nonfatal MI, or late (>3 months) revascularization over a 2-year period com-pared to a <5% rate of any cardiac event among those patients with a negative test (54).

A predischarge exercise or any pharmaco-logic stress echocardiogram 1 to 3 weeks after an uncomplicated non–Q-wave or Q-wave MI (independently of reperfusion interventions) identifies worse or new, improved, or un-changed wall-motion abnormalities within, ad-jacent or remote to the MI area with similar high sensitivity, specificity, and predictive ac-curacy (Table 3.10) (55–57). Based on these results, post-MI patients are stratified into three groups of patients with different short- and long-term prognoses. The first and most common group (about 60%) of post-MI pa-tients is constituted by those with viable but is-chemic myocardium (worsening of wall mo-tion, biphasic response, or new wall motion abnormality reflecting a residual flow-limiting infarct-related artery or remote vessel disease). The second group (about 20% to 30% of pa-

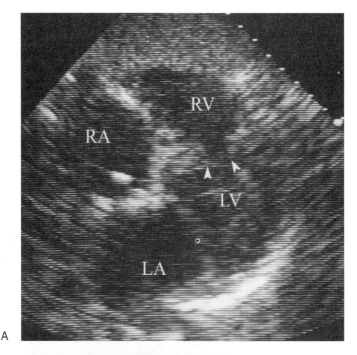

A

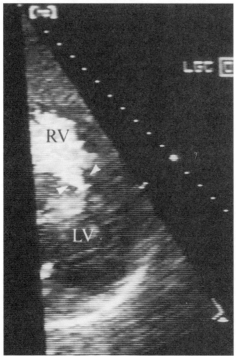

B

**FIG. 3.8. A:** Transthoracic subcostal four-chamber echocardiogram from a 77-year-old man with a recent posteroinferior myocardial infarction demonstrates a large (>1 cm) ventricular septal defect located at the base of the inferior septum *(arrowheads)*. **B:** Color Doppler demonstrates left to right communication *(arrowheads)*. Abbreviations as in previous figures. (See Color Figure 3.8B.)

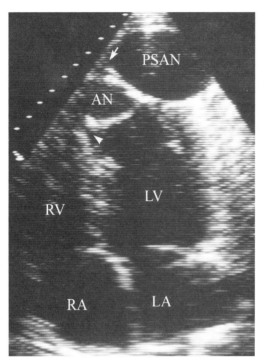
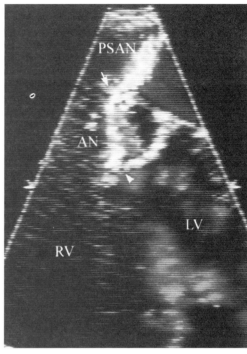

A
B

**FIG. 3.9. A:** Apical four-chamber two-dimensional echocardiogram from a 68-year-old patient with recurrent congestive heart failure and a new apical holosystolic murmur demonstrates dehiscence *(arrowhead)* of a patched apical aneurysm (AN) with subsequent rupture *(arrow)* and formation of a pseudoaneurysm (PSAN). **B:** Color Doppler demonstrate bidirectional flow between the left ventricle and aneurysm *(arrowhead)* and between the aneurysm and pseudoaneurysm *(arrow).* Abbreviations as in previous figures. (See Color Figure 3.9B.)

**TABLE 3.10.** *Diagnostic value of echocardiography for myocardial ischemia or viability and future cardiac events in patients with chest pain, unstable angina, and myocardial infarction*

| Clinical scenario/technique | Sensitivity (%) | Specificity (%) | PPV (%) | NPV (%) |
|---|---|---|---|---|
| Unstable angina/pacing transthoracic echocardiography | 88–95 | 87–91 | 95–97 | 67–87 |
| Chest pain or acute MI/resting echocardiography | 47–94 | 53–99 | 31–91 | 90–99 |
| Post-MI ischemia/exercise echocardiography | 55–82 | 67–95 | 44–94 | 83–100 |
| Post-MI ischemia/dipyridamole | 63–93 | 78–92 | 43–95 | 84–97 |
| Post-MI ischemia/DSE | 68–82 | 80–98 | 65–86 | 85–88 |
| Post-MI viability/DSE | 74–97 | 73–96 | 67–91 | 77–94 |
| Post-MI viability/low-level exercise | 81 | 92 | 95 | 73 |
| Prognosis/resting or stress echocardiography[a]: WMSI >1.5–2, ≥4 abnormal segments, myocardial viability (biphasic response), remote asynergy, LVEF <45%, or MR >2+ | 79–97 | 17–90 | 24–89 | 82–98 |

[a]Predicts death, recurrent unstable angina, or myocardial infarction (MI), heart failure, cardiogenic shock, arrhythmias, or revascularization.

DSE, dobutamine stress echocardiography; LVEF, left ventricular ejection fraction; MR, mitral regurgitation; NPV, negative predictive value; PPV, positive predictive value; WMSI, wall-motion score index.

tients) will demonstrate myocardial viability but no ischemia (wall-motion improvement reflecting open infarct-related artery and no remote CAD). The third group (10% to 20% of patients) will show no viability and no ischemia (completed transmural MI independent of patency of the infarct-related artery). Unless revascularized, patients with an ischemic response have a 5% to 10% rate of cardiac death or MI; 10% to 30% rate of unstable angina; and 20% to 40% rate of revascularization over a 1- to 2-year follow-up period (58–61).

In patients with AMI who have undergone successful reperfusion therapy (thrombolytic therapy or primary angioplasty), sustained improvement in wall motion on rest or any stress echocardiographic modality performed as early as 3 days after MI has high sensitivity (>80%), specificity (>75%), and predictive value (>80%) for a patent artery (Thrombolysis in Myocardial Infarction [TIMI] 2 or 3 antegrade flow and <30% residual stenosis), and recovery of regional wall motion and ejection fraction at 1- and 6-month follow-up resting echocardiography (62).

Therefore, in stable post-MI patients, a positive stress echocardiogram should indicate the need for cardiac catheterization and revascularization procedures. In contrast, patients with a negative test can be managed conservatively and spared from undergoing the risk and expense of invasive diagnostic and therapeutic interventions.

## Stress Echocardiography in Chronic Ischemic Heart Disease

### *Diagnosis*

Stress echocardiography is particularly useful when ECG changes of ischemia are obscured by baseline abnormalities (LV hypertrophy, LBBB, resting ST-T wave changes) or in those situations most likely to result in false-positive or uninterpretable exercise stress testing (e.g., patients receiving digoxin, women, or patients with mitral valve prolapse). In patients with chronic stable angina, exercise or pharmacologic stress echocardiography, in addition to

establishing the presence of CAD, localizes the stenosed vessel and defines the severity and extent of ischemia. This technique also is useful in identifying restenosis of a native coronary artery after angioplasty or stent placement or detecting disease of a saphenous vein or arterial bypass graft. Finally, stress echocardiography is a diagnostic alternative to routine coronary angiography for detection of cardiac allograft vasculopathy.

The overall diagnostic accuracy of the different stress echocardiographic techniques (exercise or pharmacologic) for detecting CAD probably is similar but highly variable when applied independently to populations with different clinical and angiographic characteristics. The diagnostic accuracy of these techniques is highest when high-quality images are obtained at peak stress (i.e., supine or upright bicycle exercise); in patients with previous MI; in subjects with multivessel CAD; in high-grade (>70%) vessel stenosis; in the presence of proximal LAD or RCA disease; and when ≥85% of the maximum predicted heart rate is achieved (i.e., exercise or dobutamine with atropine). Dobutamine at 30 to 40 μg/kg/min with atropine seems to have higher diagnostic accuracy than dobutamine at similar or lower doses without atropine. The sensitivity of dipyridamole echocardiography is higher with high-dose (0.84 mg/kg) compared to low-dose (0.56 mg/kg) dipyridamole. Also, adenosine echocardiography using 0.18 mg/kg/min and atropine has higher sensitivity and specificity for detecting CAD compared to 0.14 mg/kg/min (63,64). Finally, dobutamine (40 μg/kg/min) and high-dose (0.84 mg/kg) dipyridamole echocardiography, compared head to head, have demonstrated similar diagnostic value (Table 3.11) (65).

The sensitivity of stress echocardiographic techniques is low for detection of single-vessel CAD (especially for circumflex disease), in patients with LV hypertrophy, and in subjects with small ventricles.

Use of second harmonic imaging compared to fundamental imaging during dobutamine echocardiography significantly improves endocardial resolution/visualization, especially

**TABLE 3.11.** *Diagnostic value of stress echocardiography in chronic ischemic heart disease*

| Test | Overall sensitivity (%) | Sensitivity 1VD (%) | Sensitivity MVD (%) | Specificity (%) | PPV (%) | NPV (%) |
|---|---|---|---|---|---|---|
| Treadmill | 73–97 | 59–93 | 73–100 | 64–100 | 90–100 | 44–87 |
| Supine bicycle exercise | 76–93 | 70–84 | 80–100 | 80–94 | 90–96 | 58–85 |
| Upright bicycle exercise | 71–93 | 61–93 | 80–95 | 78–96 | 86–97 | 50–93 |
| Dobutamine stress echocardiography | 54–96 | 50–95 | 77–96 | 66–100 | 65–96 | 52–88 |
| Dipyridamole | 55–93 | 33–88 | 76–93 | 76–96 | 44–72 | 84–99 |
| Adenosine | 45–85 | 39–80 | 74–85 | 76–100 | — | — |
| Pacing transthoracic echocardiography | 83–95 | 75–80 | 88–95 | 76–91 | 95–97 | 67–87 |
| Pacing transesophageal echocardiography | 86–93 | 69–85 | 82–93 | 89–100 | — | — |

1VD, one-vessel disease; MVD, multivessel disease; NPV, negative predictive value; PPV, positive predictive value.

of the lateral and anterior walls; improves interobserver agreement in assessing wall motion; and increases the sensitivity of the test without affecting its specificity (66). The additive diagnostic value of second harmonic imaging should apply to any stress echocardiographic technique. Furthermore, the diagnostic value of harmonic imaging is improved further when it is used with intravenous contrast agents containing perfluorocarbon (67). However, use of these contrast agents is still uncommon in clinical practice and their cost effectiveness has not been fully evaluated.

Transesophageal dobutamine and pacing echocardiography are diagnostic alternatives in morbidly obese patients with limited precordial images and at significant risk for cardiac catheterization (68,69). Detection of aortic atheromatous disease by TEE has demonstrated high sensitivity (91% to 93%), specificity (82% to 87%), and positive (72% to 88%) and negative (90% to 95%) predictive values for detection of significant CAD (70). Finally, intraoperative TEE for assessment of wall motion and LV volumes has diagnostic and therapeutic value in high-risk patients undergoing coronary artery bypass grafting or vascular surgery, or in patients with CAD undergoing noncardiac surgery. Perioperative myocardial ischemia occurs in at least one third of these patients, and TEE has demonstrated higher diagnostic accuracy than ECG or hemodynamic monitoring (71). TEE can alter the surgical, anesthetic, or hemodynamic management of these patients.

### *Prognosis*

Development on stress echocardiography of multiple ($\geq$2) wall-motion abnormalities (e.g., akinesis or dyskinesis) at low workload, transient LV dilation, or decrease in global LV function (accompanied by severe chest pain and/or marked ST-segment depression with slow resolution, or a fall in BP) suggests severe multivessel or left main CAD, widespread ischemia, and a higher likelihood of future cardiac events.

In patients with chronic stable angina, more than ten series have demonstrated that a positive stress echocardiogram (exercise or pharmacologic) in patients (men or women) with chest pain and suspected or known CAD predicts an annual rate of 11% to 69% of unstable angina, MI, percutaneous or surgical revascularization, heart failure, or cardiac death compared to 1% to 16% among patients with a negative test. The rate of hard events (MI and death) is about 10% for a positive test (15% to 20% in patients with previous MI) and 0% to 3% if the test is negative (72–74). The predictive value of the test increases when resting wall-motion score and index and ejection fraction also are considered.

Pharmacologic stress echocardiography has important preoperative prognostic value in patients with known or suspected CAD undergoing vascular surgery. This technique has high sensitivity (up to 100%) and a good specificity (63%) for predicting nonfatal cardiovascular events and death. A positive dipyridamole or dobutamine echocardiogram in these patients has a 19% to 78% operative risk of angina, MI, coronary artery bypass grafting, or death compared to 0% to 7% in subjects with a negative test. A similar prognostic value has been demonstrated for dobutamine stress echocardiography in patients undergoing nonvascular surgery. Patients with the highest risk (>40% postoperative events) have ischemia at <60% of predicted maximum heart rate; at intermediate risk (<10% events) have ischemia at >60% of predicted heart rate; and at low risk (0% events) have no ischemia (75). Development of hypotension during dobutamine therapy appears to be an independent poor prognostic predictor in patients undergoing vascular and noncardiac surgery (76).

### Ischemic Cardiomyopathy

This clinically important condition manifests on echocardiography with multiple regional wall-motion abnormalities corresponding to a single (e.g., LAD) or multiple coronary artery distributions. The evidence of wall akinesis or dyskinesis (sometimes hypokinesis) with thinning and hyperreflectance are highly specific for CAD. However, a small proportion of patients will demonstrate global LV hypokinesis without wall thinning or hyperreflectance. In these patients, resting echocardiography cannot distinguish an ischemic from a nonischemic or mixed cardiomyopathy. Also, clinical data may not be supportive of ischemic heart disease, and patients may refuse or be at significant risk for cardiac catheterization. Dobutamine echocardiography can be of diagnostic and prognostic value in these patients. A biphasic response or enhanced wall thickening and contraction (myocardial contractile reserve) with low-dose dobutamine (5 to 10 $\mu$g/kg/min) indicate a chronically ischemic (hibernating) myocardium. These patients have poor prognosis without revascularization. Pa-

tients with myocardial contractile reserve in $\geq 5$ segments who undergo revascularization have a >90% survival at 2 to 3 years compared to 50% to 80% if they are treated medically. Patients with no myocardial viability who undergo revascularization have a similar 2-year high mortality (about 20%) compared to subjects treated medically (77,78). A resting end-diastolic wall thickness >0.6 cm has a sensitivity of 94% and a specificity of 48% for recovery of wall motion after revascularization. The combination of end-diastolic wall thickness and any contractile reserve (improvement in wall motion) during dobutamine infusion improves the specificity of the test to 77% (79). Sustained and global contractile improvement with dobutamine (>10 $\mu$g/kg/min) may suggest a nonischemic cardiomyopathy and predicts a better prognosis than in subjects with an ischemic response. Unfortunately, a small proportion of patients with LV systolic dysfunction will show a blunted response or lack of a contractile reserve. These patients can have ischemic or nonischemic cardiomyopathy and have the worst prognosis.

### SUMMARY

### Diagnostic Value of History and Physical Examination

A carefully obtained history and diligently performed physical examination are essential components in the accurate diagnosis of acute or chronic ischemic heart disease. Attention to specific details enables the astute clinician to discern between cardiac and noncardiac causes of chest pain and thus avoid the expense and potential risk of unnecessary testing. In general, transient substernal or left precordial chest discomfort described as a pressure, tightness, heaviness, squeezing, fullness, or burning or aching radiating to the neck, throat, jaw, or left shoulder and arm, brought on by the "*four Es*" (i.e., exertion, emotional stress, exposure to cold and/or hot/humid weather, or after eating a heavy meal) that is relieved promptly by rest and/or nitroglycerin favors the diagnosis of angina pectoris. When angina is new in onset and symptoms increase in intensity, frequency, and duration or occur at rest, unstable angina is said to be present. Severe, crushing, unrelenting chest pain, especially when accompanied by nausea, vomiting, diaphoresis, and profound weakness, lends support to the diagnosis of an evolving AMI.

The findings of hypertension, bruits, and/or pulse deficits of carotid, aortic, or peripheral vascular disease, or signs of hyperlipidemia (e.g., xanthomas, xanthelasmas) provide clues to the presence of underlying CAD. Patients seen during an anginal attack may develop a transient $S_4$ and $S_3$ gallop, palpable LV dyskinesia, systolic murmur of MR, or rarely a paradoxically split $S_2$ that disappears when the pain subsides. In patients who present with unstable angina or AMI, evidence of significant LV systolic dysfunction (i.e., pulmonary rales, $S_3$ gallop, pulsus alternans, jugular venous distention, new or worsening murmur of MR, hypotension, or tachycardia) portends a higher likelihood of severe underlying CAD and a high risk for an adverse clinical outcome. An $S_4$ gallop, indicative of a noncompliant LV, can be heard (or felt) in almost all patients during or shortly after the acute ischemic event. Therefore, its absence argues strongly against AMI. An $S_3$ gallop also may be present in many post-MI patients if significant LV dysfunction has developed. Distention of the neck veins, along with the Kussmaul sign, a right-sided $S_4$ and $S_3$ gallop, hypotension, and clear lung fields in patients with inferior MI, suggests the presence of concomitant RV infarction. The presence of palpable systolic bulging at or just medial and superior to the cardiac apex in anterior MI suggests the presence of an LV aneurysm. A new systolic murmur may appear when papillary muscle dysfunction or infarction causes MR or when the infarct ruptures through the septum and creates an acute VSD.

### Limitations of History and Physical Examination

Clinical history can be atypical and misleading, depending on the physician's expertise in eliciting an accurate account of the symptoms and the patient's ability, desire, or willingness (misinterpretation, denial, or secondary gain) to relay the information appropriately.

The clinical history in many patients with CAD is not always "classic," nor is it specific. Although chest pain is the hallmark of AMI, up to 25% of patients (especially the elderly or diabetic) are asymptomatic during the acute event. The diagnosis can only be made in retrospect by means of a routine ECG, myocardial isoenzymes elevation, or echocardiography.

Atypical symptoms, such as dyspnea, fatigue, lightheadedness, recurrent belching, or "indigestion," often present an easy trap for the unwary.

The presence or magnitude of symptoms does not necessarily coincide with the extent of CAD. Patients with mild anginal symptoms or even no symptoms ("silent ischemia") may have multivessel disease, whereas subjects with severe angina may have only single- or double-vessel disease. At times it can be difficult to determine symptom status because patients may scale back their activities to avoid precipitating angina. Furthermore, the terms used by the patient to describe ischemia and the threshold for eliciting it can vary considerably. Patients with CAD may, in fact, decrease or even avoid certain activities altogether in order to minimize their chances of precipitating discomfort. Even when typical symptoms do occur, <30% of patients admitted for further evaluation actually are having an acute coronary event (Table 3.5).

Patients who present with AMI occasionally may feel a sharp, stabbing, pleuritic-type of pain rather than the more typical pressure-like quality. With advancing age, chest pain declines in frequency as the presenting symptoms of AMI, such as dyspnea, syncope, acute confusion, and stroke, become more common. The presence of atypical symptoms, therefore, should not be used to exclude the possibility that an acute coronary syndrome is occurring (Table 3.4). The correlation between typical symptoms and the presence of significant CAD also varies with gender.

Studies reveal that the predictive value of classic angina pectoris is much higher in men (≥90%) than in women (≥50%). Furthermore, exercise stress testing and ambulatory ECG (Holter) monitoring suggest that the majority of ischemic episodes are never detected by the patient. Interestingly, silent ischemia has been shown to be a risk factor for an adverse clinical outcome regardless of whether or not symptomatic episodes are present.

Traditional risk factors for CAD are only weakly predictive of the likelihood of an acute ischemic event. Up to 40% of patients with AMI may have no known risk factors. The presence or absence of risk factors, therefore, should not be used to determine whether a patient with chest pain should be admitted or treated for an acute coronary syndrome.

No pathognomonic signs allow the clinician to make the diagnosis of cardiac ischemia. A paucity of abnormal findings is the rule rather than the exception in patients with uncomplicated CAD. Unless there is LV dysfunction from an MI or chronic myocardial ischemia, the cardiac examination can, in fact, be entirely unremarkable.

**Diagnostic Value of Echocardiography**

The major advantages of resting and stress echocardiography include its widespread availability, portability, versatility, reliability, noninvasive nature, relative ease with which images can be obtained, and the accurate anatomic, hemodynamic, and prognostic information it provides.

Therefore, echocardiography has become an important part of the evaluation of patients with CAD. It can be extremely useful in the triage of patients presenting to the emergency department with chest pain. Overall, echocardiographic evidence of regional wall-motion abnormalities is a rapid and accurate method for detection of AMI or myocardial ischemia in patients with prolonged chest discomfort, nondiagnostic ECGs (~50% of patients), and no prior history of MI. In contrast, normal wall motion during chest pain is consistent with a very low likelihood of an acute transmural ischemic event.

In stabilized patients with unstable angina or who are post-MI, resting or stress echocardiography, when appropriate, is valuable for detecting and defining the extent and severity of myocardial ischemia and/or infarction; assessing global and regional LV (and RV) systolic and diastolic function; defining the presence and extent of myocardial viability; evaluating the need for an acute intervention; and identifying post-MI mechanical complications. Demonstrated ischemia and LV systolic or diastolic dysfunction are powerful and independent prognostic indicators of a high complication rate and an adverse clinical outcome.

Of importance, significant LV dysfunction may be present but may not produce a detectable abnormality on physical examination. Therefore, for the patient who has a history of MI and/or Q waves on the ECG, and for the subject with clinical symptoms and signs of heart failure, echocardiographic evaluation of LV function is of significant diagnostic and prognostic importance.

Exercise or pharmacologic (for individuals unable to exercise adequately) stress echocardiography is particularly useful for patients with an intermediate pretest likelihood of CAD and for subjects with a high likelihood of a nondiagnostic and/or false-positive exercise ECG. These techniques provide valuable diagnostic and prognostic information in patients with known or suspected stable CAD and in subjects who present for preoperative evaluation.

In summary, echocardiography plays a critical role in the diagnosis, risk stratification, and definition of the most appropriate therapy in patients with acute or chronic ischemic syndromes (Table 3.12) (80).

**Limitations of Echocardiography**

The sensitivity of resting echocardiography for detecting wall-motion abnormalities progressively decreases the longer the time between resolution of chest pain and the acquisition of images. Also, absence of endocardial

**TABLE 3.12.** *Class I indications for echocardiography*[a]

In patients with chest pain
- and suspected acute myocardial ischemia, when baseline ECG is nondiagnostic, and when study can be obtained *during* pain or shortly thereafter
- and severe hemodynamic instability
- and clinical evidence of valvular, myocardial, or pericardial disease (e.g., valvular aortic stenosis, mitral valve prolapse, hypertrophic cardiomyopathy, pericarditis)

In patients with acute coronary syndromes for diagnosis, risk stratification, and prognosis
- to diagnose acute myocardial ischemia or infarction not evident by standard means
- to assess infarct size and/or extent of jeopardized myocardium
- to measure global and regional LV function
- and inferior MI with bedside evidence suggesting concomitant right ventricular infarction
- to assess post-MI mechanical complications (transesophageal echocardiography when transthoracic echocardiography not diagnostic)
- to assess the presence/extent of inducible ischemia whenever baseline ECG abnormalities are expected to compromise interpretation (exercise or pharmacologic stress echocardiography)

In patients with chronic coronary artery disease
- to diagnose myocardial ischemia in symptomatic individuals (exercise or pharmacologic stress echocardiography)
- to assess functional significance of coronary lesions (if not already known) in planning percutaneous coronary intervention (exercise or pharmacologic stress echocardiography)
- to assess ventricular function when needed to guide institution and modification of drug therapy in patients with known or suspected LV dysfunction
- to assess restenosis after revascularization in patients with atypical recurrent symptoms (exercise or pharmacologic stress echocardiography)
- to assess myocardial viability (hibernating myocardium) for planning revascularization (dobutamine stress echocardiography)

[a]Conditions for which there is evidence and/or general agreement that the study is useful and effective.
ECG, electrocardiogram; LV, left ventricular; MI, myocardial infarction.
Modified from Cheitlin MD, Alpert JS, Armstrong WF, et al. ACC/AHA guidelines for the clinical application of echocardiography. A report of the American College of Cardiology/American Heart Association Task Force on Practice Guidelines (Committee on Clinical Application of Echocardiography). Developed in collaboration with the American Society of Echocardiography. Circulation 1997;95:1686–1744.

thickening occurs when >20% of the transmural extent of a myocardial wall is involved. Therefore, echocardiography may lack sensitivity for detection of wall-motion abnormalities when a subendocardial infarction involves <20% of the myocardial thickness.

Echocardiography cannot accurately distinguish new (acute ischemia or infarction) from old wall-motion abnormalities (previous MI) or those associated with myocarditis or nonischemic cardiomyopathy. In patients with conduction disturbances (LBBB or ventricular paced rhythm), the associated paradoxic septal motion may be misclassified as ischemic wall-motion abnormality. Visual assessment of the absence of systolic endocardial thickening or thinning and scarring of the wall segment is a more specific (but not sensitive) sign of infarction or ischemia than wall-motion abnormalities.

Exercise echocardiography may fail to detect ischemia-induced wall-motion abnormalities if there is a significant delay in performing the peak stress study. About 5% to 10% of patients undergoing resting echocardiography and up to 15% of subjects undergoing stress echocardiography may have limited visualization of myocardial segments for accurate study interpretation.

Finally, application of echocardiography requires mobilization of special personnel and equipment and cannot be justified from a practical, cost-effective standpoint in all patients.

## ACKNOWLEDGMENT

The authors gratefully acknowledge the expert secretarial assistance of Ms. Mabel N. Nazzarri and Ms. Anne-Marie Collins-Hornyak in the preparation of this manuscript.

## REFERENCES

1. American Heart Association. Guidelines 2000 for cardiopulmonary resuscitation and emergency cardiovas-

cular care. Part 7: the era of reperfusion. Section 1: acute coronary syndromes (acute myocardial infarction). Circulation 2000;102[Suppl I]:I-172–I-203.

2. American Heart Association. 2001 heart and stroke statistical update. Dallas, TX: American Heart Association, 2001.

3. Ryan TJ, Anderson JL, Antman EM, et al. ACC/AHA guidelines for the management of patients with acute myocardial infarction. A report of the American College of Cardiology/American Heart Association Task Force on Practice Guidelines (Committee on Management of Acute Myocardial Infarction). J Am Coll Cardiol 1996;28:1328–1428; and Ryan TJ, Antman EM, Brooks NH, et al. 1999 update. J Am Coll Cardiol 1999;34: 890–911.

4. Gibbons RJ, Chatterjee K, Daley J, et al. ACC/AHA/ ACP-ASIM guidelines for the management of patients with chronic stable angina: a report of the American College of Cardiology/American Heart Association Task Force on Practice Guidelines (Committee on the Management of Patients with Chronic Stable Angina). J Am Coll Cardiol 1999;33:2092–2197.

5. Braunwald E, Antman EM, Beasley JW, et al. ACC/AHA guidelines for the management of patients with unstable angina and non-ST-segment elevation myocardial infarction: a report of the American College of Cardiology/American Heart Association Task Force on Practice Guidelines (Committee on the Management of Patients with Unstable Angina). J Am Coll Cardiol 2000;36:970–1062.

6. Jesse RL, Kontos MC, Tatum JL. Evaluation of chest pain in the emergency department. Curr Probl Cardiol 1997;22:149–236.

7. Willerson JT, Maseri A. Pathophysiology and clinical recognition of coronary artery disease syndromes. In: Willerson JT, Cohn JN, eds. Cardiovascular medicine, 2nd ed. Philadelphia: Churchill Livingstone, 2000:528–568.

8. Chatterjee K. Recognition and management of patients with stable angina pectoris. In: Goldman L, Braunwald E, eds. Primary cardiology. Philadelphia: WB Saunders, 1998:234–256.

9. Abrams J. Special diagnostic issues in ischemic heart disease. In: Crawford MH, DiMarco JP, eds. Cardiology. London: Mosby, 2001:5.1–5.10.

10. Chizner MA. Acute myocardial infarction and its complications: clinical spectrum, diagnosis and management. In: Chizner MA, ed. Classic teachings in clinical cardiology: a tribute to W. Proctor Harvey, M.D. Cedar Grove, NJ: Laennec Publishing, 1996:839–918.

11. Cannon CP. Diagnosis and management of patients with unstable angina. Curr Probl Cardiol 1999;24:681–744.

12. Alexander RW, Pratt CM, Ryan TJ, et al. Diagnosis and management of patients with acute myocardial infarction. In: Fuster V, Alexander RW, O'Rourke RA, et al, eds. Hurst's the heart, 10th ed. New York: McGraw-Hill, 2001:1275–1359.

13. Karliner JS. Stable and unstable angina pectoris: diagnosis and treatment. In: Chizner MA, ed. Classic teachings in clinical cardiology: a tribute to W. Proctor Harvey, M.D. Cedar Grove, NJ: Laennec Publishing, 1996: 783–818.

14. Antman EM, Braunwald E. Acute myocardial infarction. In: Braunwald E, ed. Heart disease: a textbook of cardiovascular medicine, 5th ed. Philadelphia: WB Saunders, 1997:1184–1288.

15. Murray DR, O'Rourke RA, Walling AD, et al. History and physical examination in myocardial ischemia and acute myocardial infarction. In: Francis GS, Alpert JS, eds. Coronary care, 2nd ed. Boston: Little Brown and Co., 1995:73–95.

16. O'Rourke RA, Schlant RC, Douglas JS Jr. Diagnosis and management of patients with chronic ischemic heart disease. In: Fuster V, Alexander RW, O'Rourke RA, et al., eds. Hurst's the heart, 10th ed. New York: McGraw-Hill, 2001:1207–1236.

17. Vanden Belt RJ. The history. In: Chizner MA, ed. Classic teachings in clinical cardiology: a tribute to W. Proctor Harvey, M.D. Cedar Grove, NJ: Laennec Publishing, 1996:41–54.

18. Chizner MA. Bedside diagnosis of the acute myocardial infarction and its complications. Curr Probl Cardiol 1982;7:1–86.

19. Chizner MA. Acute myocardial infarction. In: Abrams J, ed. Essentials of cardiac physical diagnosis. Philadelphia: Lea & Febiger, 1987:437–452.

20. Marriott HJL. Ischemic heart disease. In: Marriott HJL, ed. Bedside cardiac diagnosis. Philadelphia: JB Lippincott, 1993:217–228.

21. Krumholz HM, Wei JY. Acute myocardial infarction: clinical presentation and diagnosis. In: Gersh BJ, Rahimtoola SH, eds. Acute myocardial infarction, 2nd ed. New York: Chapman and Hall, 1997:123–135.

22. Armstrong WF, Pellikka PA, Ryan T, et al. Stress echocardiography: recommendations for performance and interpretation of stress echocardiography. J Am Soc Echocardiogr 1998;11:97–104.

23. Hoffmann R, Lethen H, Kuhl H, et al. Extent and severity of test positivity during dobutamine stress echocardiography. Influence on the predictive value for coronary artery disease. Eur Heart J 1999;20: 1485–1492.

24. Tousoulis D, Loukianos R, Cokkinos P, et al. Relation between exercise and dobutamine stress-induced wall motion abnormalities and severity and location of stenosis in single-vessel coronary artery disease. Am Heart J 1999;138:873–879.

25. Peteiro J, Fabregas R, Montserrat L, et al. Comparison of treadmill exercise in the evaluation of patients with known or suspected coronary artery disease. J Am Soc Echocardiogr 1999;12:1073–1079.

26. Beleslin BD, Ostojic M, Djordjevic-Dikic A, et al. Integrated evaluation of relation between coronary lesion features and stress echocardiography results: the importance of coronary lesion morphology. J Am Coll Cardiol 1999;33:717–726.

27. Badruddin SM, Ahmad A, Mickelson J, et al. Supine bicycle versus post-treadmill exercise echocardiography in the detection of myocardial ischemia: a randomized single-blind crossover trial. J Am Coll Cardiol 1999; 33:1485–1490.

28. Parodi G, Picano E, Marcassa C, et al. High dose dipyridamole myocardial imaging: simultaneous sestamibi scintigraphy and two-dimensional echocardiography in the detection and evaluation of coronary artery disease. Italian Group of Nuclear Cardiology. Coron Artery Dis 1999;10:177–184.

29. Senior R, Soman P, Khattar RS, et al. Improved endocardial visualization with second harmonic imaging compared with fundamental two-dimensional echocardiographic imaging. Am Heart J 1999;138:163–168.

30. Lewis JF, Lin L, McGorray S, et al. Dobutamine stress echocardiography in women with chest pain. Pilot phase data from the National Heart, Lung and Blood Institute Women's Ischemia syndrome Evaluation (WISE). J Am Coll Cardiol 1999;33:1462–1468.
31. Kwok Y, Kim C, Grady D, et al. Meta-analysis of exercise testing to detect coronary artery disease in women. Am J Cardiol 1999;83:660–666.
32. Koch R, Lang RM, Garcia MJ, et al. Objective evaluation of regional left ventricular wall motion during dobutamine stress echocardiography studies using segmental analysis of color kinesis images. J Am Coll Cardiol 1999;34:409–419.
33. Vitarelli A, Sciomer S, Schina M, et al. Detection of left ventricular systolic and diastolic abnormalities in patients with coronary artery disease by color kinesis. Clin Cardiol 1997;20:927–933.
34. Sabia P, Afrookteh A, Touchstone DA, et al. Value of regional wall motion abnormality in the emergency room for the diagnosis of acute myocardial infarction. A prospective study using two-dimensional echocardiography. Circulation 1991;84[Suppl I]:I-85–I-92.
35. Saeian K, Rhyne TL, Sagar KB. Ultrasonic tissue characterization for diagnosis of acute myocardial infarction in the coronary care unit. Am J Cardiol 1994;74:1211–1215.
36. Mohler ER 3rd, Ryan T, Segar DS, et al. Clinical utility of troponin T levels and echocardiography in the emergency department. Am Heart J 1998;135:253–260.
37. Shen W, Khandheria BK, Edwards WD, et al. Value and limitations of two-dimensional echocardiography in predicting myocardial infarct size. Am J Cardiol 1991;68:1143–1149.
38. Fleischmann KE, Goldman L, Robiolio PA, et al. Echocardiographic correlates of survival in patients with chest pain. J Am Coll Cardiol 1994;23:1390–1396.
39. Sabia P, Abbott RD, Afrooketeh A, et al. Importance of two-dimensional echocardiographic assessment of left ventricular systolic function in patients presenting to the emergency room with cardiac-related symptoms. Circulation 1991;84:1615–1624.
40. Gibler WB, Runyon JP, Levy RC, et al. A rapid diagnostic and treatment center for patients with chest pain in the emergency department. Am J Emerg Med 1995;25:1–8.
41. Geleijnse M, Elhendy A, Kasprzak J, et al. Safety and prognostic value of early dobutamine-atropine stress echocardiography in patients with spontaneous chest pain and a non-diagnostic electrocardiogram. Eur Heart J 2000;21:397–406.
42. Colon PJ 3rd, Guarisco JS, Murgo J, et al. Utility of stress echocardiography in the triage of patients with atypical chest pain from the emergency department. Am J Cardiol 1998;82:1282–1284.
43. Mehta SR, Eikelboom JW, Natarajan MK, et al. Impact of right ventricular involvement on mortality and morbidity in patients with inferior myocardial infarction. J Am Coll Cardiol 2001;37:37–43.
44. Moller JE, Sondergaard E, Poulsen SH, et al. Pseudonormal and restrictive filling patterns predict left ventricular dilation and cardiac death after a first myocardial infarction: a serial color-M-mode Doppler echocardiographic study. J Am Coll Cardiol 2000;36:1841–1846.
45. Neskovic AN, Marinkovic J, Bojic M, et al. Predictors of left ventricular thrombus formation and disappearance after anterior wall myocardial infarction. Eur Heart J 1998;19:908–916.
46. Chiarella F, Santoro E, Domenicucci S, et al. Predischarge two-dimensional echocardiographic evaluation of left ventricular thrombosis after acute myocardial infarction in the GISSI-3 study. Am J Cardiol 1998;81:822–827.
47. Nagahama Y, Sugiura T, Takehana K, et al. The role of infarction-associated pericarditis on the occurrence of atrial fibrillation. Eur Heart J 1998;19:287–292.
48. Crenshaw BS, Granger LB, Brinbaum Y, et al. Risk factors, angiographic patterns and outcomes in patients with ventricular septal defects complicating acute myocardial infarction. GUSTO-I (Global Utilization of Streptokinase and TPA for Occluded Coronary Arteries) Trial Investigators. Circulation 2000;101:27–32.
49. Kono T, Sabbah HN, Rosman H, et al. Mechanism of functional mitral regurgitation during acute myocardial ischemia. J Am Coll Cardiol 1992;19:1101–1105.
50. Figueras J, Cortadellas J, Evangelista A, et al. Medical management of selected patients with left ventricular free wall rupture during acute myocardial infarction. J Am Coll Cardiol 1997;29:512–518.
51. Purcaro A, Costantini C, Ciampani N, et al. Diagnostic criteria and management of subacute ventricular free wall rupture complicating acute myocardial infarction. Am J Cardiol 1997;80:397–405.
52. Stein JH, Neumann A, Preston LM, et al. Improved risk stratification in unstable angina: identification of patients at low risk for in-hospital cardiac events by admission echocardiography. Clin Cardiol 1998;21:725–730.
53. Carluccio E, Tommasi S, Bentivoglio M, et al. Usefulness of the severity and extent of wall motion abnormalities as prognostic markers of an adverse outcome after a first myocardial infarction treated with thrombolytic therapy. Am J Cardiol 2000;85:411–415.
54. Lin SS, Lauer MS, Marwick TH. Risk stratification of patients with medically treated unstable angina using exercise echocardiography. Am J Cardiol 1998;82:720–724.
55. Desideri A, Bigi R, Suzzi GL, et al. Stress echocardiography and exercise electrocardiography for risk stratification after non-Q-wave uncomplicated myocardial infarction. Am J Cardiol 1999;84:739–741.
56. Neskovic AN, Bojic M, Popovic AD. Detection of significant residual stenosis of the infarct-related artery after thrombolysis by high-dose dipyridamole echocardiography test: is it detected often enough? Clin Cardiol 1997;20:569–572.
57. Smart SC, Knickelbine T, Stoiber TR, et al. Safety and accuracy of dobutamine-atropine stress echocardiography for the detection of residual stenosis of the infarct-related artery and multivessel disease during the first week after acute myocardial infarction. Circulation 1997;95:1394–1401.
58. Golia G, Anselmi M, Tinto M, et al. Long-term prognostic value of the stenosis of the infarct-related artery and the presence of viable myocardium in akinetic ventricular regions in infarcted patients. Cardiologia 1999;44:1029–1037.
59. Franklin KB, Marwick TH. Use of stress echocardiography for risk assessment of patients after myocardial infarction. Cardiol Clin 1999;17:521–538.
60. Previtali M, Fetiveau R, Lanzarini L, et al. Prognostic value of myocardial viability and ischemia detected by dobutamine stress echocardiography early after acute myocardial infarction treated with thrombolysis. J Am Coll Cardiol 1998;32:380–386.

61. Sicari R, Picano E, Landi P, et al. Prognostic value of dobutamine-atropine stress echocardiography early after acute myocardial infarction. EDIC study. J Am Coll Cardiol 1997;29:254–256.

62. Bolognese L, Buonamicic P, Cerisano G, et al. Early dobutamine echocardiography predicts improvement in regional and global left ventricular function after reperfused acute myocardial infarction without residual stenosis of the infarct-related artery. Am Heart J 2000; 139:153–163.

63. Loimaala A, Groundstroem K, Pasanen M, et al. Comparison of bicycle, heavy isometric, dipyridamole-atropine and dobutamine stress echocardiography for diagnosis of myocardial ischemia. Am J Cardiol 1999;84: 1396–1400.

64. Miyazono Y, Kisanuki A, Toyonaga K, et al. Usefulness of adenosine triphosphate-atropine stress echocardiography for detecting coronary artery stenosis. Am J Cardiol 1998;82:290–294.

65. San Roman JA, Vilacosta I, Castillo JA, et al. Selection of the optimal stress test for the diagnosis of coronary artery disease. Heart 1998;80:370–376.

66. Franke A, Hoffmann R, Kuhl HP, et al. Non-contrast second harmonic imaging improves interobserver agreement and accuracy of dobutamine stress echocardiography in patients with impaired image quality. Heart 2000;83:133–140.

67. Cwajg J, Xie F, O'Leary E, et al. Detection of angiographically significant coronary artery disease with accelerated intermittent imaging after intravenous administration of ultrasound contrast material. Am Heart J 2000;139:675–683.

68. Madu EC. Transesophageal dobutamine stress echocardiography in the evaluation of myocardial ischemia in morbidly obese subjects. Chest 2000;117:657–661.

69. Lee CY, Pellikka PA, McCully RB, et al. Nonexercise stress transthoracic echocardiography: transesophageal atrial pacing versus dobutamine stress. J Am Coll Cardiol 1999;33:506–511.

70. Tribouilloy C, Peltier M, Colas L, et al. Multiplane transoesophageal echocardiographic absence of thoracic aortic plaque is a powerful predictor for absence of significant coronary artery disease in valvular patients, even in the elderly. A large prospective study. Eur Heart J 1997;18:1478–1483.

71. Kotoh K, Watanabe G, Ueyama K, et al. On-line assessment of regional ventricular wall motion by transesophageal echocardiography with color kinesis during minimally invasive coronary artery bypass grafting. J Thorac Cardiovasc Surg 1999;117:912–917.

72. Krivokapich J, Child JS, Walter DO, et al. Prognostic value of dobutamine stress echocardiography in predicting cardiac events in patients with known or suspected coronary artery disease. J Am Coll Cardiol 1999; 33:708–716.

73. Poldermans D, Fioretti PM, Boersma E, et al. Long-term prognostic value of dobutamine-atropine stress echocardiography in 1737 patients with known or suspected coronary artery disease: a single-center experience. Circulation 1999;99:757–762.

74. Dhond MR, Donnell K, Singh S, et al. Value of negative dobutamine stress echocardiography in predicting long-term cardiac events. J Am Soc Echocardiogr 1999;12: 471–475.

75. Das M, Pellikka P, Mahoney D, et al. Assessment of cardiac risk before nonvascular surgery: dobutamine stress echocardiography in 530 patients. J Am Coll Cardiol 2000;35:1647–1653.

76. Day SM, Younger JG, Karavite D, et al. Usefulness of hypotension during dobutamine echocardiography in predicting perioperative cardiac events. Am J Cardiol 2000;85:478–483.

77. Pasquet A, Robert A, d'Hondt AM, et al. Prognostic value of myocardial ischemia and viability in patients with chronic left ventricular ischemic dysfunction. Circulation 1999;100:141–148.

78. Senior R, Kaul S, Lahiri A. Myocardial viability on echocardiography predicts long-term survival after revascularization in patients with ischemic congestive heart failure. J Am Coll Cardiol 1999;33:1848–1854.

79. Cwajg JM, Cwajg E, Nagueh SF, et al. End-diastolic wall thickness as a predictor of recovery of function in myocardial hibernation: relation to rest-redistribution T1-201 tomography and dobutamine stress echocardiography. J Am Coll Cardiol 2000;35: 1152–1161.

80. Cheitlin MD, Alpert JS, Armstrong WF, et al. ACC/AHA guidelines for the clinical application of echocardiography. A report of the American College of Cardiology/American Heart Association Task Force on Practice Guidelines (Committee on Clinical Application of Echocardiography). Developed in collaboration with the American Society of Echocardiography. Circulation 1997;95:1686–1744.

# 4

# The Patient with Congestive Heart Failure

Bruce K. Shively

*Cardiology Division, Oregon Health Sciences University; and Echocardiographic Laboratory, Oregon Health and Science University Hospital, Portland, Oregon*

## DEFINITIONS

The diagnostic term "congestive heart failure" is used most often to refer to cardiogenic pulmonary congestion (pulmonary edema due to elevated mean left atrial pressure). Congestive heart failure connotes left ventricular contractile dysfunction for most physicians because left ventricular dysfunction is by far the most common cause of left atrial hypertension. However, congestive heart failure is not synonymous with left ventricular dysfunction, because left atrial hypertension can occur with normal left ventricular function when mitral stenosis or regurgitation is present. Congestive heart failure also can refer to a clinical syndrome due to left ventricular dysfunction that does not include pulmonary congestion. This latter is best termed "heart failure," without the qualifier "congestive," because pulmonary edema is not present. For the purposes of this chapter, congestive heart failure refers to the related clinical syndromes caused by left ventricular systolic and diastolic dysfunction.

Left ventricular dysfunction underlying congestive heart failure results in left ventricular stroke work (and, consequently, cardiac output) being less than expected for the level of left ventricular filling pressure. The abnormal relation of filling pressure to cardiac output may take the form of either normal or low cardiac output with high filling pressure, or low cardiac output with normal filling pressure. Left ventricular diastolic pressure before atrial contraction normally is <12 mm

103

Hg. Pressure after atrial contraction (end-diastolic pressure) normally is <16 mm Hg. The lower limit of normal for cardiac output is 4.5 L/min and for cardiac index is 3.0 L/min/m². In mild congestive heart failure, both cardiac output and filling pressure may be normal at rest, but with exercise cardiac output may not rise normally or filling pressure may rise abnormally in order to augment cardiac output.

The functional abnormality of the left ventricle leading to low stroke work in relation to filling pressure may be due to reduced contractility, increased chamber stiffness, or a combination of both. Reduced contractility, referred to as systolic dysfunction, is accompanied by a reduced ejection fraction. Concomitant ventricular dilation also is usually present and helps restore stroke volume toward normal despite the reduced ejection fraction. Increased left ventricular stiffness, referred to as diastolic dysfunction, tends to cause elevated filling pressure. The elevated filling pressure acts to distend the noncompliant left ventricle and, through the Frank-Starling mechanism, restores stroke volume toward normal. In most patients, both systolic and diastolic dysfunction contribute to the syndrome of congestive heart failure. However, some subjects have a severe degree of one with a minimal degree of the other. The relative degree of systolic and diastolic dysfunction is related in part to the etiology of the patient's congestive heart failure and carries major implications regarding treatment and prognosis. Furthermore, the relative contribution of systolic and diastolic dysfunction combine to determine the patient's symptoms and physical examination findings. Thus, the concepts of systolic and diastolic dysfunction serve as essential coordinates for understanding the patient's disease. Based on the history, physical examination, and echocardiographic data, the individual patient can be placed on the "map" defined by these coordinates (Fig. 4.1).

Diastolic dysfunction refers to increased stiffness of the ventricle, which may be pre-

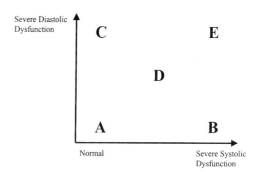

**FIG. 4.1.** Patient "mapping" by type of left ventricular (LV) dysfunction. Patient A: Normal. Patient B: Ejection fraction (EF) 10% with a severely dilated LV, left ventricular end-diastolic pressure (LVEDP) normal (15 mm Hg), and mean left atrial (LA) pressure (pulmonary capillary wedge pressure) normal (10 mm Hg). Patient C: EF 60%, normal size LV, LVEDP severely elevated (40 mm Hg), and mean LA pressure severely elevated (30 mm Hg). Patient D: EF moderately reduced (40%) with moderate LV dilation and a mildly elevated LVEDP (25 mm Hg) with mean LA pressure 20 mm Hg. Patient E: EF 20% with a severely dilated LV, LVEDP 35 mm Hg, and mean LA pressure 30 mm Hg.

sent in the absence of elevated filling pressure, as when the patient is intravascular volume depleted. However, due to the presence of diastolic dysfunction, adequate cardiac output cannot be achieved without the filling pressure rising above normal. Thus, nearly all patients with left ventricular systolic dysfunction have at least some component of diastolic dysfunction (1). The utility of the concept stems from the great variability among patients with the same degree of systolic dysfunction, who have variable levels of filling pressure necessary to achieve an adequate cardiac output. This concept of diastolic dysfunction is much broader than the more common use of the term that refers predominantly to left ventricular dysfunction characterized by elevated filling pressure with normal left ventricular systolic function.

The syndrome of right ventricular failure exists when right ventricular stroke work (and the resultant cardiac output) is reduced in relation to right ventricular filling pressure. Right ventricular failure usually develops in response to increased pulmonary artery pressure, caused by either left atrial hypertension or pulmonary disease. The signs and symptoms of right ventricular failure are considered part of the syndrome of congestive heart failure and most commonly occur in the presence of left ventricular dysfunction.

## ETIOLOGY

A wide range of diseases may cause left ventricular dysfunction and the congestive heart failure syndrome (2). The most common causes in industrialized countries are coronary artery disease, viral myocarditis (idiopathic dilated cardiomyopathy), and chronic hypertension. Certain uncommon causes also are important because they are potentially reversible. They must be recognized so that recurrent exposure of the patient to the cause can be avoided. These causes include alcoholism, persistent tachycardia (usually supraventricular), and peripartum cardiomyopathy. Also among the causes of potentially reversible left ventricular dysfunction are aortic stenosis and regurgitation, and mitral regurgitation. These lesions, if severe and not surgically corrected, eventually lead to progressive left ventricular dysfunction. In the case of aortic stenosis, the afterload reduction afforded by valve replacement leads to improvement of ejection fraction in most patients. In the case of mitral and aortic regurgitation, valve repair or replacement may not benefit the patient if severe left ventricular systolic dysfunction is established. However, if the regurgitant lesion is corrected while left ventricular systolic function is not more than mildly reduced, further deterioration can be prevented.

Most of the known causes can lead to any combination of systolic and diastolic left ventricular dysfunction. A few uncommon diseases characteristically cause predominantly diastolic dysfunction (amyloidosis, hemochromatosis, idiopathic hypertrophic cardiomyopathy). Because many causes, such as coronary artery disease, can lead to clinical syndromes in which either systolic or diastolic dysfunction predominates, there must be additional modulating factors tending to lead to one or the other. At present, these factors are not well understood.

## HISTORY

The important symptoms of the congestive heart failure syndrome are listed in Table 4.1. Neurohumoral compensatory mechanisms, activated in response to left ventricular dysfunction, tend to support cardiac output at the cost of a higher filling pressure. The high filling pressure leads to interstitial pulmonary edema and increased lung stiffness.

*Dyspnea* is the most common symptom of congestive heart failure. In mild congestive

**TABLE 4.1.** *Patient history in congestive heart failure*

| Symptom | Description |
|---|---|
| Dyspnea | Discomfort caused by an unaccustomed effort of breathing. Dyspnea should be graded when recording the history (see Table 4.2). |
| Orthopnea | Dyspnea that develops or worsens with lying down. It is characteristically relieved by elevating the upper body (as on pillows), or sitting/standing up. |
| Proxysmal nocturnal dyspnea | Dyspnea that appears within several hours after going to bed (often awakening the patient) |
| Nocturia | Awakening during the night to urinate more than once |
| Easy fatigability | Feeling of muscular or overall weakness with exertion |
| Anorexia | Loss of appetite |
| Chest discomfort | Pain, tightness, pressure, or fullness felt in the chest |
| Syncope | Transient, self-limited loss of consciousness (lasting seconds to minutes). Presyncope is a sensation of impending loss of consciousness. |
| Palpitations | Sensation of prominent (pounding), irregular, or rapid heartbeat |

heart failure, dyspnea may occur with moderate exertion only. In severe congestive heart failure, dyspnea may be marked, even at rest. The severity of the patient's functional limitation due to dyspnea is graded according to a standardized scheme (Table 4.2) (3). In taking a history, it is helpful to determine the patient's usual level of activity and recent changes in exercise tolerance. Dyspnea is not specific for heart disease; commonly it is caused by pulmonary and other disorders (e.g., anemia, uremia, deconditioning). Dyspnea in congestive heart failure also may be caused by cardiac output that is inadequate to meet the demands of activity.

*Orthopnea and paroxysmal nocturnal dyspnea* indicate moderate or severe congestive heart failure. These symptoms are caused by a shift of blood volume into the central circulation from the lower body after lying down. In the presence of left ventricular dysfunction, the increased volume raises left atrial mean pressure, leading to interstitial pulmonary edema.

*Nocturia* stems from increased urine formation at night, following a reduction of the abnormal renal arteriolar vasoconstriction required during the day to direct the limited cardiac output to working skeletal muscle. Nocturia in elderly persons is not specific for

congestive heart failure due to abnormal bladder function.

*Easy fatigability, and anorexia and weight loss* are symptoms caused by reduced perfusion to the musculature and gut, respectively. When cardiac output is reduced, adaptive neurohumoral influences act to preserve blood flow to the brain and heart, at the expense of the muscles, gastrointestinal tract, and kidneys. These symptoms appear when the other adaptive mechanisms to maintain cardiac output (elevated filling pressure, left ventricular remodeling) are not adequate; thus, they are characteristic of advanced heart failure.

*Chest pain, syncope, and palpitations* are common in patients with left ventricular disease, but are not directly related to the abnormal hemodynamics of congestive heart failure. Their occurrence should prompt a search for an additional diagnosis, such as coronary artery disease or arrhythmia. Many patients with congestive heart failure die suddenly due to ventricular arrhythmia, which can present as syncope; therefore, syncope in the context of known left ventricular dysfunction usually is treated as aborted sudden death until proven otherwise. Similarly, episodic palpitations usually warrant investigation to identify the underlying arrhythmia.

*Dizziness, nausea, and headache* are unlikely to be related to congestive heart failure.

TABLE 4.2. *Functional classification of the patient with congestive heart failure*

| Class | Description | Activity scale |
|---|---|---|
| I | Ordinary physical activity does not cause dyspnea or excessive fatigue. | Can do activities requiring no more than 7 METS, such as climbing a flight of stairs or jog/walk at 5 mph. |
| II | Slight limitations of physical activity by dyspnea or fatigue. Comfortable at rest. | Can do activities requiring no more than 5 METS, such as gardening, dancing (fox trot), walking at 4 mph, and sexual intercourse. |
| III | Marked limitation of physical activity. Comfortable at rest. | Can do activities requiring no more than 2 METS, such as showering, walking slowly (2.5 mph), and shopping. |
| IV | Symptomatic at rest, with an increase of discomfort during even minimal activity. | Cannot do activities such as those listed above. |

Adapted from Goldman L, Hashimoto B, Cook EF, et al. Comparative reproducibility and validity of systems for assessing cardiovascular class; advantages of a new specific activity scale. Circulation 1981;64:1227.

Their relevance stems from their potential as adverse effects from the medications used to treat heart failure.

## PHYSICAL EXAMINATION

As noted, many of the symptoms of congestive heart failure, such as dyspnea, are not specific for heart disease. The physical examination is essential to establish the presence of the congestive heart failure syndrome. As a first step, the examiner should attempt to differentiate between three conditions: presence of left ventricular failure in the absence of right ventricular failure, presence of both together, or presence of right ventricular failure alone (Table 4.3). Second, the severity of many ex-

amination components can be graded, and their grading usually is related to the magnitude of the underlying left and/or right ventricular dysfunction. Finally, serial examinations are extremely useful to evaluate the patient's response to treatment.

As previously noted, left ventricular disease underlying the congestive heart failure syndrome can be categorized according to the severity of systolic and diastolic dysfunction. The relative roles of these two forms of left ventricular dysfunction carry major therapeutic and prognostic implications. The physical examination often enables the clinician to characterize the predominant type of left ventricular dysfunction. Thus, the patient with severe systolic

**TABLE 4.3.** *Physical examination in congestive heart failure*

| Sign | Description | Specificity |
|---|---|---|
| Tachypnea | Respiratory rate >20 breaths/min | Nonspecific |
| Rales | Crackling or bubbling sounds heard from the lungs, especially with inspiration | LV |
| Wheezing | High-pitched, whistling sounds heard from the lungs, especially with expiration. They often are accompanied by a prolonged expiratory phase. | LV |
| Diaphoresis | Presence of perspiration | Nonspecific |
| Hypertension | Systolic blood pressure >130 mm Hg or mean arterial pressure >100 mm Hg | Nonspecific Nonspecific |
| Hypotension | Systolic blood pressure <100 mm Hg or mean arterial pressure <70 mm Hg | Nonspecific |
| Tachycardia | Heart rate >100 beats/min | Nonspecific |
| Bradycardia | Heart rate <55 beats/min | Nonspecific |
| Jugular venous distention | Estimated central venous pressure of 8 mm Hg. Estimation of venous pressure can be challenging. | RV |
| Abnormal apical impulse | Abnormal apical impulse (or point of maximal impulse [PMI]) | LV |
| $S_3$ | Third heart sound is heard at a 40- to 80-ms interval following $S_2$. It is predominately composed of low frequencies. | LV if over LV apex, RV at left sternal border, and varies with respiration |
| $S_4$ | Fourth heart sound is heard at a 40- to 80-ms interval preceding $S_1$. | LV |
| Systolic murmurs | Rushing or blowing sound heard between $S_1$ and $S_2$. They are due to high-velocity, turbulent blood flow within the heart. | Nonspecific |
| Pedal edema | Swelling of the distal lower extremities due to accumulation of interstitial fluid | RV |
| Peripheral coolness, cyanosis | Peripheral coolness is present when the extremities (usually lower) are cool to touch with the patient in a warm room. Peripheral cyanosis is a bluish discoloration of the distal extremities (usually lower) due to reduced perfusion. | Nonspecific |

LV, left ventricular dysfunction; RV, right ventricular dysfunction.

dysfunction but (relatively) normal left ventricular filling pressure is likely to present with signs referable to low cardiac output and a dilated, hypokinetic left ventricle. When systolic dysfunction is combined with diastolic dysfunction, the latter will be manifested by elevated mean left atrial pressure. Signs of pulmonary edema and a third heart sound ($S_3$) are likely to be present. When the elevated mean left atrial pressure has persisted for an extended time, evidence of elevated right atrial mean pressure is likely to be found, due to pulmonary hypertension and right ventricular dysfunction. When left ventricular diastolic dysfunction is predominant and systolic function is relatively preserved, evidence of pulmonary edema and right heart failure will be present in the absence of evidence of left ventricular dilation.

### General Appearance

The patient's general appearance, beyond the presence of specific visible signs usually is normal in early congestive heart failure. Once resting cardiac output is reduced, as in the late stages of the disease, the patient begins to look chronically ill. Weight loss due to malabsorption from gut edema may become apparent. In extreme cases, wasting of the face is noticeable. Thinning of the arms and legs from inactivity may be seen.

Diaphoresis is an important sign of a "decompensated hemodynamic state" in the patient with congestive heart failure. This implies an acute or subacute elevation of left ventricular filling pressure, lowering of cardiac output, or (usually) both. It is due to sympathetic nervous system activation, one of the "last ditch" compensatory mechanisms to maintain an adequate circulation in patients with a severe congestive heart failure syndrome. It usually indicates impending or actual cardiogenic shock and carries this implication even in the absence of corroborating signs such as tachycardia and peripheral coolness or cyanosis.

### Heart Rate and Blood Pressure

Tachycardia is another sign of sympathetic nervous system activation and carries a significance similar to that of diaphoresis. Tachycardia occurs in response to the stimulation of beta-adrenergic receptors in the heart. In chronic congestive heart failure, these receptors may be down-regulated. Thus, tachycardia may be absent or minimal despite acutely decompensated congestive heart failure. Acute congestive heart failure is one setting in which beta blockade, intended to reduce the heart rate, may be deleterious, because the tachycardia is supporting cardiac output in the presence of low stroke volume. If a patient presents with congestive heart failure and a primary rapid supraventricular tachycardia or atrial fibrillation (not a sinus tachycardia due to decompensated congestive heart failure), immediate cardioversion usually is indicated. If the supraventricular tachycardia, especially atrial fibrillation, has been of long standing, striking improvement in left ventricular function may follow restoration of a normal rhythm.

Bradycardia may be seen with congestive heart failure secondary to excessive beta blockade or as an agonal rhythm at the end stage of shock. Bradycardia as a primary arrhythmia (due to conduction block or sick sinus syndrome) may worsen the symptoms and signs of congestive heart failure; immediate and potentially long-term pacing often are helpful.

Hypertension is another sign of sympathetic nervous system activation and may be present despite low cardiac output. Hypertension contributes to the worsening spiral of acute congestive heart failure by increasing left ventricular afterload. A high afterload acts only to lower cardiac output even more, potentially driving the patient further into heart failure or cardiogenic shock (defined as cardiac index <2.0 L/min/m$^2$ due to left or right ventricular dysfunction). In patients with hypertension and left ventricular dysfunction, afterload reduction with vasodilating drugs may provide immediate and sustained benefit. Hypotension, if not due to volume depletion or excessive afterload reducing medication, is a sign of severe circulatory compromise. It is common in class III and IV failure. Hypotension may indicate an advanced stage of cardiogenic shock in which a low cardiac index is combined with the failure of physiologic mechanisms to maintain systemic blood pressure.

## Respiration

Tachypnea is the externally visible counterpart to dyspnea. When the development of congestive heart failure is insidious, the patient may be tachypneic without complaining of dyspnea. Tachypnea on conversation is the observation that the patient is unable to speak without frequent pauses to breathe. It is a sign of severe respiratory compromise and may be noted even when the patient does not otherwise appear to be short of breath. As with dyspnea, tachypnea is not specific for heart disease.

## Jugular Venous Pulse

Estimation of right atrial mean pressure is possible based on examination of the jugular venous pulse (see Chapter 1). If the jugular venous impulse is not apparent when the patient is sitting, the patient can be reclined to 45 degrees (4). If the impulse appears to be elevated, the patient should be assessed in the sitting position to avoid underestimating the height of the impulse. When the position of the impulse is located in the neck, the height (in cm) of this point from the sternal angle is determined and 5 to 10 cm is added to give an estimate of right atrial pressure in cm $H_2O$. The right atrial pressure in mm Hg is approximately 0.7 times the estimate in cm $H_2O$.

Jugular venous distention is a very important sign because it indicates the presence of an elevated mean right atrial pressure (i.e., right ventricular filling pressure) >8 mm Hg. When present to a mild degree (central venous pressure 8 to 12 mm Hg), it may occur with volume expansion due to left ventricular dysfunction, even without overt pulmonary hypertension and secondary right ventricular failure. On the other hand, mild jugular venous distention may indicate right ventricular dysfunction, and an estimated central venous pressure >12 mm Hg usually indicates secondary right ventricular dysfunction (in the absence of cor pulmonale or tricuspid valve disease).

## Pulmonary Auscultation

Rales indicate the presence of alveolar edema, the next stage in the development of pulmonary edema after interstitial edema. True rales, unlike crackles due to atelectasis, persist after a few deep coughs. Rales can be caused by noncardiogenic pulmonary edema (edema due to lung injury rather than elevated pulmonary capillary pressure). With this exception, their presence is a reliable indicator of the presence of elevated mean left atrial pressure. Basilar rales are rales limited to the basal portion of the posterior lung fields and indicate mild pulmonary edema. Rales tend to ascend to the upper lung fields with worsening pulmonary edema. They are often graded according to their upward extent (i.e., "rales one third of the way up"). Rales are more specific than sensitive for the detection of elevated left ventricular filling pressure. Rales may be absent (or minimal, or patchy) despite significant left atrial hypertension under two important circumstances: first, when pulmonary parenchymal or obstructive airway disease coexists; and second, when elevated mean left atrial and pulmonary capillary pressure of long standing has enhanced the rate of lymphatic clearance of pulmonary edema. In the latter situation, marked elevation of left atrial hypertension may be present despite the absence of pulmonary edema.

Wheezing may develop in some patients with pulmonary edema instead of or in addition to rales. Wheezes are caused by the obstruction of small airways by surrounding edema. Their presence in congestive heart failure sometimes is referred to by the oxymoron "cardiac asthma."

## Palpation

An abnormal point of maximal impulse (PMI) is caused by an abnormal left ventricle (see Chapter 1). The PMI is displaced when it is located at or lateral to the anterior axillary line. An enlarged PMI is >2 to 3 cm in diameter. A sustained PMI is a systolic motion of the PMI of longer duration than the simultaneously palpated carotid pulse. A displaced or enlarged PMI is a sign of left ventricular dilation, although enlargement without displacement can be found with concentric left ventricular hypertrophy. A sustained PMI usually indicates advanced left ventricular systolic dysfunction. In some individuals, a palpable $S_3$ or fourth heart sound ($S_4$) may be detected in the left lateral decubitus position (Fig. 1.12).

## Cardiac Auscultation

The $S_3$ often is a useful indicator of a decompensated hemodynamic state in the patient with congestive heart failure. A high mean left atrial pressure causes early diastolic transmitral left ventricular filling of high volume and velocity (see Table 4.7). The $S_3$ is produced when the in-rushing blood is abruptly decelerated in the left ventricle. Deceleration is more abrupt and the $S_3$ louder when the left ventricle is distended (on the steep portion of its pressure-volume curve). Disappearance of the $S_3$ during therapy is good evidence of falling mean left atrial pressure and reduced LV distention. Two important caveats limit the clinical utility of the $S_3$. Absence of an $S_3$ is not definitive evidence against the presence of elevated left ventricular filling pressure or congestive heart failure. The $S_3$ may fail to disappear despite effective therapy, because of persistent, although reduced, left atrial hypertension. Less often, persistence of the $S_3$ is due to markedly abnormal left ventricular diastolic properties (usually an aneurysm).

The $S_4$ is heard when the late diastolic filling wave (due to atrial contraction) is of high volume and velocity. It is likely to be heard when increased left ventricular stiffness is combined with normal or enhanced left atrial contractile function. An $S_4$ may be heard in patients with congestive heart failure when diastolic dysfunction is prominent in the disease, but is unlikely to be heard in patients with chronic LV systolic dysfunction.

Three systolic murmurs are important in patients with congestive heart failure: those of aortic stenosis, mitral regurgitation, and tricuspid regurgitation. Aortic stenosis should be ruled out by echocardiography in any patient with a suspicious systolic murmur, because aortic valve replacement may be life-saving. Echocardiography also is necessary to distinguish between mitral regurgitation as the cause of congestive heart failure versus mitral regurgitation as a complication of left ventricular dilation and dysfunction. This distinction carries major therapeutic and prognostic implications. A mitral regurgitation murmur during exacerbation of congestive heart failure usually means the mitral regurgitation is a significant contributor to the patient's symptoms. A tricuspid insufficiency murmur almost always signifies the presence of more than mild pulmonary hypertension complicating the patient's congestive heart failure. Infrequently, tricuspid insufficiency may be severe enough to contribute to the patient's peripheral edema, limit the cardiac output, and cause other complications of high central venous pressure.

Murmurs are graded by physical examination on a scale from 1 to 6. A grade 1 murmur is difficult for an experienced physician to hear, requiring 5 or more seconds of concentrated listening. A grade 2 murmur is soft but immediately recognizable. A grade 3 murmur is more prominent, and a grade 4 murmur is loud, with a palpable thrill. A grade 5 murmur is very loud, and a grade 6 murmur can be heard with the stethoscope just removed from the chest wall (4).

## Other Peripheral Manifestations

Peripheral edema is an important sign of volume expansion due to the neurohumoral mechanisms that maintain adequate cardiac output in patients with congestive heart failure. In ambulatory patients, edema will be manifest first around the ankles and ascends the legs as it becomes worse. In bedridden patients, edema is best assessed in the sacral region. Trace edema (1+) is defined as edema that is barely discernible after indentation of the skin by the examiner's fingers for approximately 10 seconds. Mild edema (2+) is readily apparent indentation (0.5 to 1.0 cm) after brief pressure by the examiner. Moderate edema (3+) allows indentation of at least 1.0 cm by the examiner and extends to the knees. Severe edema (4+) extends above the knees and will also be apparent elsewhere as anasarca. As with jugular venous distention, 1+ or 2+ edema may be present with only minimal elevation of right atrial mean pressure. Edema has other major determinants in addition to those related to heart failure. Most importantly, edema due to low plasma oncotic pressure may occur in the absence of elevated central venous pressure (5).

Peripheral coolness and cyanosis are signs of hypoperfusion. Like the symptoms of easy fatigability and anorexia, these signs suggest vasoconstriction of nonessential vascular beds to maintain an adequate blood supply to the vital organs in the face of low cardiac output.

## ECHOCARDIOGRAPHY

Echocardiography provides structural and functional information about the heart essential for the diagnosis and treatment of congestive heart failure. Echocardiographic data permit classification of the patient according to the schema shown in Fig. 4.1. This classification of the patient in turn carries important implications for optimal immediate and long-term therapy as well as prognosis.

## ECHOCARDIOGRAPHIC IMAGING

Structural features of the heart pertinent to the CHF are listed in Table 4.4.

### Left Ventricular Size and Function

Left ventricular end-diastolic size is assessed as either the short-axis linear dimension (M-mode or two-dimensional [2-D]) or volume (best determined by planimetry in two or more 2-D image planes). Left ventricular dilation (an increase in end-diastolic volume) is a compensatory mechanism to maintain normal stroke volume in the face of reduced contractile function (reduced contractility causes increased end-systolic volume, which will decrease stroke volume unless matched by an increase in end-diastolic volume). Thus, left ventricular dilation is an indirect indicator of left ventricular systolic dysfunction. Other factors, such as pre-existing concentric hypertrophy or fibrosis, may limit the degree of dilation.

### Left Ventricular Systolic Function

A more direct indicator of left ventricular systolic function is the ejection fraction. Because the volume measurements required to calculate the ejection fraction are time consuming and subject to error, it can be estimated visually (6). Semiquantitative estimation of left ventricular ejection fraction has good accuracy and is sufficient for most clinical purposes.

Visual estimation or measurement of "E point-septal separation" is helpful when estimating left ventricular ejection fraction. E point-septal separation is the distance between the septal endocardium and tip of the anterior mitral valve at the peak of early (E) filling. E point-septal separation is influenced by ventricular size and stroke volume; combined, these factors determine the ejection fraction. The absence of E point-septal separation of >0.7 cm rules out a reduced ejection fraction. In the range from 0.7 to 1.0 cm, the ejection fraction may be mildly reduced. When E point-septal separation is >1.0 cm and aortic insufficiency and mitral stenosis are ruled out, the ejection fraction is reduced. Furthermore, the degree of separation correlates with the severity of the ejection fraction reduction (7).

**TABLE 4.4.** *Echocardiographic features in CHF*

| Feature | Echocardiographic method | Comment |
|---|---|---|
| LV size (end-diastolic) | M-mode short-axis dimension | The most useful screening method for identifying LV dilation. Upper limit of normal = 5.5 cm. Subject to error due to variation in cardiac position and shape (e.g., apical aneurysm). |
| | 2-D Simpson rule: calculation of volumes from planimetry in the four- and two-chamber views | The most accurate method when ventricular geometry is abnormal (myocardial infarction). Upper limit of normal = 65 mL/M$^2$. Accurate results require validation and experience. |
| LV systolic function | M-mode fractional shortening: diastolic dimension − systolic dimension/diastolic dimension | Useful for screening. Lower limit of normal = 25%. May overestimate ejection fraction with apical infarction or underestimate with posterior infarction. |
| | 2-D Ejection fraction 2-D Simpson rule: diastolic volume − systolic volume/diastolic volume | Lower limit of normal = 55%. Errors due to underestimation of volumes, especially in end-systole. |
| | 2-D visual estimation | Sufficient for most clinical purposes. Especially accurate in the short-axis view; an experienced observer's 95% confidence interval approximates 15% (absolute EF%). |
| LV wall thickness (end-diastolic) | M-mode septal and posterior wall thickness | Identifies concentric hypertrophy. Upper limit of normal for septum = 1.1 cm, for posterior wall = 1.0 cm. Does not correlate well with LV mass, because does not consider LV size. |
| LV mass | Calculated from myocardial volume/total LV volume − LV cavity volume by an area–length geometric formula | Upper limit of normal = 130 g/M$^2$. May be greatly increased in patients with systolic dysfunction despite normal or decreased wall thickness. |
| LA size (end-systolic) | M-mode LA anteroposterior dimension | Upper limit of normal = 4.2 cm. In the absence of mitral valve disease and atrial fibrillation, dilation usually reflects elevated LV filling pressure. |
| | 2-D Simpson rule: planimetry in the four- and two-chamber views | Upper limit of normal = 28 mL/M$^2$. |
| RV size (end-diastolic) | M-mode anteroposterior dimension | With sustained elevations of LA pressure, RV dilations and failure are common, leading to "pancardiomegaly." Upper limit of normal = 3.5 cm. |

2-D, two-dimensional; LA, left atrium; LV, left ventricle; RV, right ventricle.

Another indicator of systolic function used commonly is fractional shortening of the left ventricular short axis (usually measured by M-mode). These indicators provide only an estimate of systolic function and can be misleading when preload or afterload is very abnormal. For example, in moderate or severe mitral regurgita- tion, left ventricular preload is high while after- load is low. The resultant ejection fraction may overestimate left ventricular systolic function. Under most clinical conditions, however, the left ventricular ejection fraction provides a good idea of the contribution of systolic dysfunction to the congestive heart failure syndrome.

## Left Ventricular Wall Thickness

A left ventricular wall thickness greater than normal occurs with either concentric hypertrophy (where the ratio of cavity size to wall thickness is low) or "eccentric" hypertrophy (where this ratio is normal). In concentric hypertrophy, increased wall thickness is associated with reduced left ventricular compliance and is a substrate for diastolic dysfunction. Thus, a patient with a left ventricle with normal size and ejection fraction, but thick walls, may have the congestive heart failure syndrome due to elevated left ventricular filling pressure (diastolic failure). When systolic dysfunction predominates and the left ventricle is dilated and hypokinetic, wall thickness also may be increased. This is probably an adaptive response of the myocardium to contractile failure and will tend to reduce wall stress (by Laplace's law).

## Left Ventricular Wall Motion

Certain echocardiographic features of the left ventricle can help identify the cause of the congestive heart failure. In particular, segmental left ventricular wall hypokinesis or akinesis, especially when accompanied by thinning and scar formation, is virtually diagnostic of coronary artery disease. Unfortunately, coronary disease can cause nonfocal left ventricular dysfunction; pathologic findings include nontransmural, patchy infarction and fibrosis. Thus, whereas it usually is possible to make the diagnosis of coronary disease on the echocardiogram, it is not possible to rule out this etiology. Consequently, most patients with left ventricular systolic dysfunction should undergo coronary angiography. Diffuse left ventricular hypokinesis is consistent with a wide range of diagnoses in addition to coronary artery disease, including all those mentioned in the Etiology section.

Left ventricular size, ejection fraction, wall thickness, and motion are features that provide important data for classification of the type of left ventricular dysfunction (Fig.

4.1). Patients with predominantly systolic dysfunction will have large left ventricular volumes in addition to a severely reduced ejection fraction. Wall thickness is likely to be normal or reduced. In a population of patients with severely reduced ejection fractions, those with the largest end-diastolic and end-systolic volumes had the worst prognosis (8). In a patient with a severely reduced ejection fraction but significant diastolic dysfunction, left ventricular volumes often are not greatly increased, and wall thickness may be normal. In patients with predominant diastolic dysfunction, the left ventricle may be only mildly dilated, if at all; ejection fraction may be only mildly reduced or normal; and wall thickness is usually increased. All other things being equal, a more severely reduced ejection fraction is a poor prognostic sign; the presence of high filling pressures also confers a poor prognosis. There appear to be subsets of patients with both predominant systolic or diastolic dysfunction with high short-term mortality.

## Left Ventricular Diastolic Function

The degree of diastolic dysfunction is indicated by the level of left ventricular filling pressure required to maintain stroke volume or cardiac output. Indirect indicators of elevated left ventricular filling pressure include left atrial dilation, evidence of pulmonary hypertension (e.g., right ventricular dilation and dysfunction), and right atrial and inferior vena cava dilation. Left atrial dilation can be measured as the left atrial anteroposterior dimension (by M-mode or 2-D) or estimated visually. Left atrial dilation is not a useful sign of elevated filling pressure in the presence of other processes associated with atrial dilation, such as rheumatic mitral stenosis, mitral regurgitation, or atrial fibrillation (even in the past). However, in the absence of these conditions, left atrial dimension correlates with pulmonary capillary and left ventricular end-diastolic pressure. Left atrial dimension >4.5 cm, with or without reduced left ventricular ejection fraction, is strong evidence of left ventricular diastolic dysfunction (9). Conversely, as previously noted, severely reduced left ventricular ejection fraction and a severely dilated left ventricle may be accompanied by a normal sized left atrium. In this case, left ventricular dysfunction is of the relatively pure systolic type, and pulmonary edema is a less prominent component of the congestive heart failure syndrome. In the previously noted study of patients with congestive heart failure, left atrial dilation was associated with a poor prognosis (8).

Elevation of mean left atrial pressure causes elevation of pulmonary artery diastolic and systolic pressure, thus increasing afterload for the right ventricle. Right ventricular adaptation to sustained pulmonary hypertension is limited, and right ventricular dilation and systolic dysfunction develop over a variable time course. Usually right atrial dilation is apparent as well, reflecting elevation of right ventricular diastolic pressure due to the development of right ventricular diastolic dysfunction. Thus, moderate or greater left atrial dilation, reflecting substantial elevation in mean left atrial pressure, frequently is accompanied by "pancardiomegaly" in patients with congestive heart failure. Patients with this echocardiographic picture commonly have a congestive heart failure syndrome that includes signs and symptoms of both right and left heart failure (Tables 4.1 and 4.2). This syndrome has led to the adage that the most common cause of right heart failure is left heart failure.

## Right Heart Chamber Size, Function, and Pressures

Right atrial size and right ventricular systolic function are not quantitated accurately by routine echocardiography. However, there are several useful rules of thumb. The right ventricular maximal anteroposterior dimension from the parasternal window (by either M-mode or 2-D) should not exceed 3.5 cm. The systolic excursion of the tricuspid annulus (toward the cardiac apex in the four-chamber view) should be at least 2 cm; values below 0.5 cm indicate severe right ventricular systolic dysfunction. Finally, in the four-chamber view, right atrial size, as indicated by the area of the right atrium in the 2-D image, should not exceed the left atrial area. Right atrial dilation also is present if the maximal right atrial lateral dimension (parallel to the tricuspid annulus) exceeds 4 cm.

Echocardiographic evaluation of inferior vena cava size and response to supine respiration provides a rough estimate of mean right atrial pressure (Table 4.5). The negative intrathoracic pressure generated by inspiration is normally in the range from 5 to 10 mm Hg. Because a normal right atrial pressure is within this range, inspiration normally causes the in-

**TABLE 4.5.** *Doppler echocardiographic estimation of right atrial pressure*

| Author | n | Index | Utility |
|---|---|---|---|
| Nagueh et al. (10) | 85 | Percentage collapse with sniff | <50% collapse was sensitive 72% and 76% specific for RAp <8 mm Hg (inclusion of ventilator patients likely decreased the specificity by RAp <15 mm Hg) |
| | | SFF | SFF <20% was accompanied by RAp >15 mm Hg in all cases |
| | | Mean RAp = 21.6 – 24 × SFF | Developed in an initial population (n = 35) and validated in a test population (n = 50) |
| Kircher et al. (11) | 83 | Percentage collapse with quiet inspiration | <50% was 85% sensitive and specific for RAp <10 mm Hg (excludes patients who required ventilators) |
| Cecconi et al. (12) | 114 | Percentage collapse with quiet inspiration | <45% was 80% sensitive and 90% specific for RAp >8 mm Hg (excludes patients who required ventilators) |

RAp, right atrial pressure; SFF, systolic velocity fraction (systolic forward velocity divided by sum of systolic and diastolic forward velocities).

ferior vena cava to collapse. The degree of collapse is related to mean right atrial pressure, with an inspiratory decrease in inferior vena cava dimension of >50% reliably indicating a normal right atrial pressure. If the inferior vena cava does not collapse with quiet respiration, a gentle sniff should be sufficient to cause collapse. Failure of the inferior vena cava to collapse with a sniff indicates a right atrial pressure >20 mm Hg. It should be noted that a markedly negative intrathoracic pressure with inspiration may cause inferior vena cava collapse despite an elevated right atrial pressure. These conditions include obstructive airway disease, pleural effusions, and respiratory distress of other causes. Patients on positive-pressure ventilation may not have inferior vena cava collapse despite normal right atrial pressure. Right atrial pressure also can be estimated from hepatic venous flow (page 124).

## DOPPLER FLOW DATA

Certain patterns of intracardiac flow velocities by Doppler are strongly associated with the level of filling pressure of both ventricles and pulmonary artery pressure. In addition, Doppler evaluation is important to assess the potential role of valve disease in causing or contributing to the congestive heart failure syndrome. Estimations of mean left atrial pressure and left ventricular end-diastolic pressure are important to assess the degree of diastolic dysfunction. Within certain limitations, Doppler flow patterns can identify when left ventricular filling pressures are elevated, and the approximate degree of elevation. This information can help establish the role of diastolic dysfunction in the patient's syndrome and help guide patient management.

Blood flow within the heart and great vessels is driven by pressure gradients. Transient pressure gradients at specific time points during systole and diastole are affected in characteristic ways by the levels of absolute pressure and compliances of the chambers or blood vessels. In some cases, the pressure difference (gradient) alone is important. The tricuspid regurgitation velocity, measurable in the majority of patients by Doppler, can be used to estimate the gradient between right atrial and right ventricular systolic pressure (Table 4.6). Because right ventricular and pulmonary artery systolic pressures are equal in the absence of pulmonary stenosis, an elevated tricuspid insufficiency velocity is evidence of a high pulmonary artery systolic pressure. When the right atrial pressure can be estimated clinically or from echocardiographic data, it can be added to the transtricuspid gradient to provide an estimate of absolute pulmonary artery systolic pressure. Elevated pulmonary artery pressure, in the absence of pulmonary disease, is important, albeit indirect, evidence of elevated mean left atrial pressure.

Estimation of stroke volume frequently is useful in the clinical evaluation of patients with congestive heart failure, although it is

**TABLE 4.6.** *Doppler estimation of pulmonary artery pressure and cardiac output*

| Parameter | Method | Validation |
|---|---|---|
| PAp (13) | $4 \times$ (TR velocity)$^2$ + RAp estimation | The 95% confidence interval of this method is approximately 15 mm Hg, depending in large part on RAp estimation. |
| CO[a] (14) | 0.785 × (LV outflow tract diameter)$^2$ × LV outflow velocity time integral[b] | The 95% confidence interval of this method is in the range of 20 mL. Care must be taken to avoid underestimation of outflow tract diameter. |

[a]Stroke volume (SV) = CO × heart rate. Due to compensatory tachycardia, SV is often a more sensitive indicator of poor ventricular performance. In addition, SV can be multiplied by the mean systemic pressure to estimate stroke work. The relationship between stroke work and estimated filling pressure provides the best indication of ventricular performance.

[b]The velocity time integral is the product of mean velocity and time (time in this instance is the ejection period).

CO, cardiac output; LV, left ventricle; PAp, pulmonary artery systolic pressure; RAp, right atrial pressure; TR, tricuspid regurgitation.

not needed to identify systolic or diastolic left ventricular dysfunction. Overall left ventricular performance is reflected in part by forward cardiac output (in the absence of significant valve disease). Stroke volume (cardiac output/heart rate) falls when compensatory mechanisms, such as elevated filling pressure, become inadequate. Thus, a low resting stroke volume or cardiac output is a finding in the late stages of heart failure and may contribute to dyspnea and the dysfunction of several organ systems. A low stroke volume may reflect excessive diuresis during an effort by the physician to lower or normalize filling pressure. Doppler estimation of stroke volume is possible by application of the concept that flow is the product of cross-sectional area, mean velocity, and ejection time (Table 4.6).

## Left Ventricular Filling and Estimation of Left Atrial Pressure

Diastolic flow from the left atrium to the left ventricle occurs in two pulses, the early filling (E) wave and a late (A) wave, the latter in response to atrial contraction. The E wave is driven by the pressure gradient between the left atrium and left ventricle at the time of mitral valve opening. In young people, this gradient is high because a rapidly relaxing left ventricle causes an abrupt fall in left ventricular pressure. This transient high gradient produces a relatively high-velocity E wave recorded by Doppler (Fig. 4.2).With aging or the development of heart disease, left ventricular relaxation slows and the E wave velocity falls; A wave flow then becomes predominant (Fig. 4.3). However, if the patient's heart dis-

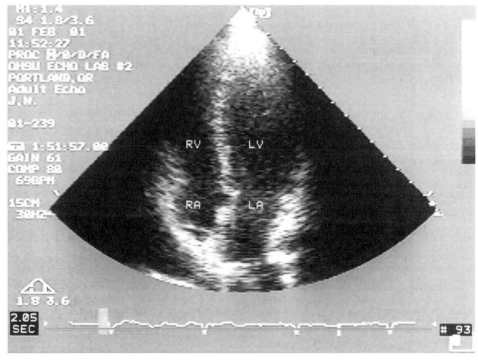

A

**FIG. 4.2.** Young normal patient. **A:** Echocardiographic four-chamber view. Note the relative size of the cardiac chambers, with the right ventricle (RV) somewhat smaller than the left ventricle (LV), and the left atrium (LA) the same size or a bit larger than the right atrium (RA).

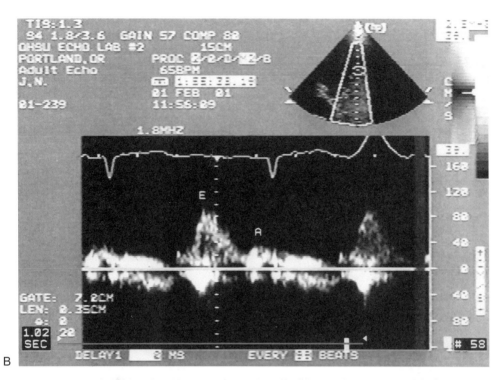

B

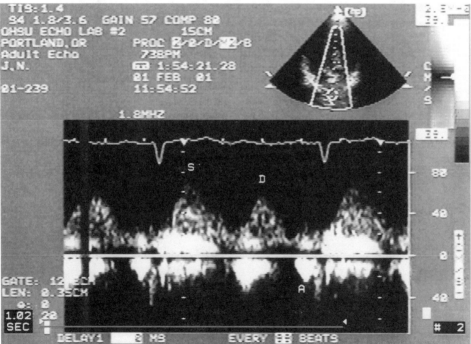

C

**FIG. 4.2.** *Continued.* **B:** Transmitral velocity recording in the same patient. Note the E wave predominance (E/A ratio >2.0, normal for a young person). **C:** Pulmonary venous flow recording in the same patient. Note the systolic forward velocity predominance (S/D ratio >1.0) and the short duration A wave.

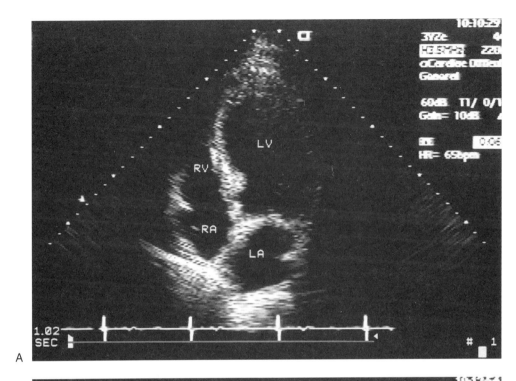

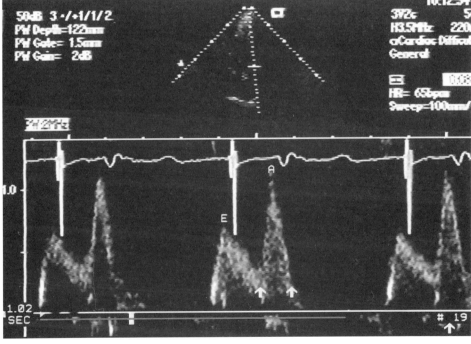

**FIG. 4.3.** Patient with predominant systolic left ventricular (LV) dysfunction. **A:** Echocardiographic four-chamber view. Note the very dilated LV. The left atrium (LA) appears mildly dilated. The right heart chambers are normal in size. **B:** Transmitral recording demonstrates A wave predominance, typical in the patient's age group (age >55 years). The E/A ratio of 0.5 renders LA hypertension extremely unlikely. *Arrows* indicate a normal A wave duration.

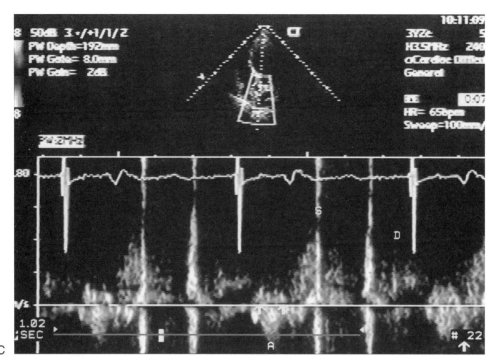

C

**FIG. 4.3.** *Continued.* **C:** Pulmonary venous recording, although technically limited, shows systolic predominance, essentially ruling out LA hypertension. The pulmonary venous A wave is shorter in duration than the transmitral A wave. Thus, the LV end-diastolic pressure probably is normal.

ease produces significant diastolic dysfunction, mean left atrial pressure may rise, increasing the left atrium–left ventricle pressure gradient at the time of mitral opening, and a high E wave velocity will be seen. Thus, in older persons or patients with heart disease, an E/A wave ratio >2:1 is a reliable indication of elevated mean left atrial pressure (Figs. 4.4 and 4.5 and Table 4.7). The presence of moderate or severe mitral regurgitation may cause a transient elevation of left atrial pressure in mid and late systole (the V wave), leading to an increased E wave velocity. Thus, in the presence of mitral regurgitation, the E wave may become prominent with lesser elevations of mean left atrial pressure.

The high E velocity seen in patients with elevated mean left atrial pressure due to left ventricular diastolic dysfunction indicates that the volume of early diastolic flow is large. When this fast-moving, high-volume flow

pulse impacts the walls of the left ventricle, an audible sound may be generated, the $S_3$. In the author's experience, when an $S_3$ is heard, the transmitral E wave almost always has a high velocity. An $S_3$ also can be heard occasionally in healthy young adults, a setting where high E velocities also are seen. An $S_3$ heard when a patient is in an exacerbation of congestive heart failure, such as pulmonary edema, is likely to be due to an acute elevation of mean left atrial pressure.

Deceleration of E wave velocity contains additional information about left ventricular filling. A short E wave deceleration time indicates the development of a force, during ventricular filling, that opposes further filling. This force appears to be a rapid rise in left ventricular diastolic pressure in response to the volume of blood contained in the E wave. For any given volume of early filling, left ventricular pressure will rise more steeply when

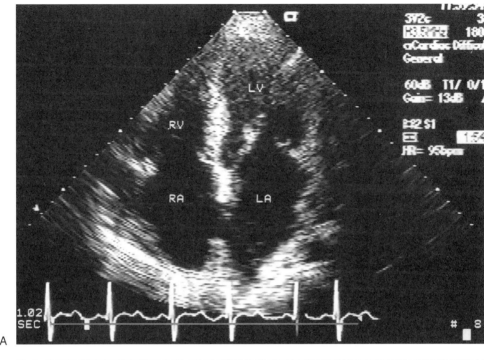

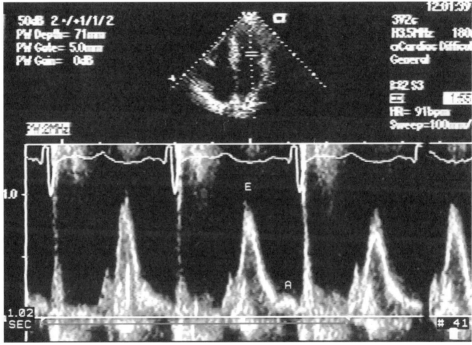

**FIG. 4.4.** Patient with predominant diastolic left ventricular (LV) dysfunction. **A:** Four-chamber view shows that the LV is normal in size, while both atria are moderately dilated. **B:** Transmitral E/A ratio is >3, which is highly specific for marked left atrial (LA) hypertension.

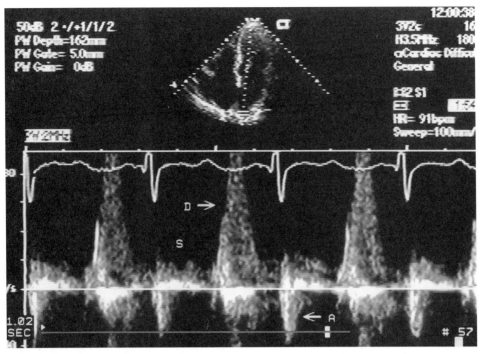

**FIG. 4.4.** *Continued.* **C:** Pulmonary venous recording shows almost no forward flow in systole, supporting marked elevation of LA mean pressure. The pulmonary venous A wave is prolonged relative to the transmitral A wave, validating the suspected elevation of left ventricular end-diastolic pressure.

the ventricular chamber is stiff. The operating stiffness of the left ventricle will be greater at higher filling pressure, so it is expected that a tall E wave and high E/A ratio are correlated with a short E deceleration time (Figs. 4.4 and 4.5). However, the E deceleration time has additional meaning, reflected in multivariate analyses, because it emerges as a strong predictor of prognosis, better than the E wave and E/A ratio, in patients with severe left ventricular dysfunction (Table 4.7).

Elevated mean left atrial pressure also alters the pattern of pulmonary venous flow into the left atrium (Table 4.7). Forward pulmonary venous flow occurs primarily in response to brief declines in atrial pressure in systole (referred to as the X descent) and in early diastole (the Y descent). In people >30 years, pulmonary venous velocity in systole is at least half of the diastolic velocity, and patients >50 years the systolic velocity is almost always greater than the diastolic velocity. Ele-

vation of mean left atrial pressure acts to suppress forward pulmonary venous flow, especially during systole (when the mitral valve is closed). Studies in adults with heart disease have shown that a systolic/diastolic velocity ratio <0.5 almost always is associated with elevated mean left atrial pressure (at least 15 mm Hg) (Figs. 4.4 and 4.5). Complete suppression of forward systolic flow is seen with marked left atrial hypertension (usually at least 25 mm Hg) or in the presence of hemodynamically significant mitral regurgitation.

Elevated left ventricular end-diastolic pressure, in the absence of elevated mean left atrial pressure, is a milder (or "earlier") form of left ventricular diastolic dysfunction. Patients with an isolated elevation of the end-diastolic pressure will not present with manifestations of pulmonary edema, low cardiac output, or biventricular failure. However, such patients may present with exertional dyspnea and often are sent to the echocardiographic

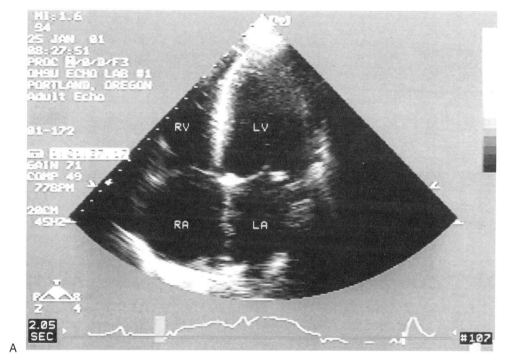

A

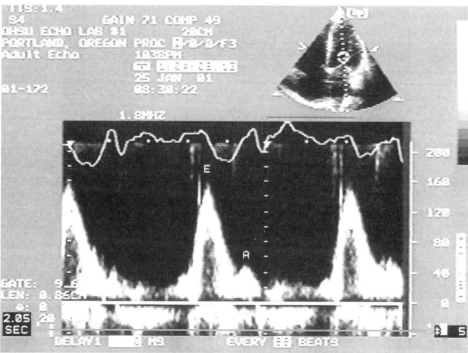

B

**FIG. 4.5.** Patient with mixed systolic and diastolic dysfunction. The pattern is the most commonly seen in patients with the congestive heart failure syndrome. **A:** There is pancardiomegaly, i.e., all four cardiac chambers are dilated. **B:** Transmitral and pulmonary venous recordings are conclusive for marked left atrial hypertension. There was moderate pulmonary hypertension as well, accounting for the right heart dilation and dysfunction.

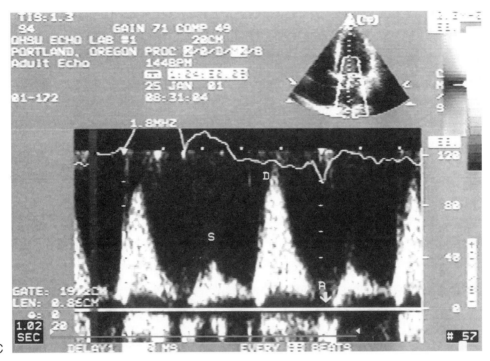

C

**FIG. 4.5.** *(Continued)* **C:** Transmitral and pulmonary venous recordings are conclusive for marked left atrial hypertension. There was moderate pulmonary hypertension as well, accounting for the right heart dilation and dysfunction.

laboratory with the request to "rule out congestive heart failure." Several indicators of elevated left ventricular end-diastolic pressure have been identified. A promising index is based on the pulmonary venous A wave. With atrial systole, blood is pushed backward into

the pulmonary veins as well as forward into the left ventricle. Normally, the backflow (pulmonary venous A wave) is brief and low in volume, but when left ventricular end-diastolic pressure is high, the pulmonary venous A wave becomes prolonged. In addition, re-

**TABLE 4.7.** *Doppler echocardiographic estimation of left ventricular filling pressures*

| Author | N | Index | Utility |
|---|---|---|---|
| Appleton et al. (9) | 70 | E/A | >1.2 was 92% sensitive, 95% specific for PCWP >10 mm Hg |
|  |  | SFPV | <50% was 85% sensitive, 95% specific for preAp >10 mm Hg |
| Brunazzi et al. (15) | 96 | SFPV | <35% was 85% specific, 90% sensitive for PCWP ≥18 mm Hg |
| Pozzoli et al. (16) | 231 | E/A | >2 was 87% sensitive, at least 80% specific for PCWP >20 mm Hg |
|  |  | SFPV | <50% was 96% sensitive, 72% specific for PCWP ≥20 mm Hg |
| Rossvoll and Hatte (17) | 45 | $PV_A$-$MV_A$ | >0 was 88% sensitive, 80% specific for LVEDP >15 mm Hg |
| Yamamoto et al. (18) | 87 | $PV_A$-$MV_A$ | >0 was 82% sensitive, 99% specific for LVEDP >20 mm Hg |
| Giannuzzi (21) | 508 | EDT | <125 ms imparts a relative risk of 2.4 for death or hospitalization, and a 45% mortality at 4 yr (vs. 13% if >125 ms) |

A, late initial filling velocity; E, early mitral filling velocity; EDT, E wave deceleration time; LVEDP, left ventricular end-diastolic pressure; PCWP, pulmonary capillary wedge pressure; preAp, pre A wave LV diastolic pressure; $PV_A$-$MV_A$, pulmonary venous A wave duration minus mitral A wave duration; SFPV, systolic fraction of pulmonary venous velocity.

sistance to forward flow acts to shorten the duration of the transmitral A wave. Studies show that when the pulmonary venous A wave is of longer duration than the transmitral A wave, the left ventricular end-diastolic pressure almost always is elevated. Currently, the utility of this sign for detecting elevations of left ventricular end-diastolic pressure in the absence of elevated mean left atrial pressure has not been thoroughly validated.

## Estimation of Right Atrial Pressure

Forward flow in the inferior vena cava is altered by the presence of right atrial hypertension in a manner analogous to the changes in pulmonary venous inflow seen with left atrial hypertension (Table 4.5). Flow velocity is best determined in the large hepatic veins that run into the inferior vena cava just below the diaphragm. A systolic proportion of total forward flow of <50% is sensitive and specific for at least mild elevation of right atrial right atrial pressure (>8 mm Hg), and <20% is specific for right atrial pressure >15 mm Hg.

## SUMMARY

### Echocardiography

As mentioned, the echocardiographic picture in patients with the clinical syndrome of congestive heart failure will vary depending on the relative importance of diastolic and systolic left ventricular dysfunction. When major systolic dysfunction is accompanied by minor diastolic dysfunction, the echocardiogram will show a very dilated, severely hypokinetic left ventricle, with normal sizes of the other chambers, normal estimated pulmonary artery pressure, and absence of evidence of elevated mean atrial pressure. At the other end of the spectrum, when left ventricular diastolic dysfunction is the predominant cause of the patient's syndrome, the echocardiogram shows a relatively normal sized LV, a relatively preserved ejection fraction, a dilated left atrium and right heart, pulmonary hypertension, and evidence of elevated mean right

atrial pressure. The vast majority of patients with congestive heart failure, however, lie between these two extremes. Most patients with congestive heart failure have significant degrees of both systolic and diastolic dysfunction, such that the ejection fraction is at least moderately reduced and filling pressures are at least mildly elevated. Thus, a typical echocardiogram in a patient with congestive heart failure will show a moderately dilated left ventricle with a moderately or severely reduced ejection fraction, at least mild left atrial dilation, evidence of left atrial hypertension, and variable degrees of pulmonary hypertension and right heart dilation and dysfunction.

## Utility and Limitations of Clinical and Echocardiographic Data

### *Diagnosis*

The symptoms listed in Table 4.1 usually lead the clinician to suspect congestive heart failure. The next diagnostic step is to attempt to confirm that the syndrome is present. The physical examination often is successful in achieving this goal and usually is sufficient to direct initial management (Table 4.3). When the patient presents with pulmonary rales combined with findings pointing to left ventricular dysfunction, such as a displaced, prominent PMI and/or $S_3$, the diagnosis of congestive heart failure is almost certain. If the findings associated with rales are only those of elevated right ventricular filling pressure, such as jugular venous distention and peripheral edema, then the diagnosis of congestive heart failure is likely but less certain. In this instance, left ventricular function may be normal, the patient may have a pulmonary disease, and the syndrome may be cor pulmonale. Unfortunately, left ventricular dysfunction may be present but the evidence may be obscured by other factors, such as the patient's body habitus. Thus, the absence of findings of left ventricular dysfunction does not rule out the congestive heart failure syndrome. On the contrary, congestive heart failure is such a common cause of rales that the diagnosis is heart failure until proven otherwise.

The diagnostic difficulty becomes greater when wheezing is present instead of rales, or when pulmonary auscultation is unremarkable. Many patients with congestive heart failure have augmented lymphatic clearance of interstitial pulmonary edema, minimizing rales, and associated pulmonary diseases may modify or obscure the auscultatory findings. Thus, the absence of rales does not rule out congestive heart failure as the cause for the patient's symptoms. Physical examination findings indicating left ventricular dysfunction may be present and confirm the diagnosis, but often they are not present.

Supplemental confirmatory evidence of congestive heart failure usually is needed. The chest x-ray almost always establishes whether or not pulmonary edema is present. When enlargement of the cardiac chambers is found, the diagnosis of heart failure is essentially confirmed. Nevertheless, in virtually all situations, at least an initial echocardiogram is required for several reasons (Table 4.8). The chest x-ray film can be misleading, and the diagnosis usually is not considered certain until it is confirmed by echocardiography. Accurate characterization of the relative roles of systolic and diastolic left ventricular dysfunction in the patient's disease often is difficult to achieve based on clinical data alone. Therapy may be guided by changes in left- and right-sided filling pressures and systolic function. The contributory role of valve disease to the patient's congestive heart failure can be suspected but not fully defined without an echocardiogram. The underlying etiology of the left ventricular dysfunction may be apparent from the echocardiogram, as when regional akinesis and scar formation indicate coronary disease. Finally, the echocardiogram often provides unique prognostic information (8).

### Management

Treatment of patients with congestive heart failure is guided by the symptoms, contribution of valve disease to the patient's syndrome, relative roles of systolic and diastolic dysfunction, and patient's prognosis. Large randomized trials have established survival benefit for patients with certain combinations of symptoms and degrees of left ventricular systolic dysfunction. Treatment of patients with left ventricular dysfunction should conform to the American Heart Association/American College of Cardiology guidelines (20).

**TABLE 4.8.** *Indications for echocardiography in patients with dyspnea, edema, or cardiomyopathy*

| Indication | Class |
|---|---|
| 1. Assessment of LV size and function in partients with suspected cardiomyopathy or clinical diagnosis of heart failure[a] | I |
| 2. Edema with clinical signs of elevated central venous pressure when a potential cardiac etiology is suspected or when central venous pressure cannot be estimated with confidence and clinical suspicion of heart disease is high[a] | I |
| 3. Dyspnea with clinical signs of heart disease | I |
| 4. Patients with unexplained hypotension, especially in the intensive care unit[a] | I |
| 5. Patients exposed to cardiotoxic agents, to determine the advisability of additional or increased dosages | I |
| 6. Reevaluation of LV function in patients with established cardiomyopathy when there has been a documented change in clinical status or to guide medical therapy | I |

[a]Transesophageal echocardiography is indicated when transthoracic echocardiographic studies are not diagnostic.

LV, left ventricle.

Reproduced from Ritchie JL, Cheitlin MD, Eagle KA, et al. ACC/AHA guidelines for the clinical application of echocardiography: a report of the American College of Cardiology/American Heart Association Task Force on Practice Guidelines (committee on clinical application of echocardiography). Circulation 1997;95:1686–1744.

The physical examination is essential for following the patient's progress on therapy. The echocardiogram can be used to follow the reduction of pulmonary artery and mean atrial pressures on diuretic therapy, but it is costly and unnecessary. Modest examination skills permit the clinician to follow the resolution of rales, reduction in peripheral edema and jugular venous pulse, and softening of $S_3$. A repeat echocardiogram is generally recommended on a yearly basis because of the importance of detecting changes, as in left ventricular ejection fraction, that may not be otherwise apparent. Repeat echocardiography often is useful when patients with known left ventricular dysfunction present with congestive heart failure exacerbations (e.g., pulmonary edema) or do not respond to treatment as expected (Table 4.8). The potential survival benefit of echocardiogram-guided lowering of filling pressure, beyond the endpoints of absence of rales and peripheral edema, has not been fully investigated. Unfortunately, patients whose filling pressures remain elevated despite diuretic therapy often develop a low cardiac output state (with pre-renal azotemia and worsening symptoms) with further attempts at volume lowering.

The prognosis of patients with congestive heart failure is influenced by multiple factors, including not only the severity of left ventricular dysfunction but also its etiology. The patient's functional status, as reflected in the functional class or objective indicators of exercise tolerance, is an important factor (Table 4.2). Studies have established that several echocardiographic features are related to the prognosis of patients with congestive heart failure. From 2-D imaging, the severity of left ventricular dilation and reduced ejection fraction are modestly associated with a poor prognosis. Thin left ventricular walls, reflecting failure of the adaptive hypertrophic response of the myocardium to contractile failure, are an adverse prognostic sign. The presence of significant inoperable valve disease greatly reduces survival of patients with congestive heart failure. Doppler data related to filling pressure and ventricular stiffness also have major prognostic importance, as well as being related to symptoms.

## REFERENCES

1. Grossman W. Diastolic dysfunction and congestive heart failure. Circulation 1990;81[Suppl III]:III-1–III-7.
2. Braunwald E, Colucci WS, Grossman W. Clinical aspects of heart failure: high-output heart failure; pulmonary edema. In: Braunwald E, ed. Heart disease: a textbook of cardiovascular medicine, 5th ed. Philadelphia: WB Saunders, 1997:445–470.
3. Goldman L, Hashimoto B, Cook EF, et al. Comparative reproducibility and validity of systems for assessing cardiovascular functional class: advantages of a new specific activity scale. Circulation 1981;64:1227.
4. Perloff JK, ed. Physical examination of the heart and circulation, 2nd ed. Philadelphia: WB Saunders, 1997.
5. Donaldson MC. Chronic venous disorders. In: Loscalzo J, Creager MA, Dzau VJ, eds. Vascular medicine, 1st ed. Boston: Little Brown and Company, 1992:1075–1098.
6. Jensen-Urstad K, Bovier, F, Hojer J, et al. Comparison of different echocardiographic methods with radionuclide imaging for measuring left ventricular ejection fraction during acute myocardial infarction treated by thrombolytic therapy. Am J Cardiol 1998;81:538–544.
7. Massie BM, Schiller NB, Ratshin RA, et al. Mitral-septal separation: a new echocardiographic index of left ventricular function. Am J Cardiol 1997;39:1008–1016.
8. Pinamonti B, DiLenarda A, Sinagra G, et al. Restrictive left ventricular filling pattern in dilated cardiomyopathy assessed by Doppler echocardiography: clinical, echocardiographic and hemodynamic correlations and prognostic implications. Heart Muscle Disease Study Group. J Am Coll Cardiol 1993;22:808–815.
9. Appleton CP, Galloway JM, Gonzalez MS, et al. Estimation of left ventricular filling pressures using two-dimensional and Doppler echocardiography in adult patients with cardiac disease: additional value of analyzing left atrial size, left atrial ejection fraction and the difference in duration of pulmonary venous and mitral flow velocity at atrial contraction. J Am Coll Cardiol 1993;22:1972-1982.
10. Nagueh S, Kopelen H, Zoghbi W. Relation of mean right atrial pressure to echocardiographic and Doppler parameters of right atrial and right ventricular function. Am J Cardiol 1996;493–496.
11. Kircher BJ, Himelman RB, Schiller NB. Noninvasive estimation of right atrial pressure from the inspiratory collapse of the inferior vena cava. Am J Cardiol 1990;66:493–496.
12. Cecconi M, LaConha G, Manfrin M, et al. Evaluation of mean right atrial pressure by two-dimensional and Doppler echocardiography in patients with cardiac disease. G Ital Cardiol 1998;28:357–364.
13. Berger M, Haimowitz A, Van Tosh A, et al. Quantitative assessment of pulmonary hypertension in patients with tricuspid regurgitation using continuous wave doppler ultrasound. J Am Coll Cardiol 1985;6:359–365.
14. Lewis JF, Kuo LC, Nelson JG, et al. Pulsed Doppler echocardiographic determination of stroke volume and cardiac output: clinical validation of two new methods using the apical window. Circulation 1984;70:425–431.

15. Brunazzi MC, Chirillo F, Pasqualini M, et al. Estimation of left ventricular diastolic pressures from precordial pulsed-Doppler analysis of pulmonary venous and mitral flow. Am Heart J 1994;128:293–300.

16. Pozzoli M, Capomolla S, Pinna G, et al. Doppler echocardiography reliably predicts pulmonary artery wedge pressure in patients with chronic heart failure with and without mitral regurgitation. J Am Coll Cardiol 1996;27:883–893.

17. Rossvoll O, Hatle LK. Pulmonary venous flow velocities recorded by transthoracic doppler ultrasound: relation to left ventricular diastolic pressures. J Am Coll Cardiol 1993;21:1687–1696.

18. Yamamoto K, Nishimura RA, Burnett JC, et al. Assessment of left ventricular end-diastolic pressure by doppler echocardiography: contribution of duration of pulmonary venous versus mitral flow velocity curves at atrial contraction. J Am Soc Echocardiogr 1997;10:52–59.

19. Ritchie JL, Cheitlin MD, Eagle KA, et al. ACC/AHA guidelines for the clinical application of echocardiography: a report of the American College of Cardiology/American Heart Association Task Force on Practice Guidelines (Committee on Clinical Application of Echocardiography). Circulation 1997;95:1686–1744.

20. Williams JF, Bristow MR, Fowler MB, et al. Guidelines for the evaluation and management of heart failure: report of the American College of Cardiology/American Heart Association Task Force on Practice Guidelines (Committee on Evaluation and Management of Heart Failure). J Am Coll Cardiol 1995;26:1376–1398.

21. Giannuzzi P, Imparato A, Temporelli PL, et al. Doppler-derived mitral deceleration time of early filling as a strong predictor of pulmonary capillary wedge pressure in postinfarction patients with left ventricular systolic dysfunction *J Am Coll Cardiol* 1994;23:1630–1637.

# 5

# The Patient with Right Heart Diseases

Robert R. Phillips, *Carlos A. Roldan, and †Jonathan Abrams

*Idaho Cardiology Associates, Boise, Idaho; *Department of Internal Medicine, University of New
Mexico School of Medicine; and Department of Internal Medicine, Veterans Affairs Medical Center,
Albuquerque, New Mexico; †Cardiology Division, University of New Mexico School of Medicine; and
Department of Internal Medicine, University Hospital, Albuquerque, New Mexico*

## DEFINITION

Right-sided heart disease encompasses a wide variety of disorders, most of which have similar clinical manifestations in their late stages. The spectrum of right heart conditions includes pulmonary hypertension of many causes, cor pulmonale, and primary tricuspid and pulmonic valve disease. Cor pulmonale, i.e., right heart disease due to pulmonary hypertension in the absence of left heart disease, implies right ventricular (RV) enlargement. The current discussion will address pulmonary hypertension, cor pulmonale, and primary right heart diseases.

## ETIOLOGY

*Pulmonary hypertension* is the major cause of RV dysfunction and is classified as vasoconstrictive, obliterative, obstructive, hyperkinetic, or passive (1). Vasoconstrictive etiologies include any cause of chronic hypoxia, such as obstructive sleep apnea, obesity hypoventilation, or the "Ondine curse." Destruction of pulmonary capillary beds, as in emphysema and $\alpha_1$ antitrypsin deficiency, leads to obliterative pulmonary hypertension. Primary pulmonary hypertension is a form of obstructive etiology. There are multiple histologic variants of primary pulmonary hypertension, which may represent the end stage of a variety of disorders, including thrombotic pulmonary arteriopathy, plexogenic pulmonary arteriopathy, and pulmonary venoocclusive disease (2). Acute and chronic pulmonary embolism is another obstructive etiology. Chronically elevated pulmonary blood flow leads to hyperkinetic pulmonary hypertension, such as with left to right shunting from an atrial septal defect (ASD), anomalous pulmonary venous drainage, and coronary to pulmonary arterial fistula. Disorders that lead to elevated left atrial (LA) pressure and pulmonary venous congestion are the most common causes of passive pulmonary hypertension. These conditions include mitral stenosis, mitral regurgitation, left ventricular (LV) dysfunction, hypertension, hypertrophic cardiomyopathy, and aortic stenosis or regurgitation.

*RV dysfunction* may occur when there is ischemia or infarction of the RV, or chronic pressure or volume overload of the RV. Arrhythmogenic RV cardiomyopathy also results from the progressive loss of RV cells. The myocardium is slowly replaced by noncontractile fibrous tissue. Chronic dilation of the RV in the absence of elevated pulmonary artery pressure can result from chronic RV volume overload. Disorders that lead to volume overload include ASD, Ebstein anomaly, partial anomalous pulmonary venous return, tricuspid regurgitation (TR), and pulmonic regurgitation (PR). The latter two conditions may be caused by endocarditis, carcinoid syndrome, iatrogenic or traumatic disorders, rheumatic valve disease, and congenital abnormalities.

## PROGNOSIS

The natural history of RV dysfunction depends primarily on the underlying cause. The most serious cause of RV dysfunction is primary pulmonary hypertension. The average age at diagnosis is 45 years. Mean survival after diagnosis is 2.5 years (2,3). Chronic pulmonary embolism carries a better prognosis if pulmonary thromboendarterectomy can be performed. The largest series reported a survival of 75% at an average 6-year follow-up (4). Passive venous congestion resulting from

left-sided heart disease, however, is the most common cause of pulmonary hypertension. In these cases, the prognosis is determined by the underlying etiology and severity of the left heart disorder.

Chronic obstructive pulmonary disease (COPD) is a major cause of pulmonary hypertension and cor pulmonale. The degree of pulmonary hypertension usually is mild to moderate. The 5-year survival rate of these patients is only 33% once cor pulmonale has developed, but it can be improved to 45% with chronic oxygen therapy (5).

Determining the impact of RV dysfunction on survival in patients with coronary artery disease is difficult because of concurrent LV dysfunction. Some, but not all, studies suggest that patients with persistent RV dysfunction following inferior myocardial infarction have decreased survival (6).

Isolated TR is relatively benign and well tolerated. Case series of patients with tricuspid valve endocarditis who underwent removal of the tricuspid valve report no significant problems for many years in the absence of RV dysfunction or pulmonary hypertension (7). These patients usually develop RV dysfunction but respond well with resolution of symptoms following valve replacement (8–10). TR is a result of elevated pulmonary artery pressure or mitral valve disease in the majority of cases.

## HISTORY

Although the spectrum of diseases associated with RV dysfunction is wide, the late stages of nearly all forms of right heart disease have similar symptoms.

Development of RV dysfunction results in fatigue, which is the most commonly reported symptom. As RV dysfunction progresses, patients may complain of a full neck (distended jugular veins), lower extremity edema, and right upper quadrant pain. Hepatic congestion may lead to ascites, and patients will complain of increasing abdominal girth. These symptoms are common to all forms of right heart disease and are not helpful for determining the specific underlying etiology.

Symptoms of coronary artery disease should be sought in patients with unexplained right heart failure. They may have a history of prior myocardial infarction or symptoms of exertional angina or dyspnea.

Pulmonary hypertension related to pulmonary venous congestion from left heart disease leads to symptoms of left-sided failure either before or concurrent with symptoms of right heart failure. Symptoms of left-sided heart failure include shortness of breath, dyspnea of exertion, orthopnea, and paroxysmal nocturnal dyspnea (PND). Symptoms of angina or a prior history of myocardial infarction are important. Patients also may complain of palpitations, PND, or fatigue due to atrial arrhythmias.

Patients with primary pulmonary hypertension or COPD have symptoms of dyspnea in the absence of significant orthopnea or PND. Severe pulmonary hypertension of any cause may be associated with chest pain, especially with exercise, that presumably is related to RV subendocardial ischemia. Syncope and presyncope are fairly common features of advanced pulmonary hypertension.

Pulmonic valvular disease may be entirely asymptomatic and only recognized on the cardiac physical examination. Cyanosis is fairly common and is reported in about 30% of cases due to shunting through a patent foramen ovale. Epistaxis and clubbing are other features of pulmonic valvular disease. Symptoms of right heart failure may occur eventually and are a poor prognostic sign.

TR may be due to RV pressure or volume overload and often results from tricuspid annular dilation. TR due to carcinoid syndrome or endocarditis, however, has distinct historical features. Most carcinoid tumors arise in the small intestine or colon. Only those that metastasize to the liver produce the valvular abnormalities and symptom complex. Symptoms include facial flushing, diarrhea, and bronchospasm. These symptoms are caused by tumor production of vasoactive amines and typically appear long before the symptoms of right heart failure from significant tricuspid or pulmonic valve disease. A history of intra-venous drug use and fever are the usual presenting historical features of tricuspid valve endocarditis.

## PHYSICAL EXAMINATION

When discussing RV dysfunction and the resulting TR, it is useful to categorize patients into those with normal pulmonary artery pressure and those with pulmonary hypertension.

### Normal Pulmonary Artery Pressure

In the absence of elevation of pulmonary artery pressure, the RV usually faces a pure volume overload. Volume overload may be the result of left to right shunting, TR, or PR. In general, the magnitude of TR is less than when pulmonary hypertension is present. The normal RV and right atrium (RA) are relatively compliant. Systemic venous distention is not seen unless severe RV volume overload results in RV dysfunction or TR is moderate to severe. With normal pulmonary artery pressure, the volume and velocity of blood refluxing from the RV into the RA and great veins due to TR generally are modest; thus, the classic tricuspid murmur and elevated jugular venous pressure with V waves may not be prominent or may even be absent. *Practical Point: An inspiratory increase in the intensity of the systolic murmur and the amplitude of venous V wave are of great diagnostic importance in patients with low-pressure TR* (Fig. 5.1). Such subjects often have no abnormal findings during inspiration. The abdominal compression test may be useful (See Chapter 1, the Jugular Venous Pulse).

### Elevated Pulmonary Artery Pressure

The RV in chronic severe pulmonary hypertension has increased systolic and diastolic pressures and volume (chamber dilation); ultimately, the tricuspid valve annulus dilates and TR develops. Decreased compliance of the hypertrophied RV will augment the magnitude of the TR. TR resulting from pulmonary hypertension tends to be more severe. In patients with

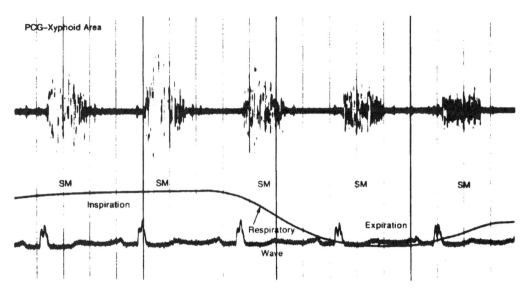

**FIG. 5.1.** Inspiratory augmentation of the murmur of tricuspid regurgitation (TR). Note the dramatic increase in amplitude of the systolic murmur (SM) during inspiration. Augmented right ventricular filling and a greater TR volume during inspiration produce a louder murmur. (From Delman AJ, Stein E. Dynamic cardiac auscultation and phonocardiography. Philadelphia: WB Saunders, 1979, with permission.)

rheumatic mitral valve disease or chronic congestive heart failure, TR generally is present in subjects with mean RA pressures >10 mm Hg.

### Arterial Pulse

There are no characteristic alterations of the carotid pulse associated with RV dysfunction. Arterial pulse amplitude may be diminutive if LV stroke volume is reduced. It is easy to confuse the dramatic swelling of the jugular veins found in patients with severe TR with the arterial pulse (Fig. 5.2). These pulsations (V waves) are systolic in timing and may be visible as well as palpable.

### Jugular Venous Pulse

Neck vein pulsations in right heart disease are of major diagnostic importance. The diagnosis of TR often can be entertained prior to auscultation by careful examination of the jugular pulse. The jugular venous pulse consists of an A wave, X descent, V wave, and Y descent. A waves occur during atrial contraction and are accentuated in several forms of right heart disease, such as tricuspid stenosis or TS; (RA contracts against the narrowed tricuspid orifice), pulmonic stenosis, and pulmonary hypertension. When there is increased RV filling pressure, the A wave increases in amplitude as the atrium must contract against high RV diastolic pressure. TS can be differentiated from other causes of elevated A wave because the obstruction in early RV diastolic filling results in a decrease in the Y descent. In addition, an opening snap and diastolic rumble are present.

A and V waves are also elevated when there is increased blood volume to the RA, with or without elevated pulmonary artery pressure, as may be seen in ASD and anomalous pulmonary venous drainage (11,12).

With increasing severity of TR, an accentuated jugular V wave appears during systole. As the severity of TR increases in magnitude, the X descent becomes attenuated and ultimately disappears (Fig. 5.2). The regurgitant V wave is systolic and simultaneous with the palpable carotid arterial pulse, although the precise timing, peak, and contour are some-

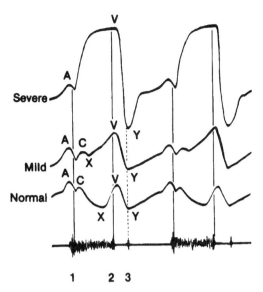

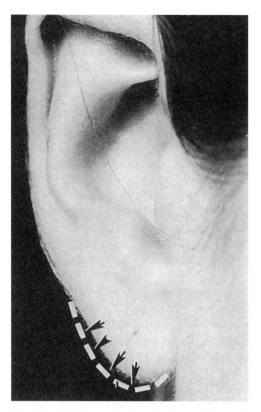

**FIG. 5.2.** Jugular venous pulse in tricuspid regurgitation (TR). Alterations of the venous contour in mild TR are depicted in the **middle tracing**. The V wave is augmented and the Y descent is more prominent; the X descent is markedly attenuated. With severe TR **(top tracing)**, there is a plateaulike systolic regurgitant C-V wave, which in part represents "ventricularization" of the right atrial and jugular venous pulses. Note the right ventricular $S_3$ coinciding with the nadir of the Y descent. A normal venous pulse is depicted in the **bottom drawing**. (From Abrams J. Prim Cardiol, 1982, with permission.)

**FIG. 5.3.** Earlobe pulsations in tricuspid regurgitation (TR). In severe TR, the jugular venous pressure is markedly elevated and the large V waves may be difficult to discern. Careful inspection of the ear lobe with the patient in the 30- to 90-degree position may reveal subtle lateral pulsations of the large systolic V waves in the right atrium throughout the proximal venous system.

what different from the arterial pulsation. The venous V wave has a more rounded contour and is somewhat sustained or plateaulike, in contrast to the brisk up-and-down motion of the arterial pulse. Furthermore, the venous pulsations usually are not palpable. With increasing degrees of TR, venous pulsation begins earlier in systole. The large systolic V wave is terminated by a sharp steep trough, the Y descent, which represents decompression of the RA as the tricuspid valve opens fully in early diastole (Fig. 5.2). The prominent Y descent is easily seen and may actually be more prominent than the swelling of the venous pulse (Y wave) preceding the Y collapse. In severe TR, the systolic venous column can be seen high in the neck and to the ear; the earlobes may move (Fig. 5.3).

In most adult patients with acquired TR due to pulmonary hypertension, the mean venous pressure will be elevated. Thus, the peak of the venous systolic wave will be high. It often is necessary to examine such subjects in the semirecumbent or sitting position. With very high venous pressures, the meniscus of the venous blood column may be invisible, as the venous system is tense and distended with blood.

The magnitude of TR increases as RV inflow increases during inspiration. As the RA distends during systole, more blood flows into the superior vena cava. This is manifest as a larger V wave, which has a higher peak and mean pressure and a more prominent Y descent during inspiration. On the other hand, occasionally severe TR can be associated with only minimal abnormality of RA pressure. Pulmonary hypertension is not likely to be present in such cases.

### Precordial Motion

In subjects with pulmonary hypertension, an abnormal systolic RV impulse typically will be present. This is a low-amplitude, sustained parasternal lift or heave. The pulmonic valve component ($P_2$) also may be palpable at the second left intercostal space (11,12). Even in the absence of pulmonary hypertension, severe TR causes prominent systolic unloading of the RV. Parasternal activity reveals a retraction wave during late systole. A brisk early systolic outward motion occurs; during the remainder of systole, the RV pulls away from the chest wall. An exaggerated early diastolic RV filling wave may be palpable (RV $S_3$).

Palpable RV activity reflects the level of pulmonary artery pressure, RV size, and severity of TR. An outward systolic impulse will be felt in most instances; it will be brief and early systolic in the non–pressure-overloaded RV and is likely to be sustained when there is major pulmonary hypertension. When the RV is large, precordial activity may produce a rocking or seesaw motion. The left anterior chest and LV apex retract as the medial RV area, adjacent to lower left sternal border, move anteriorly, and then retract during mid to late systole. A greatly enlarged RV may occupy the usual apex area, literally pushing the LV posterolaterally in the thorax, where it is no longer palpable on the chest wall.

### Heart Sounds

*First heart sound ($S_1$).* RV hypertrophy or dilation in the presence of right bundle branch block may be associated with a split $S_1$.

*Second heart sound ($S_2$).* With pulmonary hypertension, an accentuated $P_2$ often is present and may be widely transmitted over the precordium. If *both* the aortic valve component ($A_2$) and $P_2$ are audible at the apex, pulmonary hypertension is likely to be present because $P_2$ typically does not radiate to the apex. If severe RV failure is present, RV ejection will be pro-

longed and the stroke volume relatively fixed during respiration. $S_2$ will be widely split both in inspiration and expiration. This can simulate the fixed splitting of an ASD.

*Third heart sound ($S_3$).* RV $S_3$ occasionally can be heard with RV dysfunction. The $S_3$ may reflect the excessive volume of blood crossing the tricuspid valve in early diastole and/or RV decompensation associated with a large RV end-diastolic volume and decreased ejection fraction. Right-sided $S_3$ and $S_4$ typically are louder during inspiration and wane with expiration. Such sounds may be audible only in inspiration.

Right $S_3$ (or $S_4$) is best heard at the lower left sternal border and will be inaudible at the LV apex. However, if the RV is large and occupies the apical region in the left thorax, an RV $S_3$ may be readily mistaken for an $S_3$ of LV origin.

As the RV $S_3$ often is associated with high RV diastolic pressures, it may be high pitched, simulating a pericardial knock or tricuspid opening snap. The pericardial knock of constrictive pericarditis is an unusually prominent, early, and high-pitched RV filling sound (i.e., an $S_3$). As with mitral regurgitation, severe TR with a large regurgitant fraction may produce a brief diastolic flow rumble. This murmur will increase with inspiration and can simulate TS.

*Fourth heart sound ($S_4$).* A right-sided $S_4$ may be heard in patients with acute-onset TR. This is similar to the left-sided $S_4$ found in patients with acute mitral regurgitation. In such cases, the RV and the RA usually are of normal size. The regurgitant volume load results in vigorous RA contraction and produces a large increase in end-diastolic flow and pressure in the RV. Acute TR is likely to occur in a drug addict with tricuspid valve endocarditis or in a patient with traumatic rupture of a tricuspid valve cusp.

A right-sided $S_4$ may be heard in patients with RV hypertension secondary to pulmonary stenosis or idiopathic pulmonary hypertension. This results from atrial contraction into a noncompliant RV. The right-sided $S_4$ increases with inspiration. It may be quite loud and is best heard at the lower left sternal border at the fourth to fifth interspace and augments with inspiration.

*Systolic clicks or ejection sounds.* Patients with severe pulmonary hypertension may have a pulmonary artery ejection sound that is best heard at the upper left sternal border (Fig. 1.19). Respiratory variation of the click may differentiate this sound from an aortic ejection click or prominently split $S_1$.

Ejection sounds are common in valvular pulmonic stenosis. The presence of an ejection sound localizes the obstruction to the valve level. Infundibular pulmonic stenosis does not produce an ejection click. In very mild or very severe pulmonic stenosis, the pulmonic ejection click may not be heard. *Practical Point: The most characteristic attribute of the pulmonic valve ejection sound is its marked variability with respiration.* In contrast to almost all other right-sided acoustic phenomena, which become louder with inspiration, the pulmonic valve ejection click typically softens or disappears with inspiration.

With inspiration, augmented venous return to the right heart results in a more forceful RA contraction, which in turn produces a rise in RV end-diastolic pressure. RV late diastolic pressure exceeds the simultaneous pulmonary artery diastolic pressure, and the pulmonary valve cusps are pushed toward an open position during late diastole. Thus, the actual opening excursion of the pulmonic valve cusps is minimal or even absent, and the opening click is soft or not present.

In severe pulmonic stenosis, the pulmonic valve may not open fully until mid or late systole, and the click will be later in timing. The $P_2$ may be very soft to inaudible, even with a well-preserved ejection click, because of the very low pulmonary artery pressures. In addition, $P_2$ usually is delayed, which results in further difficulty in hearing this sound. In very mild pulmonic stenosis, there may not be respiratory alteration in the intensity of the click.

Pulmonic ejection clicks typically are high-frequency, sharp, discrete sounds that are at least equal in intensity to $S_1$. They are best heard with the diaphragm of the stethoscope. The later the ejection sound, the more audible it is. Ejection sounds that are distinctly separate acoustically from $S_1$ follow $S_1$ by at least 0.05 seconds. An early ejection sound may merge with $S_1$ or, more likely, is thought by the examiner to be part of the $S_1$ complex. The

more severe the valve obstruction, the earlier the click. In these cases, the ejection sound is easily confused with $S_1$.

Pulmonic ejection sounds are best heard at the second and third left interspaces and are poorly heard or inaudible at the apex. Listen with the subject in the upright position. The resultant decrease in RV venous return often results in the click becoming more audible both in inspiration and expiration.

Presence of pulmonic click in a young patient with a prominent pulmonic outflow murmur and wide splitting of $S_2$ helps identify pulmonic stenosis.

Tricuspid valve prolapse usually is not diagnosed on auscultation, although it may be detected on echocardiography. Nevertheless, the prominence of a mid to late systolic click at the lower left sternal border that becomes louder and later during inspiration should raise suspicion of tricuspid valve prolapse.

## Heart Murmurs

Heart murmurs are the cardinal manifestation of pulmonic and tricuspid stenosis or regurgitation.

### *Pulmonic Stenosis*

The pulmonic stenosis systolic murmur is mid-systolic, usually increasing in intensity with inspiration and heard best at the left second or third intercostal space. The murmur may radiate to the neck, left shoulder, or back. The murmur usually continues into late systole but stops before $P_2$. As severity increases, the murmur peaks later in systole and may even obscure the pulmonic component of the second heart sound (11,12). In most cases, there is an ejection click heard in the same location. The click becomes more faint or absent during inspiration. The response to inspiration and lack of radiation to the carotids are clues to the presence of a pulmonic stenosis murmur. Wide splitting of the second heart sound is present.

A reduction of valve orifice area to at least 70% of normal is required before there is a pressure difference across the valve in the resting state. Mildly fused or rigid cusps may not produce sufficient obstruction to result in a pressure gradient.

In general, the more significant the valve stenosis, the later peaking and the longer the murmur. The gap between the end of the sound vibrations and $S_2$ narrows with increasing obstruction of the pulmonic valve. Other associated abnormalities (abnormal precordial motion, $S_4$, ejection click, abnormal splitting of $S_2$) are likely to be prominent with increasing grades of obstruction.

### Pulmonic Regurgitation

When associated with pulmonary artery dilation and pulmonary hypertension, PR leads to an early diastolic, decrescendo murmur in the left sternal border. The murmur is called a Graham Steell murmur and usually is associated with other signs of pulmonary hypertension. The PR murmur in association with normal pulmonary pressures tends to be mid-diastolic, with a crescendo-decrescendo pattern (11). The murmur is difficult to differentiate from aortic regurgitation (AR); in one study, the examiner was correct only 25% of the time (12). Murmurs of PR usually are quite long and may be pandiastolic, continuing to $S_1$. Usually, these high-frequency murmurs are of low intensity and may be very faint in late diastole. In severe pulmonary hypertension, the high-pitched blowing Graham Steell murmur is common. This murmur invariably is associated with other signs of pulmonary hypertension, such as RV lift and increased $P_2$. Congenital PR is rare. This murmur is low to medium pitched, and usually begins after an audible pause or gap after $P_2$. It is associated with low pulmonary and RV pressures and does not mimic the high-frequency AR "blow" or Graham Steell murmur. As a rule, isolated congenital PR should not provide confusion with AR.

### Tricuspid Regurgitation

Trivial to mild TR on echocardiography is present in up to 80% of normal patients. Because the regurgitation is slight, it is audible in <20% of normal subjects. The severity of TR increases as a result of increased RV volume or pressure. The classic murmur of TR is holosystolic, increases with inspiration, and is best heard at the fourth and fifth interspaces at the lower left sternal border (Fig. 5.1). The usual TR murmur has an even, pansystolic configuration extending to $S_2$. However, it is common for the murmur to wane in late systole, often with early to mid-systolic accentuation. The possibility of TR should be actively considered in any patient with suspected pulmonary hypertension or cor pulmonale.

*Intensity.* The murmur of TR seldom is very loud and usually is of grade 2/6 or 3/6 intensity. Significant TR has been documented to be acoustically silent in some patients. Silent TR is more likely to occur with normal RV systolic pressure, as is found with traumatic or infectious damage to a previously normal valve. Making the proper diagnosis in such cases is not easy. In some patients, the murmur is heard only during inspiration, which can be misleading because it may simulate a pulmonary or pericardial process. Variation in inspiratory intensity may be difficult to detect when the tricuspid murmur is very loud.

*Frequency.* The typical TR murmur is medium frequency, but on occasion can be rough and raspy. High-frequency murmurs of TR are not common. The murmur may appear to be more high pitched at sites away from the area of maximal intensity. It is best to use both the bell and diaphragm when listening for TR.

*Tricuspid honk or whoop.* TR rarely can be associated with a vibratory, high-pitched whoop that usually demonstrates a prominent inspiratory increase. This tricuspid honk usually is intermittent and has been associated with severe pulmonary hypertension. Tricuspid valve prolapse is a likely etiologic factor.

*Location and radiation.* The TR murmur is best heard over the RV area at the lower left sternal edge at the fourth to fifth interspace. The murmur may radiate into both the right and left chest for a short distance. Transmission to the lower right sternal area is common, and one should listen carefully at the lower right sternal border whenever TR is suspected. When loud, the murmur also may be heard at the upper left sternal edge. Soft tricuspid murmurs may be well localized to a small area of the lower left sternal border.

When the RV is very large, the murmur may be heard at both the left lower sternal edge and the cardiac apex, which may be formed by the dilated RV chamber. In such cases, the murmur may be equally loud at the mid left chest and sternal edge, but it should never be loudest at the apex. It is easy to mistake the apical murmur of TR for mitral regurgitation. If the apical murmur is solely tricuspid in origin, it will not radiate into the axilla. Inspiratory augmentation should be assessed carefully.

TR murmurs often are easily detected at the xiphoid and subxiphoid areas, particularly in patients with large chests or COPD. *Practical Point: Whenever TR is suspected, listen carefully for murmur radiation to the right lower sternal border, xiphoid region, and over the superior aspect of the liver.*

*Respiratory alteration.* The inspiratory increase in the intensity of the TR murmur known as the Carvallo sign is a well-known phenomenon (Fig. 5.1). Respiratory alteration, however, is missed frequently by clinicians. The increase in murmur loudness with inspiration often is only one grade and may be a subtle finding. For optimal detection of respiratory variation, it may be useful to auscultate several centimeters *away from* the point of peak murmur intensity. With very loud murmurs, minor respiratory alterations in intensity may be difficult to detect.

One must be sure the patient is breathing deeply and smoothly without forced respirations or performance of an inadvertent Valsalva maneuver. In patients with a soft murmur, inspiration may increase the grade dramatically for only one or two beats. *Practical Point: For optimal auscultation, listen for respiratory variation over many respiratory cycles and focus on phasic alterations in peak intensity of the systolic murmur.*

*Hepatojugular reflux.* Use of the hepatojugular reflux maneuver has been shown to be helpful in identifying TR murmurs (Fig. 1.8). Firm upward pressure with the hand over the right upper quadrant of the abdomen for 10 to 15 seconds will accentuate the murmur of TR.

The maneuver is especially useful in patients with only mild to moderate TR and in the absence of pulmonary hypertension where the Carvallo sign is equivocal or not present. The tricuspid murmur typically increases in loudness for four to six beats.

*Failure to change with respiration.* In some instances, there is no detectable or consistent respiratory alteration in intensity of the TR murmur. The hepatojugular reflux maneuver should be tried in such cases. This situation is more likely to be true with mild TR and normal RV systolic pressure or, conversely, with TR associated with severe RV dysfunction and right heart failure. *Practical Point: Always have the patient sit or stand up during auscultation when TR is suspected but respiratory variation is absent.* The decrease in right heart volume and diastolic pressure caused by the diminished return in the upright posture may allow the RV to vary its stroke volume sufficiently during respiration, with a resultant increase in murmur intensity during inspiration.

*Changes with maneuvers.* Any action that increases right heart return, such as elevating the legs, squatting, the hepatojugular reflux maneuver, Müller maneuver (inhalation with the glottis closed), or exercise, will augment the systolic murmur. The TR murmur usually increases during long R-R cycles (post premature ventricular contraction beat) because there is increased RV filling during such beats.

*Variability.* Variation in the signs of TR relates to alterations in cardiovascular hemodynamics, level of pulmonary artery pressure (RV to RA pressure gradient), degree of RV dilation and dysfunction, and heart rate. In patients with pulmonary hypertension and RV failure, TR is commonly present when such patients present in a decompensated state. Severe RV failure may cause TR to be completely missed on initial examination due to marked distention of the venous system (failure to observe V wave) and absence of respiratory change in the murmur (presence of atrial fibrillation and/or severe RV failure). After therapy, the TR may become clinically evident. When treatment is optimal (e.g., conversion to normal sinus rhythm, following substantial diuresis, or rate control in atrial fibrillation), the TR may completely resolve.

An early mid-diastolic tricuspid murmur may be noted in patients with substantial TR. This murmur represents diastolic flow across the open tricuspid valve. The murmur usually is medium to low frequency. It is best heard at the lower left sternal border (fourth to fifth interspace) and follows the tricuspid opening snap or $S_3$, if present. It commonly augments with inspiration.

### Tricuspid Stenosis

In TS, the opening snap is generated by the tricuspid valve. Characteristically, this sound is best heard at the lower left sternal border and increases in intensity with inspiration. There usually is a wider $A_2$–opening snap interval than in mitral stenosis. The problem in clinical detection of the tricuspid opening snap is that virtually all patients with TS have coexisting mitral stenosis. Therefore, two opening snaps may be present, usually superimposed. Clues to tricuspid origin include respiratory variation in opening snap intensity and maximal loudness at the lower sternal border. Patients with rheumatic TS will have a tricuspid opening snap and diastolic rumble on examination. The jugular A wave should be very prominent (in the absence of atrial fibrillation). The TS rumble may be somewhat more high pitched and tends to occur earlier than the mitral rumble; it even can simulate semilunar valve insufficiency. $S_1$ may not be particularly loud in TS.

## ECHOCARDIOGRAPHY

Echocardiography plays a major role in the diagnosis of right heart disease. A complete echocardiogram also allows for differentiation between acute and chronic cor pulmonale and their differentiation from right heart disease secondary to left heart disease. With echocardiography, the diagnosis of RV enlargement, dysfunction, and hypertrophy can be made and its severity determined.

Two-dimensional (2-D) and Doppler echocardiography are the most valuable techniques, but M-mode echocardiography may play a complementary diagnostic role in a few specific situations. Transesophageal echocardiography (TEE) is used less commonly in the diagnosis of right heart disease, but it may have an important role in critically ill patients with suspected pulmonary embolism and patients with suspected right-sided masses and infective endocarditis.

### Pulmonary Hypertension and Cor Pulmonale

### M-Mode Echocardiography

M-mode echocardiography is used to determine RV dimensions and wall thickness and to evaluate septal motion patterns characteristic of RV volume or pressure overload.

Measurement of the RV dimension using M-mode echocardiography is performed from the parasternal short-axis view at the level of the tricuspid valve or from the parasternal long-axis view at the level of the mitral leaflet tips (13). This provides an estimate of RV size, but the complex shape of the RV precludes its use as an absolute determinant of RV size and volume. Because of the difficulties in determining the outer edge of the thin RV free-wall endocardium, measurements for defining degrees of hypertrophy have not been established. The normal RV free wall measures 0.2 to 0.5 cm in diastole and is considered abnormal if >0.5 cm. These measurements have a sensitivity of 93% and specificity of 95% for predicting elevated RV systolic pressure. However, in some cases, the sensitivity may be lower because the RV response to pressure overload occasionally is dilation instead of hypertrophy.

The frame rate and time resolution afforded by M-mode echocardiography makes it ideal for examination of septal motion patterns to differentiate RV enlargement or dysfunction due to volume overload from that due to pressure overload. RV pressure overload in the absence of significant volume overload leads to a shift of the septum toward the LV that is manifest during late systole and early diastole, resulting in a flattened septum that resumes its usual shape during mid and late diastole (14). Elevated RV systolic pressure leads to a prolonged RV upstroke. As a result, the pressure in the RV exceeds the pressure in the LV during late systole and into early diastole. This pattern of motion is seen predominantly in patients with moderate and severe degrees of RV hypertension (pulmonary artery pressure >45 mm Hg). However, it may be absent in patients with elevated LV end-diastolic pressure. It is important to keep in mind that in chronic pressure overload, the RV response also is dilation and TR that can lead to a mixed pattern of volume and pressure overload.

M-mode motion pattern of the pulmonic valve may help differentiate whether RV hypertension is secondary to outflow obstruction or pulmonary hypertension. Pulmonary hypertension leads to mid-systolic closure of the pulmonic valve and loss of the normal A wave. This is seen in approximately 30% to 60% of cases, but has a specificity >90%. In contrast, in pulmonic valve stenosis the A wave is increased (>7 mm) and the mid-systolic closure of the valve is absent.

### Two-Dimensional Echocardiography

Two-dimensional echocardiography allows for differentiation between acute and chronic cor pulmonale. With acute cor pulmonale, the RV commonly has normal dimensions and wall thickness. Usually there is RV dysfunction characterized by global decrease in contractility. The two most common etiologies of acute RV dysfunction are pulmonary embolism and RV infarction. If acute RV dysfunction is suspected, the LV must be examined carefully for concomitant LV dysfunction. The RV and RA must be examined carefully for the presence of thrombus, which is seen occasionally in patients with pulmonary embolism.

Chronic pressure overload may lead to RV hypertrophy and dilation over time. Distortion of the interventricular septum during systole is seen with severe pressure overload. This leads to a D-shaped LV during late systole in the parasternal short-axis view (Fig. 5.4). With purely volume overload, distortion of the septum is seen during diastole. The increased

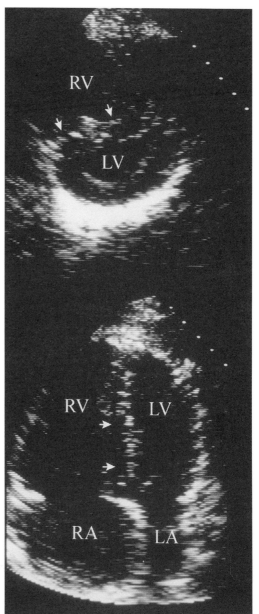

A

FIG. 5.4. Severe cor pulmonale. **A:** Transthoracic short-axis and four-chamber views in a 32-year-old woman with chronic recurrent pulmonary embolism demonstrate severe dilation of the right heart chambers and abnormal septal motion *(arrows)* consistent with right ventricular pressure overload (estimated pulmonary artery systolic pressure 75 mm Hg). After successful pulmonary thromboendarterectomy, pulmonary hypertension and right heart enlargement and dysfunction significantly improved to near normal values.

*(continued on next page)*

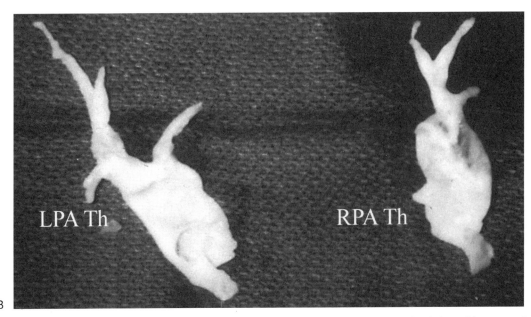

B

**FIG. 5.4.** *Continued.* **B:** Note the large, branching, multiple, and well-organized thrombi removed from the left (LPA Th) and right (RPA Th) pulmonary arteries. (See Color Figure 5.4B.)

volume returning to the RV leads to flattening or inversion of the septum and a diastolic D-shaped LV. During systole, the distortion of the septum is corrected and there is rapid anterior movement of the septum. This is analogous to the paradoxic septal motion seen by M-mode echocardiography.

RV hypertrophy, predominantly of the RV free wall, can be seen with 2-D imaging. Two-dimensional imaging is less reliable than M-mode imaging for assessment of RV hypertrophy because of its slower frame rate and decreased endocardial resolution.

Chronic pulmonary hypertension will lead to dilation of the pulmonary artery (>3 cm). In these patients, the pulmonary artery usually is visualized easily in the parasternal short-axis view.

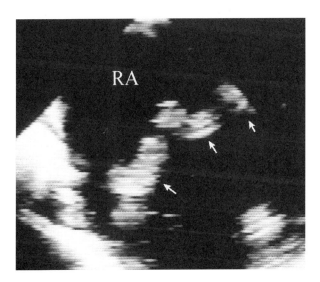

**FIG. 5.5.** Free-floating right atrial thrombi. Transesophageal echocardiographic four-chamber view focused on the right atrium (RA) demonstrates multiple and freely mobile (swirling) thrombi *(arrows)*. This patient had associated severe RA and right ventricular enlargement and dysfunction and multiple lung perfusion defects consistent with pulmonary embolism.

Two-dimensional echocardiography plays an important role in the detection of RA or RV thrombi. The presence of thrombi in the right heart, especially in the RA, has two important etiologies: (i) venous thromboembolism and (ii) *in situ* formation. Venous thromboembolism is characterized by a migrating or transient thrombus seen in the RA, RV, or pulmonary arteries. These thrombi are mobile, irregular, and free-floating masses (often prolapsing across the tricuspid valve) (Fig. 5.5). They generally do not have a point of attachment, but rarely are attached to a Chiari network. Thrombi can be visualized across a patent foramen ovale, leading to paradoxic embolism (these patients generally have pulmonary and RA hypertension and evidence of cor pulmonale).

*In situ* thrombus formation has two principal mechanisms: (i) blood stasis and (ii) endocardial damage. Blood stasis occurs in atrial fibrillation, RA dilation and dysfunction, and cardiomyopathies involving the RV. Endocardial damage occurs with placement of central venous and Swan-Ganz catheters, ventriculoatrial shunts, and temporary or permanent pacing or automatic implantable cardioverter-defibrillator electrodes. An *in situ* thrombus usually is a minimally or nonmobile mass. The thrombus has distinct margins with a broad base and is adhered to the atrial wall or catheter (Fig. 5.6). Uncommonly, RA thrombi can form around indwelling right heart catheters or wires (Fig. 5.7). Awareness of the presence and echocardiographic characteristics of normal right heart variants, such as the eustachian valve, Chiari network, and the moderator band, should avoid misinterpretation of these structures as abnormal right heart masses or thrombi (15).

### Continuous and Pulsed Wave Doppler

Determination of transvalvular gradients using continuous wave Doppler peak velocities allows for quantification of pressure differences between adjacent chambers or structures. Pulsed and continuous wave tracings

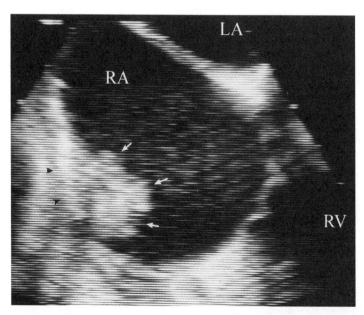

**FIG. 5.6.** *In situ* right atrial wall thrombus. Transesophageal echocardiographic four-chamber view focused in the right atrium (RA) demonstrates a large mass *(arrows)* attached to the RA lateral wall *(arrowheads)*. This patient had an RA catheter tip extending to the atrial wall and mass. Pulmonary perfusion scan was of low probability for pulmonary embolism. This mass was confirmed to be an organized thrombus. LA, left atrium; RV, right ventricle.

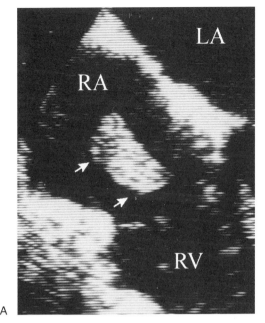

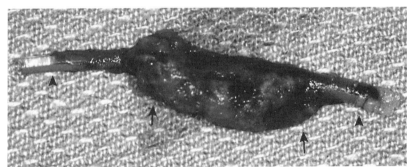

**FIG. 5.7.** Right atrial thrombus attached to an indwelling catheter. **A:** Transesophageal echocardiographic four-chamber view in a patient with a central venous catheter demonstrates a large and elongated mass *(arrows)* in the right atrium. A linear echolucency across the long axis of the mass consistent with the catheter lumen was demonstrated (not well appreciated in this figure). **B:** A well-organized thrombus *(arrows)* attached to and surrounding a catheter *(arrowheads).* The patient had a high-probability perfusion scan for pulmonary emboli. Abbreviations as in previous figures. (See Color Figure 5.7B.)

also are helpful for locating intracardiac shunts, assessing stenotic valves, and evaluating RV diastolic function.

Pulmonary hypertension can be quantified using a variety of Doppler techniques. The most common and most accurate method uses the simplified Bernoulli equation ($\Delta P = 4V^2$, where P = pressure and V = peak TR velocity) to determine the gradient between RV and RA (16). This calculated pressure is added to an estimate of RA pressure to obtain the RV systolic pressure, which is equal to the pulmonary artery systolic pressure in the absence of pulmonary artery or valve stenosis. Because TR is present in up to 80% of normal individuals and in >90% of those with pulmonary hypertension, pulmonary artery systolic pressure can be estimated in the majority of patients (17).

If TR is not present or the TR continuous wave tracing is not well defined, the time to peak velocity of the pulmonary outflow (acceleration time) or the RV isovolumic relaxation time can be used as indicators of pulmonary hypertension. There is a linear relationship between mean pulmonary artery pressure and time to peak velocity. An acceleration time <80 ms is highly predictive of pulmonary hypertension. This method is uncommonly used because it is less reliable. Many clinicians find it most useful if acceleration time is normal (>110 ms). The pulmonary artery flow velocity curve may show a mid-systolic reduction in flow that correlates with the mid-systolic closure of the pulmonary valve seen by M-mode echocardiography.

Serial postoperative echocardiographic studies are valuable for follow-up of patients after pulmonary thromboendarterectomy to assess reduction in pulmonary artery pressures. Serial studies also are performed during medical treatment of primary pulmonary hypertension to evaluate the response to vasodilator therapy.

### *Transesophageal Echocardiography*

Transesophageal imaging of the main and right or left pulmonary arteries allows for identification of large pulmonary emboli in patients who are hemodynamically compromised with evidence of RV dysfunction by transthoracic imaging. The percentage of patients with a massive pulmonary embolism that will be detectable by TEE imaging is not known, but in one series thrombi were detected in 44 of 56 patients (18). TEE is superior to transthoracic echocardiography (TTE) for detection and characterization of RA masses and their differentiation from normal variants (Figs. 5.5–5.7).

### **Right Ventricular Systolic Dysfunction and Dilation**

#### *M-Mode Echocardiography*

RV volume overload leads to striking changes in septal motion. The increase in volume leads to increased RV diastolic pressure. This causes displacement of the septum toward the LV as the LV diastolic pressure is ex-

ceeded and produces the characteristic flattened septum during mid diastole. During systole, the pressure difference reverses and the septum resumes its normal contour. Therefore, there is a paradoxic posterior diastolic motion and systolic anterior motion of the septum. This pattern of septal motion will be less prominent when pressure and volume overload occur in combination. Because of the septal interdependence on right- and left-sided diastolic pressures, it usually is not seen with mild volume overload and is seen in only about 50% of those with moderate volume overload.

### *Two-Dimensional Echocardiography*

Two-dimensional echocardiography using multiple views is the most accurate method for evaluating both RV size and systolic function, as well as for assessing the tricuspid and pulmonic valves.

The RV has a complex shape that makes it difficult to obtain simple measurements that can be used to calculate its size and volume. Therefore, the RV must be examined in multiple views and a visual estimate of its size made. The LV provides a valuable comparison in the apical four-chamber view. One method compares RV area to LV area in the four-chamber view (Fig. 5.4). With mild dilation, RV area remains less than LV area. In severe dilation, RV area exceeds LV area. The apex of the RV should be located short of the LV apex by approximately one third of the distance from the base to the apex. Any alteration from this pattern suggests the possibility of RV enlargement. False-positive results can occur if the transducer probe is not located over the LV apex. False-negative results can occur when the LV is concurrently enlarged.

Systolic RV function is more commonly visually estimated than calculated. Difficulties measuring RV volume have made methods for measuring ejection fraction inaccurate. Using nuclear techniques, the normal RV ejection fraction is ≥40%. One method utilizes the excursion of the tricuspid valve annulus in systole. RV function is considered normal if systolic annular excursion toward the RV apex is >2 cm. This method has a good correlation with ejection fraction determined by nuclear methods ($R = 0.92$). RV annular systolic excursion ≤5 mm indicates significant RV dysfunction. Precise RV ejection fraction is rarely determined by echocardiography, and normal values are not standardized.

Two-dimensional echocardiography provides useful diagnostic and prognostic information in patients with suspected RV infarction complicating LV posteroinferior myocardial infarction. Recent data suggest that patients with posteroinferior infarcts and RV dysfunction have a higher incidence of cardiogenic shock, complete heart block, recurrent myocardial infarction, and mortality. The poor prognosis of these patients appears to be independent of LV function (6,19).

RA enlargement occurs with volume overload and chronically elevated RA pressure. An estimate of RA pressure can be made using the diameter and degree of inspiratory collapse of the inferior vena cava (IVC) (20). RA pressure is <5 mm Hg if the IVC is small (<1.5 cm) and collapses with inspiration; 5 to 10 mm Hg if the IVC measures 1.5 to 2.5 cm and collapses >50% with inspiration; 10 to 15 mm Hg if the IVC is of normal size and collapses <50% with inspiration; 15 to 20 mm Hg if the IVC is >2.5 cm and collapses <50%; and >20 mm Hg if the hepatic veins are dilated and the IVC does not collapse with inspiration. Failure of the IVC to collapse with a sniff indicates RA pressure >20 mm Hg. This method is not accurate if the patient is using positive-pressure ventilation. Also, patients with severely elevated RA pressure often show doming of the atrial septum toward the LA. RA hypertension also may lead to coronary sinus dilation. Anomalies such as ASD, persistent left superior vena cava, and unroofed coronary sinus are associated with a dilated coronary sinus and may lead to elevated RA pressures.

In patients with unexplained RV dilation, an ASD should be considered. False-positive results are common in the apical four-chamber view, due to echo dropout at the level of the fossa ovalis. This is the result of the fossa ovalis being parallel to the echo beam. The subcostal view allows imaging of the atrial septum in a perpendicular plane, but image resolution is inadequate for diagnosing small or moderate size septal defects. Therefore, the specificity of the technique for diagnosing ASD is decreased. Color Doppler interrogation of the septum is a useful adjunct.

### Continuous and Pulsed Wave Doppler

Doppler evaluation in the presence of chronic RV dilation and dysfunction is primarily useful for evaluation of pulmonary hypertension. Pulsed wave interrogation of the hepatic veins can be used to estimate RA pressure in a manner similar to pulmonary venous inflow for estimation of LA pressure. Principles used for evaluation of LV diastolic function can be applied to the RV. With pulmonary hypertension and RV hypertrophy, there will be a decrease in the E wave and increase in the A wave velocity consistent with abnormal RV relaxation. With further progression, the E wave becomes elevated until a restrictive pattern with an elevated E wave and a decreased A wave is seen (21). Systolic, diastolic, and atrial reversal of hepatic vein inflow in patients with RA hypertension will show changes similar to those seen in pulmonary vein inflow of patients with LA hypertension. Pulsed wave Doppler also can be used to confirm the presence of interatrial shunting through a patent foramen ovale or ASD.

### Color Doppler

Color Doppler often is used as the initial screening technique to determine whether significant valvular regurgitation or stenosis is present in patients with RV dilation. Color Doppler also is a useful technique for detecting ASD or patent foramen ovale. False-positive results are not uncommon with color flow because IVC flow is directed along the interatrial septum. Suspected patent foramen ovale or ASD should be confirmed with agitated saline contrast evaluation.

### Stress Echocardiography

Stress echocardiography is rarely helpful for diagnosis of cardiac ischemia in patients with RV dysfunction. Patients with pulmonary hypertension secondary to mitral stenosis can be evaluated with stress echocardiography to determine whether an increase in pulmonary artery pressure warrants mitral valvuloplasty or replacement.

## Pulmonic Valve Stenosis

Pulmonic stenosis is primarily congenital and, therefore, usually diagnosed in childhood. Occasionally patients will be followed for years with the diagnosis of benign murmur that later is diagnosed by echocardiography as pulmonic stenosis as the severity increases.

### M-Mode Echocardiography

Pulmonic valve stenosis, in contrast to pulmonary hypertension, usually has an exaggerated A wave and no mid-systolic closure of the pulmonic valve. When these findings are seen in the presence of other signs of RV pressure overload, pulmonic stenosis should be suspected. The major limitation of these findings is the frequent inability to visualize the pulmonary valve.

### Two-Dimensional Echocardiography

Imaging of the pulmonic valve from the transthoracic approach is limited. The best images are obtained from the parasternal short-axis view with the imaging plane parallel to the RV outflow tract. Detected abnormalities include pulmonic valvular stenosis, pulmonary arterial bands, RV dynamic outflow obstruction, and pulmonary arterial dilation. Imaging resolution limitations of this technique decrease its sensitivity and speci-

ficity in the detection of these conditions. There are multiple variants of congenital pulmonic valvular stenosis. The most common form of isolated pulmonic stenosis is a central orifice with either a single or no commissures. This valve shows parallel movement of the leaflet tips during early systole as opposed to the leaflet tips moving away from each other, as in a normal valve. During systole, the valve has a domed appearance with either a central or concentric orifice. In the Noonan syndrome, the valve and proximal pulmonary artery may be dysplastic, with thickened deformed leaflets and a concentric orifice. Pulmonary valves also may be unicuspid, bicuspid, or quadricuspid. The stenotic valve in carcinoid disease will appear fixed in position, with thickened and retracted leaflets (22).

The pulmonary artery should be evaluated for the presence of pulmonary artery dilation. It is not uncommon for patients to develop left pulmonary artery dilation because the poststenotic jet is directed toward the left. This dilation usually is of little clinical significance but may lead to rupture and the need for repair.

### Continuous and Pulsed Wave Doppler

The severity of pulmonic valve stenosis is defined by the presence of a pressure gradient across the pulmonic valve. The pulmonic valve gradient is determined by applying the simplified Bernoulli equation to the continuous wave Doppler peak velocity (Fig. 5.8A). Mild pulmonic stenosis is defined as a peak gradient <30 mm Hg. The stenosis is severe when the gradient exceeds 50 mm Hg. Treatment with balloon valvotomy or surgery is recommended for patients with cardiac symptoms and for asymptomatic patients with gradients >50 mm Hg (23). There is disagreement about the treatment of asymptomatic patients with valve gradients between 30 and 50 mm Hg. Determining the area of a stenotic pulmonic valve can be performed using the continuity equation. The peak pulmonic flow velocity using continuous wave Doppler and

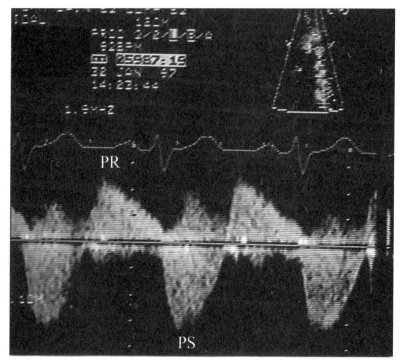

A

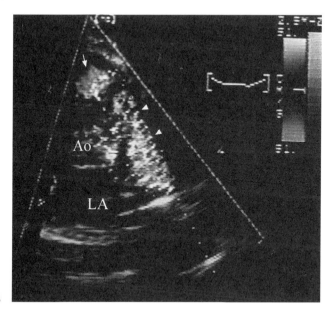

B

**FIG. 5.8.** Pulmonic stenosis and regurgitation due to carcinoid syndrome. **A:** At the pulmonic valve level, the continuous wave Doppler pattern confirms the presence of significant pulmonary stenosis (peak velocity 3.5 m/sec and gradient 49 mm Hg) and regurgitation (short pressure half-time). **B:** Color Doppler recordings from the basilar short-axis view at the pulmonic valve level demonstrate an acceleration zone *(arrow)* at the right ventricular (RV) outflow tract and high-turbulence mosaic color Doppler pattern above the pulmonic valve *(arrowheads)*. These features suggest pulmonic valve stenosis. (See Color Figure 5.8B.)

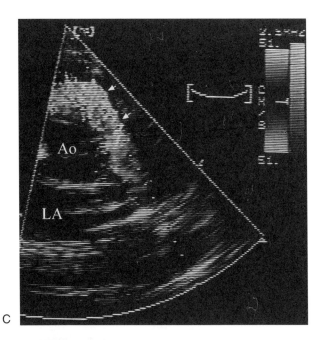

C

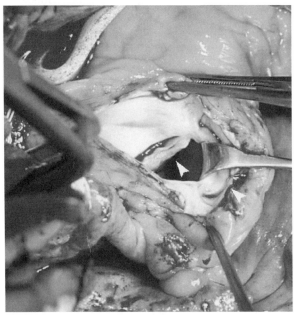

D

**FIG. 5.8.** *Continued.* **C:** At the pulmonic valve level, the color Doppler short-axis view demonstrates a regurgitant jet width that occupies the entire RV outflow tract. This feature is consistent with severe pulmonary regurgitation. **D:** At surgery, the pulmonic valve demonstrated a shaggy appearance with severe thickening, marked stiffness, and incomplete closure *(arrowhead)*. (See Color Figures 5.8C and 5.8D.)

the velocity in the RV outflow tract using pulsed wave Doppler usually are obtained from the basal parasternal short-axis view. The largest source of error occurs in measuring the diameter of the RV outflow tract because of the dropout in the anterior portion of the pulmonary artery. Therefore, the pulmonic valve area usually is not used to determine the severity of pulmonic valve stenosis.

It is not uncommon for patients with pulmonic stenosis to have a dynamic RV outflow tract gradient, which results from RV hypertrophy secondary to chronic pressure over-load. The dynamic gradient can be diagnosed with pulsed wave interrogation of the RV outflow tract. A dagger-shaped signal also can be seen commonly with continuous wave Doppler tracing.

### Color Doppler

Color Doppler is useful for identifying an acceleration zone, the vena contracta (the narrowest jet height or width), and a poststenotic jet (Fig. 5.8B). Occasionally the pulmonic valve is not well visualized, and not uncommonly an assessment of the valve structure is made during surgery or postmortem (Fig. 5.8D). Identification of these color Doppler parameters of a stenotic jet complements the pulse and continuous wave Doppler findings. Color Doppler can be helpful for localizing pre- and postvalvular stenosis secondary to bands that are difficult to visualize with 2-D echocardiography.

## Pulmonic Regurgitation

### Two-Dimensional Echocardiography

Mild and moderate PR are characterized by normal RV dimensions and systolic function. Hemodynamically significant PR will lead to RV dilation. Chronic RV volume overload from severe PR eventually will lead to RV systolic dysfunction and TR.

### Pulsed and Continuous Wave Doppler

Doppler evaluation of the pulmonic valve is useful to characterize the pattern of pressure decay between the pulmonary artery and RV and to determine regurgitant volume. The continuous wave signal of the PR jet will display a slow decay in mild to moderate regurgitation. As the regurgitation becomes more severe, the pulmonary artery and RV pressures become nearly equal at end-diastole, leading to a steeper decay slope and shorter pressure half-time (Fig. 5.8A). A decay slope

>3 m/s is associated with significant regurgitation (24).

The pulsed wave signal can be utilized to determine RV stroke volume. In the absence of significant left-sided valvular disease, LV stroke volume determined from the LV outflow tract can be subtracted from the RV outflow tract stroke volume to obtain the regurgitant volume. Because of difficulties in measuring the diameter of the RV outflow tract, this method is seldom used and values for severity have not been determined.

### Color Doppler

Severity of PR is assessed by comparing the relative diameter of the regurgitant jet to the diameter of the RV outflow tract at the pulmonary valve (Fig. 5.8C). The length of the jet also is taken into consideration. One study suggested that a jet length <20 mm was unlikely to be heard on physical examination, and only jets >20 mm were likely to be associated with significant heart disease. Another method that has correlated well with calculated regurgitant fraction is the regurgitant jet area indexed to body surface area. Mild regurgitation was associated with an index $<0.64 \pm 0.60$ cm/m$^2$ and severe with an index of $2.2 \pm 1.67$ cm/m$^2$. Finally, continuous wave Doppler velocity decay slope >3 m/s has correlated with significant PR defined as regurgitant jet length >20 mm or jet area >1.5 cm$^2$ (24). It is important to remember that trace to mild PR is seen in 78% to 92% of normal subjects.

## Tricuspid Regurgitation

### Two-Dimensional Echocardiography

Transthoracic imaging of the tricuspid valve is important for determining the etiology of tricuspid valve disease. Tricuspid vegetations can be seen in either the TTE parasternal or transgastric TEE RV inflow view or from the TTE or TEE four-chamber view. From these views, significant thickening or calcification of the annulus or leaflets and congenital anomalies such as tricuspid valve dysplasia or Ebstein anomaly can be detected.

TR is most often functional due to RV and annular enlargement, but also may occur secondary to conditions affecting the valve structure. Structural abnormalities often are detectable with TTE. Tricuspid vegetations and/or perforations often are seen from the RV inflow and four-chamber views. Rheumatic heart disease leads to thickened leaflets and commissural fusion causing both stenosis and regurgitation. The leaflets may be tethered from papillary or chordal thickening and retraction leading to more severe TR. With carcinoid disease, the leaflets appear thickened and retracted, with a fixed orifice that is stenotic and regurgitant (Fig. 5.9A).

Several factors are related to the severity of regurgitation, including annular dimension, magnitude of apical leaflet displacement, chordal tethering, malcoaptation, and incomplete coaptation. These factors should be considered in addition to the Doppler data for determining regurgitant severity.

### Pulsed and Continuous Wave Doppler

Pulsed wave Doppler interrogation of tricuspid valve inflow and hepatic vein flow patterns can be useful for evaluating diastolic RV function and assessing the severity of regurgitant flow.

When evaluating the severity of TR, the hepatic vein flow can be utilized. In moderate TR, there will be a reduction in normal systolic flow; in severe TR, systolic flow will be absent or reversed. Finally, the TR signal in severe TR will be as dense as the diastolic in-

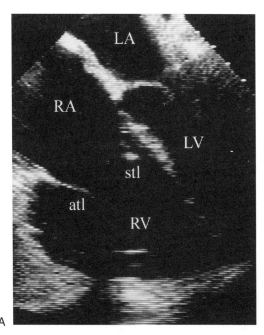
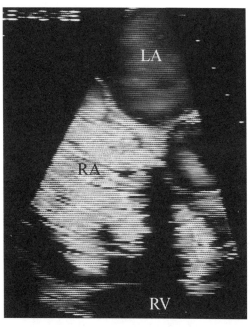

A                                                                                             B

**FIG. 5.9.** Tricuspid regurgitation due to carcinoid syndrome. **A:** Transesophageal echocardiographic four-chamber view during systole (note the closed mitral valve) demonstrates severe dilation of the right heart chambers, and thickened and fixed open anterior (atl) and septal (stl) tricuspid leaflets. **B:** Color Doppler four-chamber view demonstrates a large regurgitant jet occupying the entire atria, consistent with severe tricuspid regurgitation. (See Color Figure 5.9B.)

flow signal, and there will often be a V wave or early reduction in velocity during the latter half of systole as the RV and RA pressures equalize (25).

### Color Doppler

When assessing the severity of TR, the indexes of severity used for the mitral valve cannot be applied directly. The size and length of a regurgitant jet are related to momentum, which is the product of mass and velocity. Velocity is increased relative to the pressure gradient across the valve. Because the RV is generally a lower pressure chamber, regurgitation of a similar volume of blood will appear smaller in the RA than in the LA. Conversely, in the presence of severe pulmonary hypertension, a jet may appear larger and longer in relation to the RA despite a smaller volume of regurgitation (26). With this in mind, it is clear that the color Doppler flow area should not be the sole determinate of the severity of TR. Previously described features, such as valvular morphology, atrial size, hepatic vein flow, and pulmonary artery pressure, should be included in the assessment.

The optimal method for determining the severity of TR should be widely applicable and allow the reader to differentiate between large and small regurgitant volumes. RV angiography is not the optimal gold standard because the catheter may increase the severity of TR. Grossman et al. compared the jet area and proximal flow convergence to RV angiography as the gold standard for differentiating between mild to moderate (grade 1 to 2) and severe (grade 3) TR. They found that the proximal isovelocity surface area radius (PISA) at an aliasing velocity of 28 or 41 cm/s was comparable to either jet area or jet length, but all were better than the ratio of jet area to RA area. All were 87% accurate, but the jet area percentage was only 79% accurate. Cutoff values for severe regurgitation were a PISA radius of 10.6 mm for a Nyquist limit of 28 cm/s;

PISA radius of 6.8 mm for a Nyquist limit of 41 cm/s; jet area of 10.6 cm$^2$; and jet length of 5.3 cm (27). It has been shown that a TR jet to RA area <34% has not required annuloplasty or replacement in 95% of cases. A jet to RA area ratio >40% denotes severe TR (Fig. 5.9B). These latter criteria are identical to those used for assessment of MR severity. A recent study demonstrated that vena contracta width ≥6.5 mm detects severe TR with 88.5% sensitivity and 93% specificity (28).

### Transesophageal Echocardiography

TEE is useful primarily for further determination of the etiology of TR if it is not well defined by TTE. TEE imaging of the tricuspid valve is superior to TTE imaging in some cases where vegetations and valve perforations are the suspected causes.

## Tricuspid Stenosis

### Two-Dimensional Echocardiography

TS is most commonly due to rheumatic heart disease. Two-dimensional imaging demonstrates thickening, retraction, and tethering of the tricuspid leaflets similar to that seen in rheumatic mitral stenosis (Fig. 5.10A) (29). The RA is enlarged in cases of at least moderate TS and if there is significant coexisting TR. Because of the anterior location of the tricuspid valve, determining the valve area by planimetry by 2-D imaging is difficult and unreliable as a measure of severity. Doppler information about the transvalvular gradient is essential because valves that appear to have severe stenosis in 2-D imaging may have low gradients. With carcinoid syndrome, the leaflets may appear thickened and shortened, with significant immobility. In severe cases, they may remain fixed in a partially open position throughout the cardiac cycle (Fig. 5.9A). Loeffler disease also will cause thickening of the tricuspid valve, resulting in stenosis and regurgita-

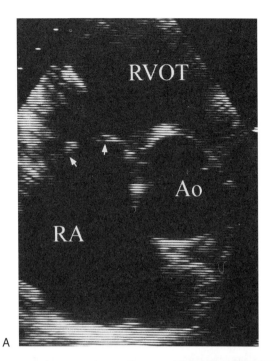

A

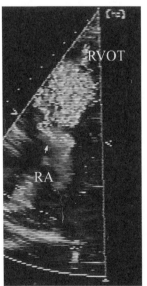

B

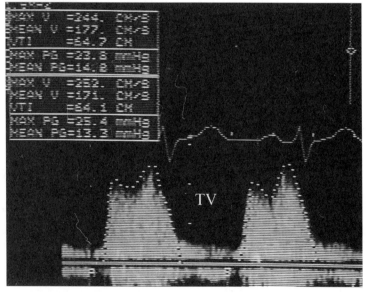

C

**FIG. 5.10.** Tricuspid stenosis due to carcinoid syndrome. **A:** Transthoracic short-axis view demonstrates diffuse thickening, retraction, and doming mobility *(arrows)* of the anterior and septal tricuspid leaflets. Associated severely dilated right atrium is noted. Color Doppler demonstrated moderate tricuspid regurgitation. **B:** Color Doppler image at the tricuspid valve level demonstrates a large acceleration zone *(arrow)* and highly turbulent (mosaic pattern) tricuspid valve inflow. **C:** Continuous wave Doppler tracing confirmed the presence of severe tricuspid stenosis, with peak and mean gradients of 25 and 13 mm Hg, respectively. (See Color Figure 5.10B.)

tion. However, the specificity of 2-D echocardiography for determining the presence and severity of valve thickening, especially if mild, is unknown and probably limited. Differentiating the cause of tricuspid valve stenosis based on appearance alone is difficult and requires knowledge of clinical data.

Because >90% of TS cases are associated with rheumatic mitral valve stenosis, RV and RA dilation due to pulmonary hypertension frequently are present.

### Pulse and Continuous Wave Doppler

Continuous wave Doppler has replaced right heart catheterization for determining the hemodynamic consequences and severity of TS. The transvalvular mean gradient across a stenotic tricuspid valve is calculated using the continuous wave time velocity integral of the tricuspid valve inflow. LV outflow tract diameter and left-sided stroke volume can be used to estimate tricuspid valve area by the continuity equation. Mean gradient and valve area are utilized to determine severity and whether the patient should be referred for valvuloplasty or replacement. In general, TS is significant if mean transvalvular gradient is ≥4 mm Hg (Fig. 5.10C). Valve area is used less often for determination of severity, but an area <1.3 cm$^2$ is generally considered significant. The tricuspid inflow pattern also should show a prolonged deceleration of the E wave slope (29,30).

### Color Doppler

Color Doppler echocardiography for assessment of tricuspid valve stenosis is not as impor-tant as for assessment of TR. An acceleration zone and highly turbulent inflow are suggestive of underlying valve stenosis (Fig. 5.10B).

### Transesophageal Echocardiography

TEE is sometimes superior to TTE for characterizing the etiology of TS. Transthoracic imaging usually is adequate, but occasionally TEE may be needed when the valve cannot be well visualized. Better imaging will allow the echocardiographer to determine whether the patient is a candidate for percutaneous valvuloplasty.

### SUMMARY

Right heart disease includes a wide variety of diagnostic possibilities. Clues found on physical examination are helpful to characterize a specific etiology, but they often are subtle, nonspecific, and frequently only present in advanced disease. Based on a careful history and physical examination, echocardiography should be considered (Table 5.1). Echocardiography will allow for better characterization of a specific abnormality and accurate determination of its severity (Table 5.2).

**TABLE 5.1.** *Class I indications for echocardiography*

1. Suspected pulmonary hypertension
2. Pulmonary emboli and suspected clots in the right atrium or ventricle or main pulmonary artery branches
3. To distinguish cardiac vs. noncardiac etiology of dyspnea in patients in whom clinical and laboratory clues are ambiguous
4. Evaluation and follow-up of pulmonary artery pressure in patients with pulmonary hypertension to evaluate response to treatment
5. Lung disease with clinical suspicion of cardiac involvement (suspected cor pulmonale)
6. Edema with clinical signs of elevated central venous pressure when a potential cardiac etiology is suspected or when central venous pressure cannot be estimated with confidence and clinical suspicion of heart disease is high
7. Dyspnea with clinical signs of heart disease
8. Patient with unexplained hypotension, especially in the intensive care unit
9. Diagnosis and assessment of hemodynamic severity of valvular stenosis, or regurgitation
10. Assessment of left ventricular and right ventricular size, function, and/or hemodynamics in a patient with valvular stenosis or regurgitation
11. Assessment of changes in hemodynamic severity and ventricular compensation in patients with known valvular stenosis or regurgitation during pregnancy
12. Reevaluation of asymptomatic patients with severe stenosis or severe regurgitation
13. Reevaluation of patients with mild to moderate valvular regurgitation with changing symptoms
14. Reevaluation of patients with mild to moderate valvular regurgitation with ventricular dilation without clinical symptoms
15. Assessment of the effects of medical therapy on the severity of regurgitation and ventricular compensation and function

**TABLE 5.2.** *Stratification of right heart diseases*

| Condition | Mild | Moderate | Severe |
|---|---|---|---|
| Right atrial hypertension | Pressure 10–15 mm Hg if IVC 1.5–2.5 cm and collapses >50% | 15–20 mm Hg if IVC >2.5 cm and collapses <50% | >20 mm Hg if IVC is >2.5 cm and does not collapse. Hepatic veins are dilated. |
| Pulmonary hypertension | Pressure 35–45 mm Hg | 46–60 mm Hg | >60 mm Hg |
| Pulmonic stenosis | Peak gradient <30 mm Hg | 30–50 mm Hg | >50 mm Hg |
| Pulmonic regurgitation | Jet length <10 mm | 10–20 mm | >20 mm |
| Tricuspid stenosis | Mean gradient <2 mm Hg | 2–5 mm Hg | >5 mm Hg |
| Tricuspid regurgitation | Jet/right atrial area <20% | 20%–40% | >40%; jet area >10 cm$^2$; jet length >5.3 cm; PISA radius ≥10 mm for a Nyquist limit of 30 cm/s; PISA radius ≥7 mm for a Nyquist limit of 40 cm/s; vena contracta width ≥6.5 mm |

IVC, inferior vena cava; PISA, proximal isovelocity surface area.

## Pulmonary Hypertension

By the time symptoms develop, the process often is advanced. The early signs are primarily an accentuated $P_2$ and RV heave. At the time of diagnosis, most patients also will exhibit a TR murmur. By the time peripheral edema and cyanosis appear, the process is quite advanced.

Pulmonary artery systolic pressure can be estimated accurately by echocardiography, and the severity of right heart disease can be related to PA pressure. Signs of advanced pulmonary hypertension, including RV dysfunction and dilation, RA dilation, and pulmonary artery dilation, are identified readily. Progression of the disease process and response to therapy can be followed with serial examinations.

## Right Ventricular Dysfunction

RV dysfunction may occur with pulmonary hypertension, TR, PR, and PS or with RV infarction or cardiomyopathy. Physical findings associated with RV dysfunction include elevated neck veins, peripheral edema, and RV $S_3$. RV $S_3$ is differentiated from that of left heart disease by its location adjacent to the lower sternum and because its intensity increases with inspiration. Ascites may be present with advanced dysfunction. Most patients with significant RV dysfunction will have a TR murmur secondary to dilation of the tricuspid annulus. Echocardiography accurately detects moderate or worse degrees of RV dilation and systolic or diastolic dysfunction.

## Pulmonic Stenosis

The most common physical findings in pulmonic stenosis include a crescendo-decrescendo murmur that becomes late peaking with increased severity. The murmur may become louder with inspiration and is heard best in the left upper sternal border. With disease progression, $S_2$ may become widely split, with the systolic murmur continuing through $A_2$. An RV heave may be palpable. RV $S_3$ and elevated A wave are seen only in advanced cases. A pulmonic ejection click that *decreases* with inspiration almost always is present.

The most important findings on echocardiography include valve morphology and a high velocity jet with continuous wave Doppler corresponding to the gradient across the pulmonic valve. Stenosis severity is based upon the transvalvular gradient. Valvuloplasty is recommended in patients with a gradient $\geq$50 mm Hg.

## Pulmonic Regurgitation

PR is characterized on physical examination by a decrescendo diastolic murmur at the second to third left interspace. In nonpulmonary hypertensive PR, the low gradient between PA and RV results in a soft murmur that can be missed easily. Severe PR, although rare, leads to volume overload, and RV dilation and dysfunction. In the late stages, signs of RV failure, including RV $S_3$, TR murmur, and elevated neck veins, will be present.

Mild and moderate PR often is diagnosed first by echocardiography. Color Doppler demonstrating a diastolic regurgitant jet in the RV outflow tract is the most helpful finding for making the diagnosis and is the basis for determination of severity. Other signs of severe PR include dilation of the RV and RA.

## Tricuspid Regurgitation

The physical findings of significant TR include a holosystolic murmur along the left heart border. The murmur typically increases in intensity with inspiration. A prominent V wave is seen on the jugular venous examination, and a pulsatile liver, peripheral edema, or ascites may be present. An RV heave is common if pulmonary hypertension is also present.

Two-dimensional echocardiography is most valuable for evaluating TR etiology. The valve can be examined for the presence of thickening, vegetations, chordal structure and integrity, and congenital abnormalities. Color Doppler is utilized most often for determining the presence and severity of TR. Jet area, ratio of jet to RA area, PISA length, and vena contracta width are the parameters used most commonly to assess TR severity. Other parameters of TR severity include RA enlargement, RA hypertension, abnormal hepatic vein flow patterns, and RV dilation or dysfunction.

## Tricuspid Stenosis

The physical findings associated with TS include an elevated jugular A wave (if the patient remains in sinus rhythm) with a decreased Y descent. A diastolic rumble at the lower sternal border can be heard that increases with inspiration. Peripheral edema and ascites may be present in advanced cases.

The echocardiographic findings can be readily overlooked. TS is associated with rheumatic mitral valve disease in >90% of cases; thus, a diagnosis of mitral or aortic rheumatic disease should prompt careful inspection of the TV valve. Findings include a thickened valve with restricted movement. Continuous wave Doppler forms the basis for determining the severity of stenosis. Patients with significant TS will have RA enlargement and often will demonstrate TR.

## Limitations

The main limitation of the physical examination for assessment of right heart disease is its lack of specificity. During the late stages, many right heart diseases have similar manifestations. Advanced right heart disease from multiple etiologies will lead to RV dilation, RV dysfunction, tricuspid annular dilation, significant TR, and elevated central venous pressures. Therefore, it becomes difficult to determine the primary etiology of disease in its late stages. In this respect, echocardiography is of important complementary diagnostic value to the physical examination.

Two-dimensional imaging of the RV and right-sided valves is limited by the anterior location and shape of the RV. It is difficult to estimate RV volumes because of the complex shape of the RV. This also makes it difficult to estimate RV ejection fraction; therefore, RV function is estimated qualitatively. The right-sided valves are more difficult to image than the left-sided valves. The pulmonary valve is especially difficult to image from any location. The tricuspid valve usually, but not always, is seen better by TEE. The pulmonary valve is equally difficult to image by TEE and TTE.

The most common source of error in estimating pulmonary artery pressure is failure to obtain the true peak TR velocity due to non-coaxial alignment of the Doppler sample and the regurgitant jet. This lead to the underestimation of pressure.

Color Doppler is commonly used to estimate the severity of TR. It is important to remember that there is a wide variation in RV systolic pressure. Because the area of the TR jet is related to the jet momentum, a similar volume of regurgitation will appear as a larger jet if RV pressure is elevated. This is much less of a problem for the LV because there is almost always a large pressure gradient between LV and LA. Other factors, such as the RV systolic pressure and hemodynamic consequences of regurgitation, must be considered when grading the severity of TR. Adjunctive data should include hepatic vein pulsed wave Doppler flow.

## REFERENCES

1. Krowka MJ. Pulmonary hypertension: diagnostics and therapeutics. Mayo Clin Proc 2000;75:625–630.
2. Rich S. Primary pulmonary hypertension. In: Fauci, Braunwald E, Isselbacher KJ, et al., eds. Harrison's principles of internal medicine, 14th ed. New York: McGraw-Hill, 1998;1466–1468.
3. Moraes D, Loscalzo J. Pulmonary hypertension: newer concepts in diagnosis and management. Clin Cardiol 1997 20:676–682.
4. Archibald CJ, Auger WR, Fedullo PF, et al. Long term outcome after pulmonary thromboendarterectomy. Am J Respir Crit Care Med 1999;160:523–528.
5. Criner GJ. Effects of long-term oxygen therapy on mortality and morbidity. Respir Care 2000;45:105–118.
6. Konomi S, Hideaki Y, Hiroaki K, et al. Prognostic significance of persistent right ventricular dysfunction as assessed by radionuclide angiography in patients with inferior wall acute myocardial infarction. Am J Cardiol 2000;85:939–944.
7. Arbulu A, Asfaw I. Tricuspid valvulectomy without prosthetic replacement: ten years of clinical experience. J Thorac Cardiovasc Surg 1981;82:684–691.
8. Pelligrini A, Colombo T, Donatelli F, et al. Evaluation and treatment of secondary tricuspid insufficiency. Eur J Cardiothorac Surg 1992;6:288–296.
9. McGrath LB, Chen C, Bailey BM, et al. Early and late events following tricuspid valve replacement. J Card Surg 1992;7:245–253.
10. Scully HE, Armstrong CS. Tricuspid valve replacement: fifteen years of experience with mechanical prostheses and bioprostheses. J Thorac Cardiovasc Surg 1995;109:1035–1041.
11. Marriott HJL. Bedside cardiac diagnosis. Philadelphia: JB Lippincott, 1993.
12. Greenberger NJ, Hinthorn DR. History taking and physical examination: essentials and clinical correlates. St. Louis: Mosby, 1993.
13. Schiller NB, Shah PM, Crawford MH, et al. Recommendations for quantitation of the left ventricle by two-dimensional echocardiography: American Society of Echocardiography Committee on Standards, Subcommittee on Quantitation of Two-Dimensional Echocardiograms. J Am Soc Echocardiogr 1989;2:358–367.
14. Louie EK, Rich S, Levitsky S, et al. Doppler echocardiographic demonstration of the differential effects of right ventricular pressure and volume overload on left ventricular geometry and filling. J Am Coll Cardiol 1992;19:84–90.
15. Stoddard M, Liddell N, Longaker R, et al. Transesophageal echocardiography: normal variants and mimickers. Am Heart J 1992;124:1587–1598.
16. Currie PJ, Seward JB, Chart K-L, et al. Continuous-wave Doppler determination of right ventricular pressure: a simultaneous Doppler-catheterization study in 127 patients. J Am Coll Cardiol 1985;6:750–756.
17. Singh JP, Evans JC, Levy D. Prevalence and clinical determinants of mitral, tricuspid, and aortic regurgitation (the Framingham heart study). Am J Cardiol 1999;83:892–902.
18. Wittlich N, Raimund E, Andreas E, et al. Detection of central pulmonary emboli by transesophageal echocardiography in patients with severe pulmonary embolism. J Am Soc Echocardiogr 1992;5:515–524.
19. Bowers TR, O'Neill WW, Goldstein JA, et al. Effect of reperfusion on biventricular function and survival after right ventricular infarction. N Engl J Med 1998;338:933–940.
20. Kircher BJ, Himelman RB, Schiller NB. Noninvasive estimation of right atrial pressure from the inspiratory collapse of the inferior vena cava. Am J Cardiol 1990;66:493–496.
21. Ozer N, Tokgozoglu L, Coplu L, et al. Echocardiographic evaluation of left and right ventricular diastolic function in patients with chronic obstructive pulmonary disease. J Am Soc Echocardiogr 2001;14:557–561.
22. Lundin L, Landelius J, Andren B, et al. Transesophageal echocardiography improves the diagnostic value of cardiac ultrasound in patients with carcinoid heart disease. Br Heart J 1990;64:190–194.
23. Bonow RO, Carabello AC, De Leon AC, et al. ACC/AHA guidelines for the management of patients with valvular heart disease. J Am Coll Cardiol 1998;32:1486–1588.
24. Lei MH, Chen JJ, Ko YL, et al. Reappraisal of quantitative evaluation of pulmonary regurgitation and estimation of pulmonary artery pressure by continuous wave Doppler echocardiography. Cardiology 1995;86:249–256.
25. Schiller NB. Echocardiographic evaluation of the severity of tricuspid valve regurgitation: 29 considerations useful in recognizing hemodynamically important lesions. Isr J Med Sci 1996;32:853–867.
26. Nagueh SF. Assessment of valvular regurgitation with Doppler echocardiography. Cardiol Clin 1998;16:405–419.

27. Grossman G, Stein M, Kochs M, et al. Comparison of the proximal flow convergence method for the assessment of the severity of tricuspid regurgitation. Eur Heart J 1998;19:652–659.

28. Tribouiloy CM, Enriquez-Sarano M, Bailey KR, et al. Quantification of tricuspid regurgitation by measuring the width of the vena contracta with Doppler color flow imaging: a clinical study. J Am Coll Cardiol 2000; 36:472–478.

29. Pearlman AS. Role of echocardiography in the diagnosis and evaluation of severity of mitral and tricuspid stenosis. Circulation 1991;84[Suppl I]:I-193–I-197.

30. Blaustein AS, Ramanathan A. Tricuspid valve disease. Cardiol Clin 1998;16:551–672.

# 6

# The Patient with Mitral Regurgitation

Phoebe Ashley, *Carlos A. Roldan, and †Jonathan Abrams

*Department of Internal Medicine, University of New Mexico School of Medicine; and Department of
Internal Medicine, Veterans Affairs Medical Center, Albuquerque, New Mexico; *Department of Internal
Medicine, University of New Mexico School of Medicine; and Department of Internal Medicine, Veterans
Affairs Medical Center, Albuquerque, New Mexico; †Cardiology Division, University of New Mexico
School of Medicine; and Department of Internal Medicine, University Hospital, Albuquerque, New Mexico*

## INTRODUCTION

Mitral regurgitation (MR) is the most diverse of all acquired valvular lesions. The functional anatomy of mitral valve closure is complex; abnormal valve function may result from disease or distortion of the mitral leaflets, the valvular suspensory or supporting "apparatus," or the left ventricle (LV) itself. In addition, multiple pathologic conditions can affect the mitral valve, making MR the most common valve lesion in adults. The presence of MR may be acute, transient, or chronic, and the subsequent hemodynamic sequelae may wax and wane in severity.

## NORMAL ANATOMY AND FUNCTION OF THE MITRAL VALVE

The mitral valve has two major leaflets or cusps: a large anterior leaflet and a smaller posterior leaflet (Fig. 6.1). The anterior leaflet is longer and more mobile than the posterior leaflet; however, the posterior leaflet has a larger area of attachment to the mitral annulus. The two mitral cusps are anchored by a complex network of chordae tendineae that insert at or near the free edges of the leaflets and also attach to the commissural aspects of the valve (Fig. 6.1). The chordae arise from either of the two major papillary muscles in a cascading network of

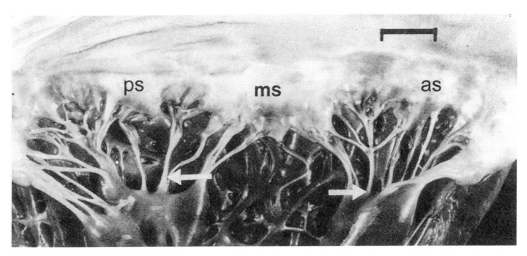

**FIG. 6.1.** Normal mitral valve. Autopsy specimen of a patient with a normal heart. Note the complexity of the chordae tendineae and their fine structure. *Arrows* indicate the cascade of chordae tendineae giving rise to one or more valve scallops. as, anterior scallop; ms, middle scallop; ps, posterior scallop of the posterior mitral leaflet. (From Luca RV, Edwards JE. The floppy mitral valve. Curr Probl Cardiol 1982;7:1, with permission.)

individual chords. The chordae are smooth, delicate strands of connective tissue and are vulnerable to stretching, thickening, foreshortening, and rupture. The papillary muscles are specialized extensions of the LV muscular trabeculae. There is an anterolateral and a posteromedial papillary muscle. *Practical Point: The posteromedial papillary muscle is more vulnerable to ischemia fibrosis, contraction, or rupture.*

## ETIOLOGY

There are a variety of causes of MR (Table 6.1) (1). The major etiologies of acute and chronic MR include myxomatous degeneration of the valve, mitral valve prolapse (MVP), chordal rupture, ischemic heart disease with associated papillary muscle dysfunction, and rheumatic heart disease.

### Myxomatous Mitral Valve Disease and Mitral Valve Prolapse

MVP, usually associated with myxomatous degeneration, affects up to 2% to 3% of adults in industrialized countries, with a 2:1 female predominance. Myxomatous degeneration of the mitral valve is the most common cause of MR in the United States.

The myxomatous appearance of the leaflets in MVP is due to a loss or dissolution of the normal dense collagen fibers (fibrosa), with replacement and invasion of a less sturdy type of connective tissue (spongiosa). The leaflets, chordae tendineae, and annulus all may be affected by myxomatous proliferation. The leaflets are thickened and redundant, and the chordae tendineae become elongated (Fig. 6.2). Both mitral leaflets can be affected in MVP, but the posterior leaflet is more commonly involved.

Prolapse represents abnormal superior systolic displacement of the mitral valve leaflets; one or both of the leaflets extend beyond the normal systolic coaptation point, allowing MR to occur. During systole, individual scallops or an entire leaflet may billow excessively into the left atrium (LA). For severe MR to be present, both leaflets must be affected or one leaflet may be flail, such as in the case of a ruptured chordae tendineae. The stress on the ballooning

**TABLE 6.1.** *Etiologies of acute and chronic mitral regurgitation*

| Acute | Chronic |
|---|---|
| Mitral annular disorders<br>  Infective endocarditis (abscess formation)<br>  Trauma (valvular heart surgery)<br>  Paravalvular leak resulting from interruption<br>    (surgical technical problems of infective<br>    endocarditis) | Inflammatory<br>  Rheumatic heart disease<br>  Healed infective endocarditis<br>  Systemic lupus erythematosus<br>  Ankylosing spondylitis<br>  Scleroderma |
| Mitral leaflet disorders<br>  Myxomatous degeneration<br>Infective endocarditis (perforation or interference<br>  with valve closure by vegetation)<br>Rheumatic heart disease<br>Trauma (tear during percutaneous mitral balloon<br>  valvotomy or penetrating chest injury)<br>Tumors (atrial myxoma)<br>Systemic lupus erythematosus (Libman-Sacks<br>  lesion) | Degenerative<br>  Myxomatous degeneration of leaflets (Barlow click-<br>    murmur syndrome, prolapsing leaflet, mitral valve<br>    prolapse)<br>  Marfan syndrome<br>  Ehlers-Danlos syndrome<br>  Pseudoxanthoma elasticum<br>  Sclerosis and calcification of mitral valve leaflets<br>    and annulus |
| Rupture of chordae tendineae<br>  Idiopathic (e.g., spontaneous)<br>  Myxomatous degeneration (mitral valve prolapse,<br>    Marfan syndrome, Ehlers-Danlos syndrome)<br>  Infective endocarditis<br>  Acute rheumatic fever<br>  Trauma (percutaneous balloon valvotomy, blunt<br>    chest trauma) | Infective<br>  Infective endocarditis affecting normal, abnormal,<br>    or prosthetic mitral valves |
| Papillary muscle disorders<br>  Coronary artery disease (causing dysfunction<br>    and, rarely, rupture)<br>  Acute global left ventricular dysfunction<br>  Infiltrative diseases (amyloidosis, sarcoidosis)<br>  Trauma (blunt chest trauma) | Structural<br>  Ruptured chordae tendineae (spontaneous or<br>    secondary to myocardial infarction, trauma, mitral<br>    valve prolapse, endocarditis)<br>  Rupture or dysfunction of papillary muscle<br>    (ischemia or myocardial infarction)<br>  Dilation of mitral valve annulus and left ventricular<br>    cavity (congestive cardiomyopathies, aneurysmal<br>    dilatation of the left ventricle) |
| Primary prosthetic mitral valve disorders<br>  Porcine cusp perforation (endocarditis)<br>  Porcine cusp degeneration<br>  Mechanical failure (strut fracture)<br>  Immobilization disk or ball of the mechanical<br>    prosthesis by thrombus or pannus | Congenital<br>  Mitral valve clefts or fenestrations<br>  Parachute mitral valve abnormality in association<br>    with<br>      Endocardial cushion defects<br>      Endocardial fibroelastosis<br>      Transposition of the great vessels<br>      Anomalous origin of the left coronary artery |

Adapted from Braunwald E. Braunwald heart disease. A textbook of cardiovascular medicine, 5th ed. Philadelphia: WB Saunders, 1997:1018.

leaflets during ejection may result in additional stretching of the valve tissue and chordae. Thus, prolapse may beget greater prolapse.

The spectrum of MVP ranges from an isolated systolic click in an asymptomatic individual to full-blown, severe myxomatous MR necessitating valve replacement. Serious complications associated with MVP include infective endocarditis, embolic phenomenon, transient cerebral ischemic attacks, gradual progression of MR, LV dilation and dysfunction, atrial fibrillation, congestive heart failure, rupture of a mitral valve chordae, and sudden death (<1% per year).

Most common is an idiopathic abnormality of mitral valve tissue that appears to have its

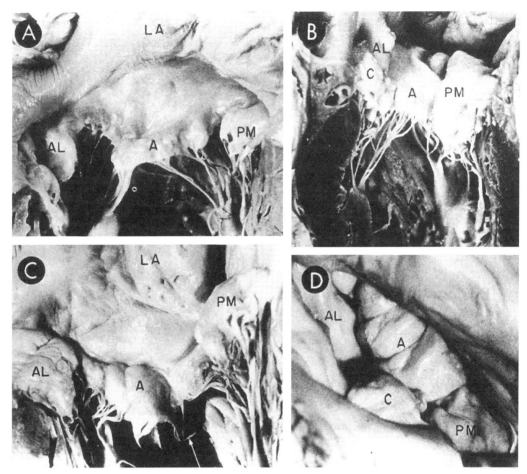

**FIG. 6.2.** Anatomy of mitral valve prolapse. **A:** Note bulging of the outer portion of the anterior leaflet and hooding of the posteromedial and anterolateral scallops of the posterior leaflet. **B:** More advanced degree of prolapse with hooding of the anterior leaflet as well as hooding of all three scallops of the posterior leaflet. **C:** Hooding of the anterior leaflet, and the posteromedial and anterolateral scallops. Two ruptured chordae are attached to the anterior leaflet, with elongated and thinned chordae elsewhere. **D:** Same specimen as in **B** with the mitral valve viewed from the atrium. A, anterolateral leaflet; AL, anterolateral scallop; C, central scallop; LA, left atrium; PM, posteromedial scallop. (From Luca RV, Edwards JE. The floppy mitral valve. Curr Probl Cardiol 1982;7:1, with permission.)

onset after childhood. Primary MVP may be familial. It is commonly associated with thoracic skeletal abnormalities, such as straight spine and pectus excavatum.

Rupture of a chordae tendineae is the most common cause of acute severe MR. Chordal rupture may occur independent of any underlying disease, or it may occur secondary to a variety of disorders, including MVP, endocarditis, connective tissue diseases, rheumatic heart disease, and trauma. Spontaneous rupture of a chordae is most commonly associated with the posterior leaflet. Endocarditis can disrupt chordal function either in the setting of acute valve infection or months to years after bacterial eradication.

Blunt or penetrating trauma can result in acute MR if the mitral leaflets or supporting apparatus are damaged or disrupted; chordal or papillary muscle rupture occurs frequently.

The chordae to one or both leaflets or individual scallops may be involved. The most severe sequelae of ruptured chordae tendineae are experienced in patients with a previously normal heart, with resultant severe acute MR (flail mitral leaflet). If the chordae to only one valve cusp are disrupted, only one of the mitral leaflets or scallops may protrude into the LA. The portion of the valve that prolapses into the atrium may produce a hoodlike deformity, which directs the regurgitant stream opposite to the site of valve prolapse. This "eccentric" jet of blood may produce unusual patterns of murmur radiation.

### Papillary Muscle Dysfunction

A variety of conditions leading to fibrosis, ischemia, or contractile dysfunction of the papillary muscles and surrounding LV muscle can result in MR. Myocardial ischemia is the most common cause of papillary muscle dysfunction, most commonly involving the posteromedial papillary muscle. Papillary muscle dysfunction may be associated with LV dilation and dysfunction, mitral annular dilation, and trauma. Discoordinate LV contractility contributes to the development of ischemic MR. Severe LV wall-motion abnormalities, global LV dilation, or an overt ventricular aneurysm also are likely to involve one of the papillary muscles (the posteromedial most commonly), resulting in MR. The papillary muscles are literally pulled laterally away from their normal alignment in the LV cavity and lose the optimal angle for generation of wall tension, producing prolapse of the mitral valve leaflets (Fig. 6.3).

### Papillary Muscle Rupture

Papillary muscle rupture is a rare complication of acute myocardial infarction (MI)

that generally occurs during the second or third day following infarction. Rupture of the posteromedial papillary muscle is two to three times more common than rupture of the anterolateral papillary muscle. Traumatic papillary muscle rupture is a rare cause of acute severe MR. Acute mitral valve rupture or chordal rupture is uncommon; it usually is found in association with other significant cardiac injury. In the setting of mitral valve injury, rupture of the papillary muscle is the most likely, followed by rupture of the chordae tendineae and avulsion of the valve itself. Papillary muscle rupture may be complete, involving the whole belly of the muscle, or partial, involving one or more apical heads. Early recognition of acute MR, regardless of the cause, is crucial to patient survival.

### Rheumatic Heart Disease

In developing countries, rheumatic heart disease is the primary cause of MR. In the setting of acute rheumatic fever, a diffuse inflammatory reaction involving connective tissue and collagen leads to a pancarditis. In the setting of acute rheumatic fever, MR may result from LV dilation, restricted leaflet mobility, annular dilation, or leaflet prolapse. In the chronic phase of rheumatic valvular heart disease, thickening of the valve leaflets and edges, commissural fusion, as well as tethering of the chordae, prevent the leaflets from reaching the coaptation point, leading to significant MR and often mitral stenosis.

### PATHOPHYSIOLOGY

The pathophysiology of MR may be divided into three stages: acute, chronic compensated, and chronic decompensated. Acute MR is poorly tolerated and frequently results in profound clinical deterioration. When acute, MR results in abrupt or rapid-onset volume overload of the left heart. The preexisting size and compliance of the LA are para-

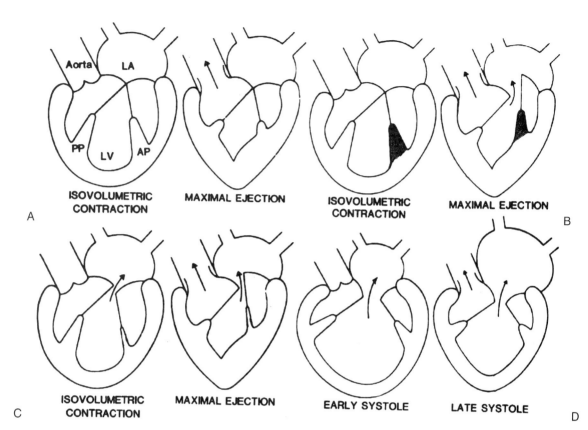

**FIG. 6.3.** Mechanism of mitral regurgitation (MR) caused by papillary muscle dysfunction. **A:** Normal heart. The papillary muscles contract during systole as left ventricular (LV) cavity size diminishes. An intact mitral apparatus prevents reflux of blood from the LV into the left atrium (LA). **B:** Papillary muscle dysfunction. In this diagram, the posterolateral papillary muscle is functionally abnormal (ischemia or infarction) and is unable to maintain valvular apposition during peak systole when LV cavity size is at its nadir. The mitral leaflet(s) protrudes into the LA and mid to late mitral regurgitation occurs. The mitral valve typically remains competent in early systole; therefore, there is no murmur during the first third of systole. **C:** Papillary muscle scarring. In this example, the papillary muscle is fibrotic and/or atrophic, such that even during isovolumic systole it is unable to prevent reflux of blood into the LA because of an inadequate tethering effect on the chordae tendineae. The MR may worsen during ejection. **D:** In this example of a markedly dilated LV, the papillary muscles are displaced laterally and lose their normal alignment within the LV cavity. This may result in inability of the mitral valve to adequately coapt because of abnormal tension on the displacement of the mitral valve apparatus. The resultant murmur of MR is believed to be related to distortion of papillary muscle-ventricular anatomy rather than true dysfunction. (From Burch GE, Depasquale MP, Phillips JH. The syndrome of papillary muscle dysfunction. Am Heart J 1968;75:399, with permission.)

mount in determining the resultant signs and symptoms. A large volume of regurgitation into a normal, noncompliant atrium results in high LA pressures. The LV does not tolerate an acute volume load when compensatory mechanisms of dilation and hypertrophy do not have time to develop; LV diastolic and LA pressures increase markedly. The clinical course of such patients may rapidly decline and result in death.

In the setting of chronic MR, a mild degree of regurgitation produce little derangement in LV function. Moderate and even severe MR, when chronic, may be surprisingly well tolerated for years. In chronic severe MR, LV volume load occurs as the refluxing blood in the

clicks typically sounds like a faint crackling or rustling noise. The clicks often appear to be disassociated from the murmur and may have a metallic quality. When several clicks are present in succession, the resultant sound may be mistaken for a scratchy systolic murmur or friction rub. Finally, clicks often are very faint. Acoustically, they are dissimilar to the far more common low-frequency cardiac sounds (e.g., $S_3$, $S_4$). Most physicians are not accustomed to listening to sounds in the high-frequency range. Multiple clicks do not have a prognostic or diagnostic implication different from that of a single mid-systolic click. *Practical Point: Many patients with MVP have only a mid-systolic click or multiple clicks without a late or holosystolic murmur.*

### Timing of the Click

The mid-systolic click of MVP, in contradistinction to an ejection click, bears no relationship to ejection of blood from the heart. The clicks coincide with prolapse of a leaflet or scallop, after LV systolic size has decreased considerably. Thus, the click normally is found in *mid to late systole* and not during early systole. Some authors favor the term "nonejection click" to emphasize the difference between an ejection click and a sound produced by a stiffened or stenotic semilunar valve. Nevertheless, the click of MVP may occur just after $S_1$, when the onset of the prolapse occurs very early in systole.

When maneuvers that accentuate the discrepancy between the size of the mitral valve and the LV cavity are carried out, the prolapse will appear earlier and the click will move closer to $S_1$. When very early prolapse occurs, the click can move into $S_1$ and a separate sound may not be audible; $S_1$ will appear to be increased in intensity. Whenever one hears a loud "$S_1$" in conjunction with a holosystolic murmur, it should suggest the diagnosis of holosystolic mitral leaflet prolapse. The click moves closer to $S_1$ in the upright posture; the systolic murmur lengthens and the murmur vibrations extend toward $S_1$. Squatting decreases the duration and extent of mitral prolapse by increasing LV volume; both the click and murmur are heard later in systole.

### Opening Snap

Contrary to popular belief, an opening snap occasionally may be present in patients with pure rheumatic MR. This probably is related to thickened, stiff, and distorted mitral leaflets. The opening snap coincides with the opening motion of the anterior leaflet. The presence of an audible opening snap raises the question of coexisting mitral stenosis. In such cases, the intensity of $S_1$ and the presence and length of the diastolic rumble require special attention.

### Systolic Whoops and Honks

Occasionally, patients with MVP develop peculiar loud vibratory or musical systolic murmurs known as whoops or honks. Usually, these murmurs come and go in an intermittent fashion and may suddenly appear and disappear during auscultation. Changes in body position, such as standing or leaning forward, often initiate these murmurs. Typically, the patient will have the classic acoustic findings of mid-systolic MVP, which abruptly becomes more pronounced, initiating a whoop. These murmurs can be so loud that the patient may hear them.

### Murmur of Mitral Regurgitation

The typical murmur of MR is a continuous systolic murmur beginning immediately with $S_1$ and extending to $S_2$. The murmur usually is of medium–high frequency, best heard at the LV apex, and radiates clearly into the left axilla. *Practical Point: Auscultation in the left lateral decubitus position (Fig. 1.11) usually will augment the murmur of MR and often increase its intensity by one to two grades.* This maneuver occasionally accentuates the holosystolic nature of a late tapering murmur. This position should be used routinely when an apical systolic murmur is of low amplitude and long duration.

*Shape and Duration*

The typical MR murmur is holosystolic or pansystolic (Fig. 6.5A–D) with an even intensity throughout systole (Fig. 6.5A). The murmur of MR may taper or augment in late systole. The most common variant is mid- to late systolic accentuation of the murmur. Sound vibrations may fan out during the last third of systole (Fig. 6.5B). In more severe MR, the murmur is more likely to have mid-systolic accentuation, giving it an ejection quality (Fig. 6.5C). In all these situations,

careful auscultation usually will identify sound vibrations at the *beginning* and at the *end* of systole, which confirm that the murmur is truly regurgitant in quality as opposed to a more common systolic ejection murmur.

The least common variant of the MR murmur is one that tapers or decreases in intensity in late systole (Fig. 6.5D). This configuration is more likely to be found in trivial degrees of MR. In severe, recent-onset MR, the murmur often is decrescendo in late systole due to rapid equilibration of LV and LA pressures (Fig. 6.5D). This murmur may take on ejection characteristics (Fig. 6.5E). Such attenuation in late systole does not occur in chronic MR.

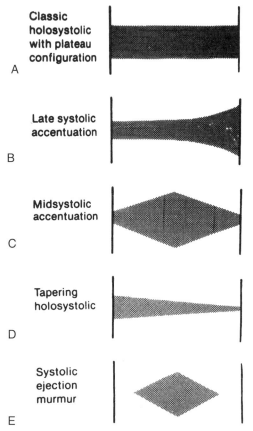

A  Classic holosystolic with plateau configuration

B  Late systolic accentuation

C  Midsystolic accentuation

D  Tapering holosystolic

E  Systolic ejection murmur

**FIG. 6.5.** Variable contours of the murmur of mitral regurgitation (MR). **A–D:** Holosystolic murmurs with differing configuration (see text). Note that sound vibrations extend to S₂ in each example. **E:** Typical systolic ejection murmur shown for comparison purposes. Note the sound-free interval immediately following S₁ and, most importantly, at the end of the murmur. (From Abrams J. Prim Cardiol 1983, with permission.)

*Intensity*

In general, the louder the murmur of MR, the greater the degree of reflux. Patients with moderate to severe MR and a large regurgitant fraction usually have grade III to IV/VI systolic murmurs. Thus, a systolic apical thrill is common in severe MR. However, there are important exceptions to this rule; certain conditions predispose to a murmur of decreased amplitude even when the degree of regurgitation is significant. On occasion, the murmur may be barely audible in the setting of severe regurgitation. *Practical Point: The most important factor affecting murmur intensity is the state of LV function. With preserved LV contractility and vigorous systolic function, the velocity and volume of blood flow are high and the murmur is loud. If LV dysfunction develops, the murmur will become softer even though the degree of MR is severe.*

The most common cause of a soft murmur is a mild degree of MR. The intensity of the murmur of MR does not vary with changes in cycle length (e.g., in atrial fibrillation, post-premature ventricular contraction [PVC] beats). This is in contradistinction to ejection or flow murmurs that augment in intensity following a long diastolic filling period, particularly following a PVC.

*Frequency or Pitch*

In mild cases of MR, the murmur is high pitched. Thus, firm pressure with the diaphragm of the stethoscope routinely should be used in auscultation for MR.

With increasing degrees of regurgitation, LA pressure increases and the gradient between the LV and the LA decreases. This change produces a murmur with lower-frequency vibrations. In many patients with a substantial degree of MR, the murmur has mixed frequencies, reflecting both a large gradient and high flow. The typical MR murmur has a whirring, somewhat musical pitch. In severe MR, the murmur may be harsh in quality.

*Location and Radiation*

MR of any etiology is best appreciated at the LV apex. In some individuals, the murmur may be louder just inside the apical impulse. In tall thin subjects with small hearts, the murmur and apical impulse can be medial, near, or adjacent to the left sternal edge. The murmur of chronic MR rarely is best heard away from the apical impulse.

The classic murmur radiates leftward into the axilla and often is well heard at or beneath the left scapula in the posterior chest. When the LA is large, the murmur may be audible over the thoracic vertebral column.

Occasionally, loud MR murmurs radiate rightward and are heard readily at the lower sternal border. These murmurs may occur in patients with a large LV; in such cases, one must be sure there is no coexisting TR. With a markedly dilated LV, the murmur may be louder in the axilla than at the apex.

In auscultation of systolic murmurs, concentration on the last third of systole is important. *Practical Point: In almost all cases of MR, sound vibrations in late systole continue until S₂, although the murmur may have a variable contour.*

Unique characteristics of the various MR murmurs occur. Table 6.2 outlines some of the differentiating features of the various forms of MR.

### Murmur of Mitral Valve Prolapse

*Shape and Duration*

The mid- to late systolic, crescendo or crescendo-decrescendo murmur of MVP is characteristic, although there is considerable variability in the timing of murmur onset related to different body positions and various physical maneuvers. A prolapse murmur that begins in early systole or is clearly holosystolic suggests moderate to severe MR. A pansystolic murmur in MVP occurs in approximately 10% of the subjects with MVP. The term "floppy valve syndrome" has been loosely applied to patients with MVP and severe MR.

*Intensity*

In the setting of MVP, the degree of MR when present usually is mild and the systolic murmur typically is soft. However, the late systolic component occasionally displays considerable accentuation and may be quite prominent. *Practical Point: The intensity of the MVP murmur is extremely variable. In some persons, the murmur may be inaudible in one position but grade II to IV/VI intensity in another position. The murmur also may vary several grades with various maneuvers.*

**TABLE 6.2.** *Physical examination characteristics of mitral regurgitation*

| Valve abnormality | Left ventricular impulse | Murmur |
| --- | --- | --- |
| Mitral valve prolapse | Normal | Mid to late systolic |
| Chordal rupture | Hyperkinetic; laterally displaced in chronic MR | Decrescendo |
| Papillary muscle dysfunction/rupture | Bifid or sustained | Early to mid systolic |
| Rheumatic valve disease | Hyperkinetic; laterally displaced in chronic MR | Holosystolic |

MR, mitral regurgitation.

### Murmur of Chordal Rupture

*Shape and Duration*

Usually, in the setting of chordal rupture, MR occurs in the presence of a noncompliant LA. Consequently, moderate to severe MR will commonly result in a substantial elevation of atrial pressure. In the latter third of systole, the LV–LA pressure gradient decreases as the reflux into the LA decreases (Fig. 6.5D). This results in a tapering of sound vibrations and a decrescendo configuration to the murmur. Often, the peak mid-systolic intensity produces a crescendo-decrescendo systolic murmur. *Practical Point: Although the murmur of ruptured chordae tendineae commonly simulates a systolic ejection murmur, careful auscultation invariably will detect sound vibrations extending to $S_2$. In fact, such a murmur often obliterates $A_2$.*

*Intensity*

In patients with a ruptured chordae and normal LV function, the amount of the regurgitant volume is likely to be large, the murmur typically is harsh, loud (grade III to IV/VI intensity), and accompanied by a thrill.

*Location and Radiation*

Often chordal rupture causes eccentric localization and radiation of the murmur as the protrusion of one of the leaflets directs the regurgitant jet in a well-localized stream. Incompetence of the posterior leaflet tends to deflect the refluxing torrent of blood toward the medial LA wall and LV outflow tract. The sound vibrations radiate toward the proximal aorta, and the murmur may have its maximal intensity at the second left or right interspace, and simulate aortic stenosis. A deformity of the anterior leaflet directs the blood posterolaterally to produce a murmur that is loudest at the apex and left posterior thorax. *Practical Point: When the murmur of a posterior ruptured chordae tendineae has a crescendo-decrescendo shape, it is easily mistaken for aortic stenosis. To avoid the error of confusing MR with aortic stenosis,* one must pay attention to the length of the systolic murmur at both the aortic area and apex as well as the quality of the carotid upstroke.

### Murmur of Papillary Muscle Dysfunction/Papillary Muscle Rupture

*Shape and Duration*

The classic murmur of papillary muscle dysfunction is a *late systolic crescendo murmur* extending up to $S_2$ (Fig. 6.5B). When papillary muscle contraction is altered, the mitral leaflets prolapse, resulting in reflux of blood into the LA, during the last half of systole, which produces late accentuation of the murmur. When there is severe global contractile dysfunction and/or marked fibrosis and shortening of the papillary muscles, the resultant MR may be *holosystolic*; in such situations, the murmur often retains late systolic accentuation. Frequently, papillary muscle murmurs have mid-systolic accentuation and take on ejection characteristics.

*Intensity*

Papillary muscle rupture produces acute, severe MR. The murmur may be silent or very soft or can be loud and harsh. An $S_4$ and $S_3$ are common, and the patient is likely to be in acute pulmonary edema with or without hypotension. Late systolic tapering of the murmur may be present as a result of a decreasing LV–LA pressure gradient in end-systole (Fig. 6.5D).

As LV function improves, the murmur of papillary muscle dysfunction may disappear or may get louder as contractile force increases. *Practical Point: Variability in the amplitude of the murmur is a common feature of papillary muscle dysfunction.*

### Murmur of Rheumatic Valve Disease

*Shape and Duration*

The murmur associated with rheumatic valve disease typically is holosystolic. The murmur does not always plateau in intensity and may taper or augment in late systole. In chronic rheumatic MR, the murmur may wane in late systole if the degree of reflux decreases during the latter third of systole due to a large LV with foreshortened chordae tendineae. The smaller cavity size in late systole allows more complete coaptation of the mitral leaflets, and the degree of late systolic regurgitation is diminished.

### Intensity

In general, the louder the murmur of rheumatic MR, the greater degree of regurgitation. Patients with moderate to severe MR usually have grade III to IV/VI systolic murmurs unless there is systole dysfunction in which case the murmur can be soft.

### Location and Radiation

As with most forms of MR, the murmur is best appreciated at the LV apex and radiates to the left axillae.

### Assessment of Severity

Table 6.3 lists various findings on physical examination that help to separate mild, moderate, and severe chronic MR.

### Differential Diagnosis of the Systolic Murmur of Mitral Regurgitation

The murmur of mild MR can be readily mistaken for an *ejection murmur* with apical radiation, particularly if the mitral murmur is decrescendo in quality. The critical question relates to the *length* of the murmur in late sys-

tole. Attention to post-PVC beats may be of aid in this differential diagnosis. Ejection murmurs will augment in intensity, whereas the loudness of the MR murmur will remain unchanged.

*TR* may be difficult to separate from MR when there is significant RV enlargement. In this setting, the "apical" murmur may arise from the right heart and reflect TR. Careful attention to respiratory variation is essential. In the presence of atrial fibrillation, changes in murmur intensity with respiration may be virtually undetectable.

A *ventricular septal defect* murmur can simulate MR, although its maximal location at the lower sternal border should readily differentiate the two (see Chapter 13). However, in patients with small hearts or long chests, the MR murmur can be medial and easily confused with a ventricular septal defect murmur.

In *hypertrophic cardiomyopathy*, MR is commonly present. A long systolic ejection murmur is typical in these patients, and often it is difficult to be sure that there is a *separate* murmur of MR. The typical radiation pattern of the regurgitant murmur often is absent in hypertrophic cardiomyopathy. Careful assessment of the response of the systolic murmur to positional changes, maneuvers, and pharmacologic agents may be helpful.

Patients with cardiac decompensation or massive cardiomegaly often have a murmur of MR in the absence of intrinsic disease of the mitral valve. Frequently, the holosystolic murmur disappears or softens after treatment of congestive heart failure and clinical improvement. This murmur has been described as *functional* MR.

**TABLE 6.3.** *Physical examination features of chronic mitral regurgitation*

| Physical examination finding | Mild MR | Moderate MR | Severe MR |
|---|---|---|---|
| Carotid upstroke | Normal | Brisk, jerky, small volume | Quick rising, poorly sustained, low amplitude |
| Left ventricular impulse | Normal/hyperdynamic | Normal/hyperdynamic | Sustained |
| S$_2$ | Normal | Widely split | Split during expiration; widely split during inspiration |
| S$_3$ | Absent | Generally absent | Present |
| Mid-diastolic murmur | Absent | Absent | Present |
| Murmur | Soft to absent | Medium pitched | Very loud or soft to absent if poor LV function |

MR, mitral regurgitation.

It is believed that most of these murmurs result from dilation of the mitral annulus.

## ECHOCARDIOGRAPHY

### Introduction

The mitral annulus, anterior and posterior leaflets, chordae tendineae, papillary muscles, LV myocardium underlying the papillary muscles, and LA wall comprise the mitral valve apparatus. Echocardiography plays a pivotal role in the evaluation of the various components of the mitral valve as well as MR. It provides information about the etiology, severity, and progression of valvular lesions as well as the atrial and ventricular response to the resulting volume overload. Additionally, echocardiography can be used to assess the hemodynamic impact of MR by determining the presence or absence of LA and pulmonary hypertension. Echocardiography can accurately separate a normal variant of MR (usually trivial or mild) from a pathologic one. The presence of thickening, sclerosis, or calcification as well as decreased mobility of the valve leaflets, chordae tendineae, or annulus define an abnormal valve. Based upon the pattern of structural abnormality, mitral valve morphology can be categorized as degenerative, myxomatous (with or without MVP), ischemic, rheumatic, or infectious. Also, alteration of the geometry of the mitral valve apparatus due to LV dilation or dysfunction leading to functional MR can be identified. M-mode, two-dimensional (2-D), and color Doppler echocardiography are the most currently used techniques to define the etiology, mechanism, severity, and hemodynamic impact of MR. Table 6.4 describes the class I indications for echocardiographic studies in patients with suspected or known MR according to the American College of Cardiology and the American Heart Association (2).

The severity of MR should be viewed in terms of both the regurgitant volume and the effect of that volume on the cardiovascular system. Current echocardiographic parameters used in defining the severity of MR should include the assessment of LV size and systolic function, LA size and pressure, and pulmonary artery pressures.

When transthoracic image quality is suboptimal, transesophageal echocardiography (TEE) should be considered to evaluate valve morphology, cardiac structure, and MR severity. TEE also is of important value for assessment of eccentric color flow jets and flow patterns of the pulmonary veins. Transesophageal imaging is especially effective in evaluating mitral prosthetic insufficiency, and it is invaluable intraoperatively before and after mitral valve repair or replacement. In the setting of acute MR, TEE assessment may be more accurate than transthoracic echocardiography (TTE) (3). With TEE, the etiology of acute MR, such as vegetations, valve perforation, or

**TABLE 6.4.** *Class I indications for transthoracic and transesophageal echocardiography in mitral regurgitation*

1. For baseline evaluation to quantify severity of MR and LV function in any patient suspected of having MR
2. For delineation of mechanism of MR
3. For annual or semiannual surveillance of LV function (estimated by ejection fraction and end-systolic dimension) in asymptomatic severe MR
4. To establish cardiac status after a change in symptoms
5. For evaluation after mitral valve replacement or mitral valve repair to establish baseline post-operative status
6. Intraoperative TEE to establish the anatomic basis for MR and to guide repair
7. TEE for evaluation of MR patients in whom transthoracic echocardiography provides nondiagnostic images regarding severity or mechanism of MR, and/or status of LV
8. Diagnosis, assessment of hemodynamic severity of MR, leaflet morphology, and ventricular compensation in patients with physical signs of MVP
9. To exclude MVP in patients who have been given the diagnosis when there is no clinical evidence to support the diagnosis

LV, left ventricle; MR, mitral regurgitation; MVP, mitral valve prolapse; TEE, transesophageal echocardiography. Reproduced from Bonow RO, Carabello B, De Leon, AC, et al. ACC/AHA guidelines for the management of patients with valvular heart disease. J Am Coll Cardiol 1998;32:1486–1588.

rupture of a chordae tendineae or papillary muscle, can be easily differentiated.

## Echocardiographic Appearance

### *M Mode*

M-mode analysis of the mitral valve usually is performed from the 2-D parasternal long- and short-axis views. From this view, the motion of the anterior mitral leaflet appears as an M and the motion of the posterior leaflet appears as a blunted W. A variety of measurements can be made from the mitral valve M-mode recording, including leaflet opening and closing patterns, leaflet excursion, separation, and thickness. Although leaflet thickness frequently is visually defined, this measurement has limited specificity for mild degrees of leaflet thickening. TEE M-mode analysis from the four- and two-chamber views gives a less than 20-degree misalignment with the mitral leaflets; therefore, it provides accurate assessment of leaflet thickness (4). Color M-mode echocardiography is useful for evaluating the timing of the MR. Additionally, M-mode echocardiography is useful for assessing LV size and mass, but assessing LA size may be limited due to the asymmetric shape of the LA cavity. However, an LA diameter of 4.5 cm on M-mode images correlates highly with LA hypertension, which may result from significant MR.

*Infective vegetations* attached to the valve leaflet, chordae, or ventricular endocardium can be discrete sessile masses or pedunculated. By M-mode echocardiography, the majority of vegetations appear as shaggy, irregular masses attached to the valve leaflets, with a characteristic independent chaotic or rotary motion. However, this technique has low sensitivity and specificity for detection of valve vegetations.

The echocardiographic diagnosis of *MVP* can be made from M-mode recordings (Fig. 6.6). The most common finding is prominent mid-systolic posterior displacement (>2 mm) of the mitral leaflets. M-mode demonstration of early systolic anterior motion of the mitral leaflets followed by late systolic posterior mo-

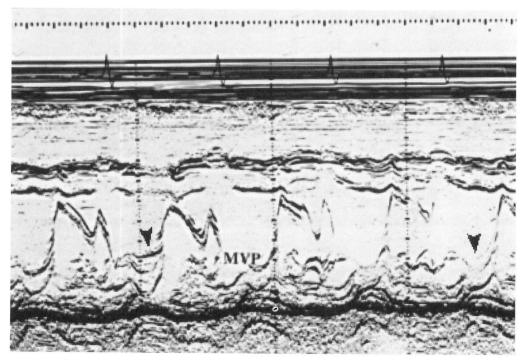

**FIG. 6.6.** M-mode analysis of the mitral valve in a patient with mitral valve prolapse (MVP). Note the prominent mid- to late systolic posterior displacement of the mitral leaflets *(arrowheads).*

tion of the leaflets corresponds to the systolic murmur of MVP. Occasionally, the systolic prolapse may be holosystolic. M-mode echocardiography has low sensitivity but high specificity for diagnosis of MVP.

With a *flail mitral valve*, part of the valve extends into the LA during systole. The flail leaflet also may be seen in the LV as a thickened valve or tissue meshwork during diastole on M-mode analysis. Generally during systole, the tip of the flail leaflet points toward the LA; this differentiates a flail leaflet from a severely prolapsed leaflet (where the leaflet tip of the latter points toward the LV).

*Mitral annular calcification* (MAC) can lead to MR and be associated with coronary artery disease. This abnormality can be accurately detected by M-mode echocardiography. It appears as a highly echo-reflectant linear structure that moves parallel and anterior to the LV posterior wall in the long- and short-axis views.

### *Two-Dimensional Echocardiography*

Two-dimensional echocardiography provides accurate assessment of LV and LA size, and of the mitral valve morphology and its supporting apparatus.

The mitral annulus area normally is smaller during systole than during diastole. *MAC* increases the rigidity of the annulus and impairs systolic contraction, which in turn leads to MR. Calcification of the mitral annulus is a common finding in elderly subjects, whereas premature calcification of the mitral annulus is seen more frequently in patients with hypertension, renal failure, and coronary artery disease. On 2-D imaging, MAC appears as an area of increased echogenicity on the ventricular side of the annulus near the insertion of the posterior leaflet. In the short-axis views, MAC may involve a focal area of the annulus, or it may involve the entire U-shaped posterior annulus. *Age-related degenerative changes* of the mitral leaflets often occur both with and without MAC. The leaflets typically appear irregular and thickened, with increased areas of echogenicity. MAC is considered mild when the degree of sclerosis in the cross-sectional views appears <5 mm, moderate if 5 to 10 mm, and severe if >10 mm.

*Myxomatous mitral valve disease* is characterized by leaflet thickening (>5 mm) with soft tissue echo-reflectance, redundant chordae, and billowing of the leaflets into the LA during systole. The severity of disease varies from mild displacement of the leaflets into the LA, such as in MVP, to complete prolapse or flail of a portion of the leaflet into the LA.

The diagnosis of MVP by 2-D echocardiography is based on late systolic posterior displacement of the mitral leaflet into the LA of at least 2 mm or more beyond the mitral annulus in the parasternal long-axis view. The posterior displacement of the mitral valve in late systole corresponds with the systolic click and late systolic murmur.

Patients with hyperkinetic ventricles or volume depletion who demonstrate MVP are considered to be normal variants of MVP or pseudo-MVP. Additionally, patients with mild to moderate billowing of one or both nonthickened leaflet(s) toward the LA with the leaflet coaptation point on the ventricular side of the mitral annulus and with minimal or no MR by Doppler echocardiography probably are normal.

On TEE images, systolic protrusion of a scallop of the posterior leaflet or segment of the anterior leaflet into the LA suggests MVP. TEE from the four- and two-chamber views is accurate in assessing the thickness and redundancy of the mitral leaflet (4).

A flail mitral valve often is detected with 2-D echocardiography. In systole, part of the valve extends into the LA. The criterion used to differentiate a flail mitral leaflet from severe MVP is the direction in which the leaflet points. During systole, the tip of the flail leaflet points toward the LA; the tip points toward the LV in the setting of severe MVP.

The most common cause of a flail mitral leaflet is rupture of a chordae tendineae. A flail leaflet and the free chordae may be seen "dancing" about in the ventricle. When the chordae are not visible, the diagnosis rests on the pattern of leaflet motion. Marked leaflet deformities suggest chordal or papillary muscle rupture. Generally, a noticeable separation of the anterior and posterior leaflets can be identified in the parasternal long-axis and apical four-chamber views. Three signs of flail mitral leaflet secondary to ruptured chordae have been identified: noncoaptation of the anterior and posterior mitral leaflets; systolic fluttering of the valve in the LA; and diastolic chaotic motion of the leaflet.

TEE is superior to TTE for diagnosis of ruptured chordae tendineae (Fig. 6.7). TEE has a sensitivity and specificity of 100% for detection of ruptured chordae, compared to a sensitivity of 35% and a specificity of 100% using TTE (5). On TEE, a ruptured chordae produces abnormal systolic echoes in the LA and almost always is associated with significant and eccentric MR (Fig. 6.8).

In addition to chordal rupture, papillary rupture (partial or complete) may lead to a flail mitral leaflet. Two-dimensional echocardiography is particularly useful in the diagnosis of *papillary muscle rupture*. Often the detached papillary muscle head can be visualized swing-

ing freely with the flow of blood from the ventricle to the atrium (Figs. 6.9 and 3.7). Typically the portion of the mitral leaflet attached to the ruptured papillary muscle is flail and Doppler analysis demonstrates severe, eccentric, and frequently diastolic MR (due to severe LV end-diastolic pressure). Because of the associated highly eccentric MR jet, TTE may underestimate the severity and mechanism of MR. Therefore, TEE should be promptly performed in patients suspected of having a ruptured papillary muscle.

Partial papillary muscle rupture may also occur. Generally in this setting normal mitral leaflet coaptation is maintained. As in the case of chordal rupture, TEE is often superior to TTE for the evaluation of partial or complete papillary muscle rupture.

In patients with *papillary muscle dysfunction*, both abnormal leaflet motion and sys-

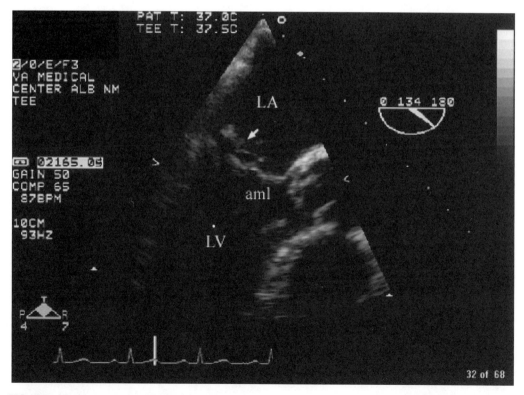

**FIG. 6.7.** Myxomatous mitral valve disease with chordal rupture and flail posterior leaflet. Longitudinal transesophageal echocardiographic view demonstrates myxomatous thickening of the anterior (aml) and posterior (pml) mitral leaflets. Note the flail posterior leaflet *(arrow)* prolapsing into the left atrium (LA). LV, left ventricle.

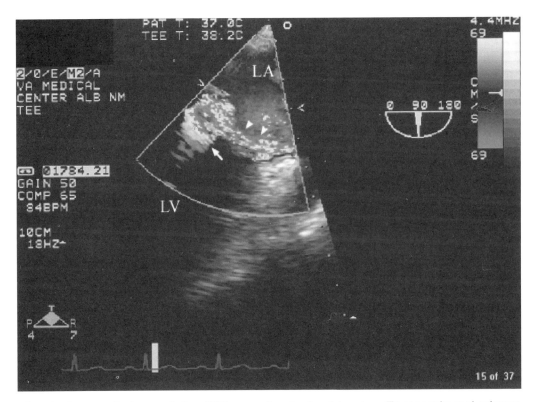

**FIG. 6.8.** Severe mitral regurgitation (MR) secondary to chordal rupture. Transesophageal echocardiogram demonstrates severe MR with a large (>1.5 cm) flow convergence zone *(arrow)* and a highly eccentric MR jet *(arrowheads)*. Abbreviations as in Fig. 6.7. (See Color Figure 6.8.)

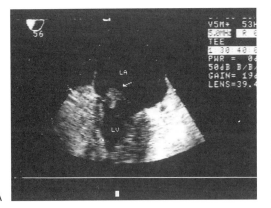
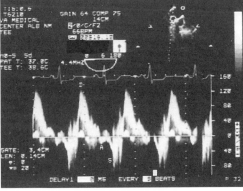

A                                                                                               B

**FIG. 6.9.** Ruptured papillary muscle. **A:** Transesophageal two-chamber view demonstrates a ruptured posteromedial papillary muscle freely prolapsing into the left atrium *(arrow)*. Note the incomplete coaptation of the anterior and posterior mitral leaflets, which resulted in torrential mitral regurgitation (MR). **B:** Pulsed Doppler imaging of the pulmonary veins demonstrates predominance of the diastolic flow (D), a brief period of flow reversal coincident with atrial systole (A), and dramatic flow reversal during systole (S) characteristic of severe MR.

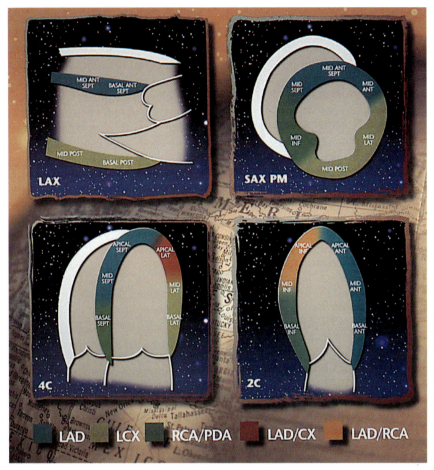

**COLOR FIGURE 3.4.** Diagram demonstrating the 16 wall segments of the left ventricle and their corresponding coronary artery supply. (Courtesy of Biosound, Inc.)

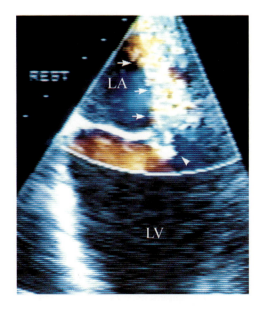

**COLOR FIGURE 3.6. B:** Severe mitral regurgitation demonstrated by color Doppler with a highly eccentric and posterolaterally directed jet extending to the pulmonary veins *(arrows)*. Abbreviations as in previous figures.

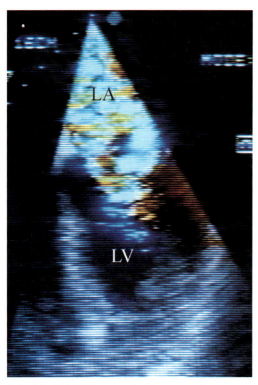

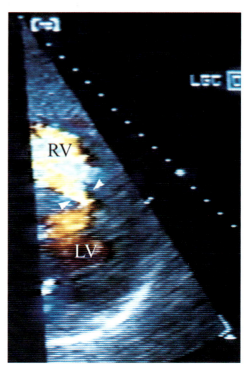

COLOR FIGURE 3.7. C: Four-chamber trans-esophageal echocardiograms demonstrate a flail anterior mitral leaflet with a portion of the posteromedial papillary muscle attached *(arrow)* and associated severe mitral regurgitation by color Doppler.

COLOR FIGURE 3.8. B: Color Doppler demonstrates left to right communication *(arrowheads)*. Abbreviations as in previous figures.

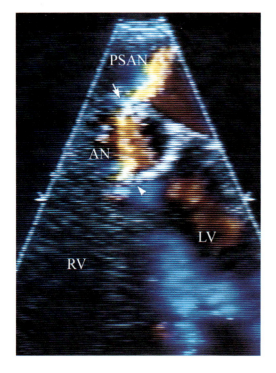

COLOR FIGURE 3.9. B: Color Doppler demonstrate bidirectional flow between the left ventricle and aneurysm *(arrowhead)* and between the aneurysm and pseudoaneurysm *(arrow)*. Abbreviations as in previous figures.

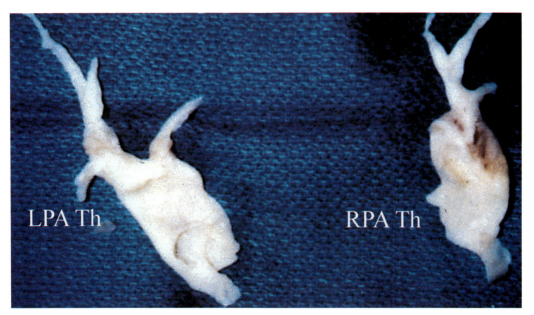

**COLOR FIGURE 5.4.** Severe cor pulmonale. **B:** Note the large, branching, multiple, and well-organized thrombi removed from the left (LPA Th) and right (RPA Th) pulmonary arteries.

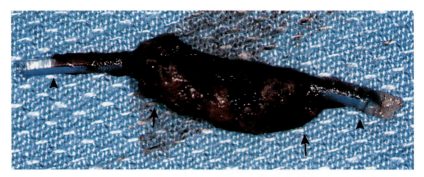

**COLOR FIGURE 5.7.** Right atrial thrombus attached to an indwelling catheter. **B:** A well-organized thrombus *(arrows)* attached to and surrounding a catheter *(arrowheads)*. The patient had a high-probability perfusion scan for pulmonary emboli. Abbreviations as in previous figures.

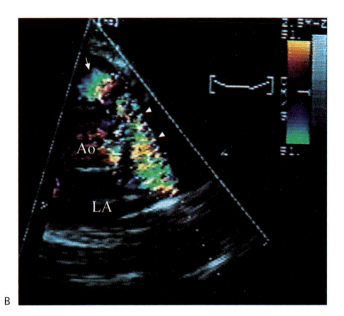

B

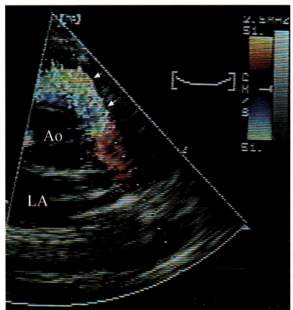

C

**COLOR FIGURE 5.8.** Pulmonic stenosis and regurgitation due to carcinoid syndrome. **B:** Color Doppler recordings from the basilar short-axis view at the pulmonic valve level demonstrate an acceleration zone *(arrow)* at the right ventricular (RV) outflow tract and high-turbulence mosaic color Doppler pattern above the pulmonic valve *(arrowheads)*. These features suggest pulmonic valve stenosis. **C:** At the pulmonic valve level, the color Doppler short-axis view demonstrates a regurgitant jet width that occupies the entire RV outflow tract. This feature is consistent with severe pulmonary regurgitation.

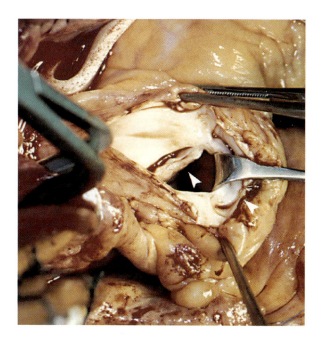

**COLOR FIGURE 5.8. D:** At surgery, the pulmonic valve demonstrated a shaggy appearance with severe thickening, marked stiffness, and incomplete closure *(arrowhead)*.

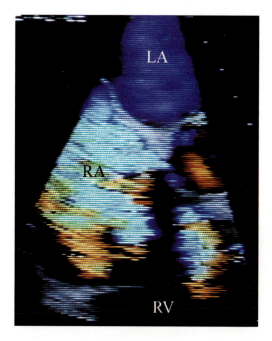

**COLOR FIGURE 5.9.** Tricuspid regurgitation due to carcinoid syndrome. **B:** Color Doppler four-chamber view demonstrates a large regurgitant jet occupying the entire atria, consistent with severe tricuspid regurgitation.

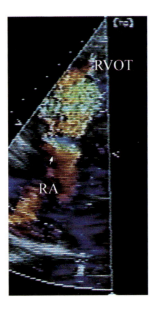

**COLOR FIGURE 5.10.** Tricuspid stenosis due to carcinoid syndrome. **B:** Color Doppler image at the tricuspid valve level demonstrates a large acceleration zone *(arrow)* and highly turbulent (mosaic pattern) tricuspid valve inflow.

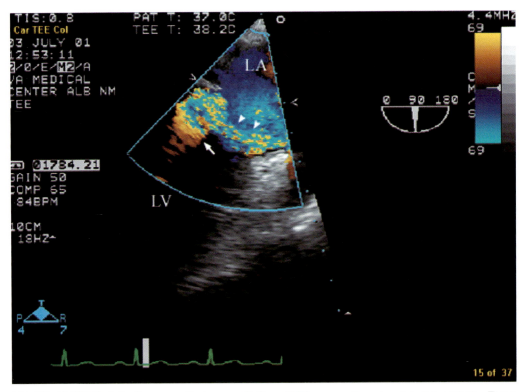

**COLOR FIGURE 6.8.** Severe mitral regurgitation (MR) secondary to chordal rupture. Transesophageal echocardiogram demonstrates severe MR with a large (>1.5 cm) flow convergence zone *(arrow)* and a highly eccentric MR jet *(arrowheads)*. Abbreviations as in Fig. 6.7.

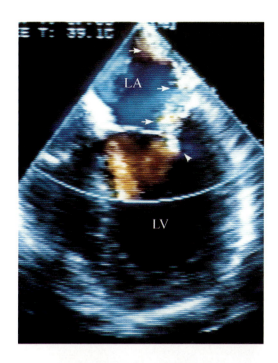

**COLOR FIGURE 6.11.** Ischemic mitral regurgitation (MR). Transesophageal echocardiographic two-chamber view with color Doppler imaging in a patient after inferior myocardial infarction with anterior mitral leaflet pseudoprolapse demonstrates a highly eccentric MR jet *(arrows)* with a vena contracta of 4 mm and a flow convergence zone of 7 mm *(arrowhead)*.

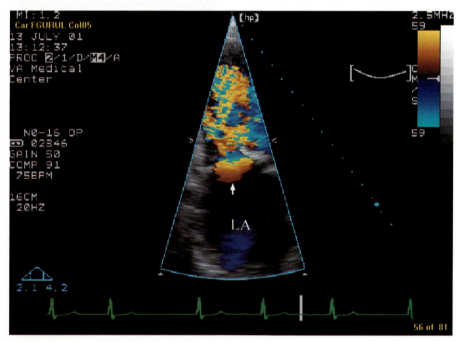

**COLOR FIGURE 7.7.** Color Doppler assessment of mitral stenosis. **B:** Large flow convergence zone *(arrow)* is noted proximal to the mitral orifice. The mitral valve area calculated with the proximal isovelocity area was 0.9 cm$^2$ and correlated well with that calculated by the pressure half-time and continuity equation. Abbreviations as in Fig. 7.5. (Courtesy of the Albuquerque New Mexico Veterans Affairs Medical Center Echocardiography Laboratory.)

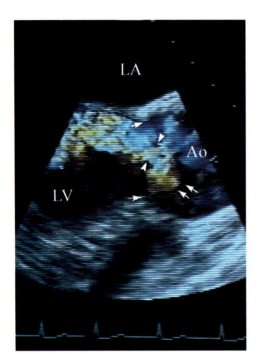

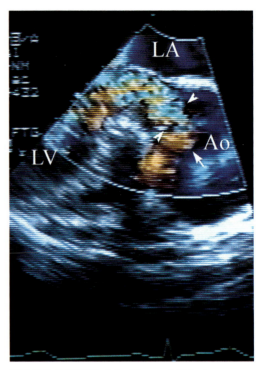

**COLOR FIGURE 9.7.** Ankylosing spondylitis and symptomatic severe aortic regurgitation in a 43-year-old man. **B:** Transesophageal echocardiographic longitudinal view with color Doppler imaging demonstrates moderate to severe aortic regurgitation as judged by a large (>6 mm wide) vena contracta *(arrowheads)*. Note a large flow convergence zone *(arrows)*. Using the flow convergence area method, the effective regurgitant orifice area was calculated as 1.2 cm$^2$. Ao, aorta; LA, left atrium; LV, left ventricle; ncc, noncoronary cusp.

**COLOR FIGURE 9.8.** Sinus of Valsalva aneurysm and symptomatic aortic regurgitation in a 58-year-old patient. **B:** Transesophageal echocardiographic longitudinal view of the aortic valve with color Doppler imaging demonstrates a large flow convergence zone *(arrow)*, vena contracta width of 7 mm *(arrowheads)*, and ratio of the color jet height to outflow tract height >75%. Because of the eccentricity of the regurgitant jet, adequate continuous wave Doppler tracings for assessing pressure half-time were not obtained by transthoracic echocardiography. Abbreviations as in previous figure.

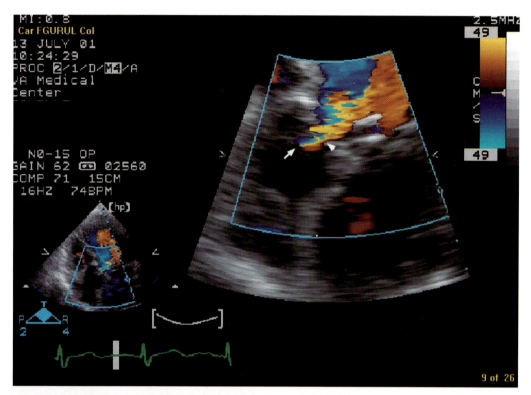

**COLOR FIGURE 9.9.** Degenerative aortic valve disease with mild aortic regurgitation and stenosis. **B:** Apical transthoracic echocardiographic close-up view of the aortic valve with color Doppler interrogation demonstrates a small flow convergence zone *(arrow)* and a small vena contracta width of 3 mm *(arrowhead)*.

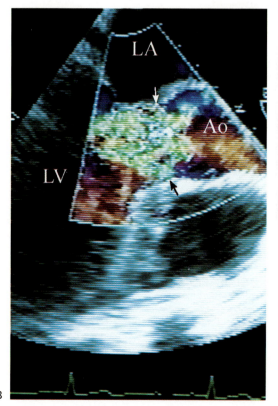

B

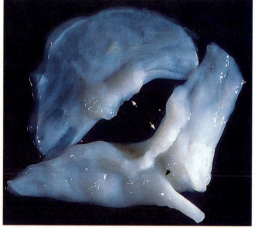

C

**COLOR FIGURE 9.10.** Bicuspid aortic valve and severe aortic regurgitation in a symptomatic 46-year-old man. **B:** Transesophageal echocardiographic longitudinal view of the aortic valve with color Doppler imaging demonstrates severe aortic regurgitation as judged by a ratio of jet height and LV outflow tract height *(arrows)* >65% as well vena contracta width >6 mm. **C:** This surgically resected bicuspid aortic valve shows moderate thickening of the tip portion of the aortic cusps *(arrows)* with incomplete coaptation and an apparent large regurgitant orifice (>1 cm²). Note the raphe of the posteriorly located cusp *(black arrow)*.

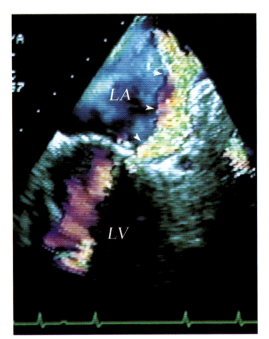

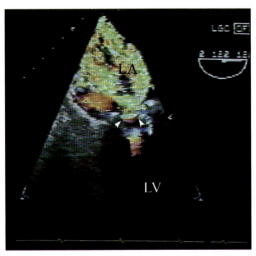

COLOR FIGURE 10.8. B: Color flow Doppler image showing severe mitral regurgitation centrally through the leaflets. Note the large jet width and acceleration zone *(arrowheads)* consistent with severe regurgitation.

COLOR FIGURE 10.6. Transesophageal four-chamber view showing a St. Jude mitral valve in the open position. C: Color Doppler flow image showing perivalvular leak *(arrowheads)* in systole.

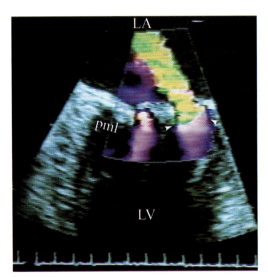

COLOR FIGURE 11.2. Mitral valve infective endocarditis due to *Staphylococcus aureus* in a 43-year-old woman with underlying mitral stenosis. B: Color Doppler demonstrates a wide regurgitant jet through a perforation *(arrowheads)*.

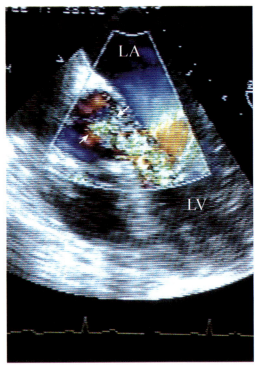

COLOR FIGURE 11.5. Aortic and metastatic mitral valve infective endocarditis due to *Staphylococcus aureus* in a 57-year-old man with underlying mild aortic stenosis. B: Both mitral valve lesions resulted from jet lesions due to severe aortic regurgitation as demonstrated by color Doppler. *Arrows* delineate a large jet width. RA, right atria; RV, right ventricle.

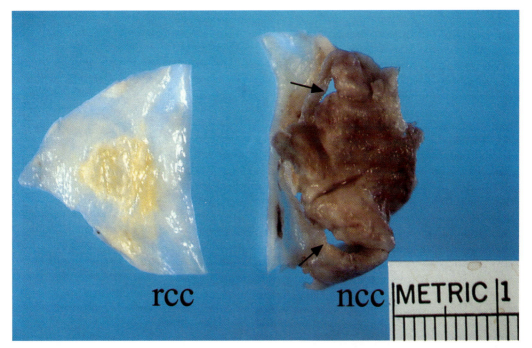

**COLOR FIGURE 11.3.** Aortic valve infective endocarditis due to β-hemolytic streptococcus in a 63-year-old man. **B:** Note the thickening and distortion of the ncc with two discrete perforations *(arrows)*. Also note the contrasting minimal sclerosis of the rcc. Other abbreviations as in previous figures.

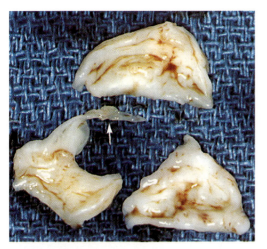

**COLOR FIGURE 11.7.** Aortic valve excrescence in a noninfected 47-year-old man with chronic symptomatic aortic regurgitation. **B:** Diffuse myxomatous thickening of the three aortic valve cusps is noted with a thin and lucent excrescence attached to the tip of the right coronary cusp *(arrow).* Abbreviations as in previous figures.

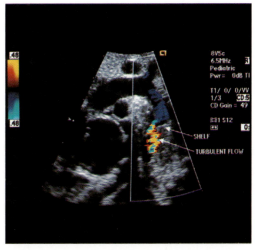

**COLOR FIGURE 13.9.** Two-dimensional and Doppler images of the aorta and a coarctation. **B:** Turbulence of flow begins at the shelf.

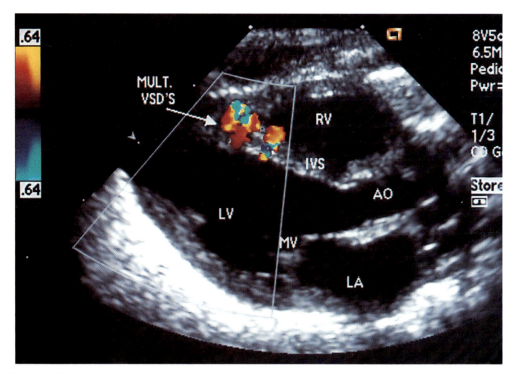

**COLOR FIGURE 13.5.** Parasternal long-axis view of multiple muscular ventricular septal defects in a newborn baby. These defects will likely close spontaneously. Note the lack of left atrial or left ventricular dilation and the minimal turbulence by color Doppler. The left to right shunt volume is small because pulmonary vascular resistance has not yet fallen. AO, aorta; IVS, interventricular septum; MV, mitral valve; RV, right ventricle.

tolic leaflet position are seen. Frequently, akinesis or dyskinesis of the corresponding wall of attachment of one or both papillary muscles is noted. Calcification, fibrosis, and thinning of the papillary muscles may be identified, particularly in the setting of an old MI. In these patients, the characteristic pattern of abnormal leaflet motion is failure of one or both leaflets to reach the normal peak systolic position relative to the mitral annulus. This is best visualized in the apical four-chamber view. MR in post-MI patients is defined as ischemic when primary valve pathology cannot be identified. Its incidence is about 20% and similar in anterior and inferior MI. In patients with inferior MI, the ischemic or infarcted posteromedial papillary muscle causes tethering and decreased mobility predominantly of the posterior mitral leaflet leading to leaflet malcoaptation, and relative anterior leaflet prolapse or

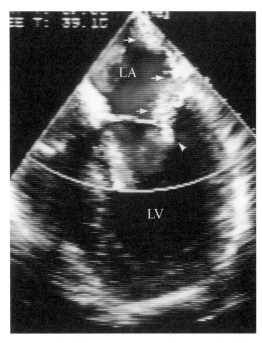

**FIG. 6.11.** Ischemic mitral regurgitation (MR). Transesophageal echocardiographic two-chamber view with color Doppler imaging in a patient after inferior myocardial infarction with anterior mitral leaflet pseudoprolapse demonstrates a highly eccentric MR jet *(arrows)* with a vena contracta of 4 mm and a flow convergence zone of 7 mm *(arrowhead)*. (See Color Figure 6.11.)

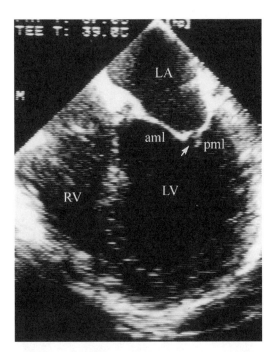

**FIG. 6.10.** Ischemic mitral valve pseudoprolapse. Transesophageal two-chamber view of a patient with a large inferior myocardial infarction demonstrates incomplete mitral leaflet coaptation and anterior mitral leaflet pseudoprolapse *(arrow)*. RV, right ventricle.

pseudoprolapse (Fig. 6.10) (6). The anterior mitral pseudoprolapse explains the characteristically eccentric and posterolaterally directed MR jet (Fig. 6.11). In patients with anterior MI, LV dilation and dysfunction lead to downward and lateral displacement of the papillary muscles. The mitral leaflets undergo incomplete but symmetric malcoaptation; therefore, the MR jet is central (6).

The mitral valve itself usually appears normal in MR that is secondary to *LA or LV dilation* of any cause or in cases of MR due to *ischemic heart disease*, especially after anterior MI. LA dilation is common in moderate or severe MR, but wide variation exists in the relationship between MR severity and LA size. In severe MR, right heart chamber dilation and inferior vena cava plethora due to pulmonary hypertension are observed fre-

quently. In cases of acute MR due to ischemia, MI, infective endocarditis, or papillary muscle trauma, the LA frequently is normal in size.

*Rheumatic MR* is characterized by thickening and sclerosis (increased echo-reflectance), primarily of the leaflet tips (Fig.
6.12). Characteristically the leaflet tips have a
"hockey stick" appearance demonstrated by a
90-degree angle from the chordae to the tip of
the leaflet. Frequently the posterior mitral
leaflet is more involved than the anterior
leaflet. Often, incomplete leaflet coaptation is
noted at one of the commissural margins during early systole. The degree of regurgitation
is related to the area of incomplete leaflet closure. Severe MR is seen in cases of incomplete closure of a single leaflet and in cases of
incomplete closure of both leaflet margins or
the entire closure line.

In the setting of acute rheumatic fever, focal nodular thickening of the leaflet tips and
body of the leaflet may be identified. These
nodules are seen in patients with a first attack
of rheumatic fever as well as in patients with
recurrent rheumatic fever (7). These nodules
measure 1 to 5 mm, have a soft tissue echo-reflectance, and are located more commonly at
the leaflet coaptation point. Unlike the infective endocarditis vegetations, these nodules
do not exhibit chaotic mobility and are not
visible on follow-up studies. In some cases,
prolapse of the anterior leaflet may be identified, more commonly in cases of recurrent
rheumatic fever (7).

In cases of endocarditis, the leaflets appear
thickened and deformed. The mitral valve is
involved more frequently in *infective endocarditis* than is any other cardiac valve. Vegetations may involve either the anterior or pos-

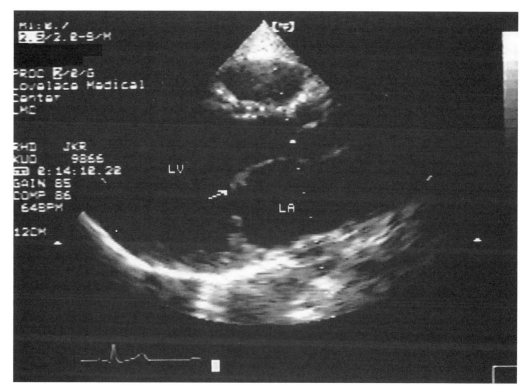

**FIG. 6.12.** Rheumatic mitral valve disease. Transthoracic parasternal long-axis view demonstrates
thickening predominantly of both posterior and anterior mitral leaflet tips *(arrow)*. Note the diastolic
doming deformity of the leaflets suggesting commissural fusion and subvalvular involvement.

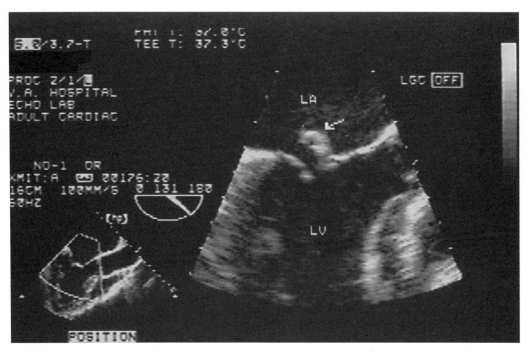

**FIG. 6.13.** Mitral valve endocarditis with chordal rupture and flail anterior leaflet. Transesophageal long-axis view of the mitral valve demonstrates a flail anterior mitral leaflet with a vegetation *(arrow)*. Note the incomplete coaptation of the leaflets.

terior leaflet and occur most often on the atrial side and at the leaflet coaptation point (Fig. 6.13). Freely mobile vegetations may prolapse into the LA during systole and may fall into the LV during diastole. Rarely, large vegetations may cause obstruction of the mitral valve and mimic mitral stenosis clinically or echocardiographically.

Valve vegetations appear as circumscribed, soft tissue echo-reflective masses that generally arise from the leaflet tips. These masses may appear as irregular areas of leaflet thickening or as discrete pedunculated or fixed masses. In acute endocarditis, the vegetations appear soft and friable, with varying degrees of independent motion, whereas chronic or healed vegetations appear fixed and echo-dense.

By TTE, mitral valve vegetations must be differentiated from a variety of other valvular disorders, including LA and valvular tumors, myxomatous degeneration of the valve, and rheumatic valvulopathy. A prolapsing atrial tumor is generally differentiated from an endo-carditic lesion based upon the point of origin of the prolapsing mass. Myxomatous degeneration of the valve is associated with leaflet redundancy and diffuse leaflet thickening, whereas most vegetations are localized to the leaflet tips. Restricted motion and fixation of the posterior leaflet usually suggest a rheumatic valve rather than endocarditis of the valve.

TEE is clearly superior to TTE for identifying valvular vegetations and differentiating them from other lesions (8), valvular ring abscesses, sinus of Valsalva and mycotic aneurysms, subaortic aneurysm from mitral-aortic intervalvular fibrosa, and rupture of a subaortic aneurysm into the LA (9).

### *Color Doppler*

Color Doppler is more sensitive than pulsed or continuous wave (CW) Doppler techniques because it is less likely to miss small or eccentric jets. Color Doppler provides a method for detecting the direction and extent of MR jets into the LA. Color Doppler also detects changes in the velocity of blood flow at the regurgitant orifice. MR causes a high-velocity Doppler signal that is detected at the leaflet coaptation point during systole on the LV side. The apical four- and two-chamber as well as the parasternal long- and short-axis views are useful in developing a three-dimensional view of the MR jet.

### Color Doppler Parameters Used To Estimate Severity of Mitral Regurgitation

*Color Jet Area and Jet Area to Left Atrial Area Ratio.* Independent of the etiology of MR, the geometry of the mitral valve apparatus dictates the shape and direction of the MR jet. In the presence of a central jet, as seen in cases of LV or mitral annular dilation, the area of the regurgitant jet or the expression of jet area in relation to the LA size correlate well with the severity of MR as assessed by angiography. MR is mild when the jet area is <3 cm$^2$, moderate when 3 to 6 cm$^2$, and severe when >6 cm$^2$ (10). Based on the jet area to LA area ratio (11), MR is mild when the ratio is <20%, moderate if 20% to 40%, and severe if >40% (Fig. 6.14). These two methods have demonstrated high diagnostic accuracy and high correlation with an-

giographic parameters. However, in the presence of an eccentric jet (as in MVP, flail leaflet, or ischemic MR), the degree of MR may be underestimated because the jet hugs the wall of the LA, producing a deceptively small area of color flow. Eccentric jets frequently are identified when the posterior leaflet is abnormal, resulting in an anteriorly directed jet, or when an anterior leaflet or papillary muscle is dysfunctional and the jet is directed posteriorly.

*Color Jet Length.* The length of the regurgitant jet can be used in the assessment of MR severity. Unlike the jet area to LA ratio, jet length and height correlate poorly with angiography. Severe MR is suggested when the jet length occupies more than half the length of the atrium, whereas MR is mild when the jet is limited to the space immediately behind the leaflet coaptation point. Typically, mild MR is denoted by a jet length <1.5 cm, moderate if 1.5 to 2.7 cm, moderately severe if 3.0 to 4.4 cm, and severe MR if >4.4 cm (12).

*Color Jet Width/Vena Contracta.* In addition to the jet area and length, the size of the vena contracta, the narrowest portion of the proximal regurgitant jet, relates well to the regurgitant orifice area and is a reliable indicator of the severity of MR. This method is particularly useful with eccentric MR jets. A

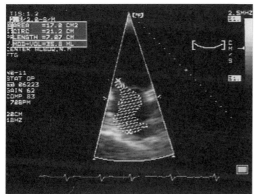
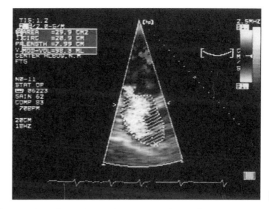

A                                                                                                    B

**FIG. 6.14.** Systolic frames of transthoracic apical two-chamber views demonstrating mitral regurgitation (MR) jet and left atrial area. **A:** Area of regurgitant flow within the left atrium. **B:** Area of regurgitant flow compared to the left atrial area. The regurgitant area of 17 cm$^2$ and area ratio of 56% are consistent with severe MR.

width <0.3 cm favors mild MR, whereas a vena contracta >0.5 cm suggests severe MR (Fig. 6.11). *Practical Point: An important hemodynamic determinant of the size of the MR jet is the transvalvular pressure gradient. Thus, a patient's blood pressure should be noted during an echocardiographic study. For similar size jets, a normotensive patient is more likely to be indicative of a larger regurgitant orifice than that found in a hypertensive patient.*

*Proximal Isovelocity Surface Area.* The aforementioned color Doppler evaluations are all considered semiquantitative in the evaluation of MR. A quantitative method of evaluation of MR severity is the proximal isovelocity surface area (PISA). PISA allows assessment of regurgitant volume and effective regurgitant orifice area using the concept of the continuity equation and flow convergence. The flow proximal to the regurgitant orifice, on the ventricular side of the mitral annulus, is equal to the flow that passes through the regurgitant orifice into the LA. Acceleration of flow occurs proximal to the regurgitant orifice. Flow approaches the regurgitant orifice in hemispheric shells. The flow passing through each shell is identical to the flow that finally passes through the orifice. At the outer edge of the convergence zone, the area is large and the velocity is low; as the jet approaches the regurgitant orifice it becomes smaller in size and higher in velocity (13). The larger the radius of the shell, the greater the severity of MR (Figs. 6.8 and 6.11). *Regurgitant flow* in a convergent jet can be calculated as the *PISA area × jet velocity (aliasing velocity).* The PISA area of a hemisphere is $2\pi r^2$, where r is the radius of the hemispheric shell. By adjusting down the Nyquist limit (the color Doppler velocity scale) usually to 30 cm/s, a measurable radius at the point of aliasing can be achieved. The area of this hemisphere is multiplied by the Nyquist velocity and then divided by the peak MR velocity (assessed by CW Doppler). These provide an instantaneous area of the mitral valve regurgitant orifice. Areas >0.3 $cm^2$ indicate a large mitral regurgitant orifice and severe MR (14).

### Pulsed Wave Doppler

#### Regurgitant Flow and Regurgitant Fraction

The pulsed wave Doppler technique has a sensitivity of at least 90% and a specificity of ≤95% for detection of MR (15). Pulsed wave Doppler provides another marker of MR. Pulsed wave Doppler can be used to assess MR severity by allowing calculation of regurgitant flow and regurgitant fraction. This method is accurate but time consuming (16). *Total flow can be calculated as the mitral valve orifice area × the time velocity integral of flow across the mitral valve. Forward flow* is determined at a nonregurgitant orifice (aortic most commonly used) and *is calculated as the product of outflow tract area × the systolic time velocity integral.* By subtracting the forward flow from total flow, the regurgitant flow can be obtained. The regurgitant fraction is equal to the regurgitant flow divided by the total flow. The larger the regurgitant fraction, the more severe is the MR. MR is denoted as mild by a regurgitant fraction <20%, moderate 20% to 40%, moderately severe 40% to 60%, and severe >60% (17).

#### Pulmonary Veins Inflow Parameters

Perhaps the most useful pulsed wave Doppler information for assessment of the severity of MR is gleaned from pulsed wave Doppler interrogation of pulmonary veins flow. As the MR increases in severity, LA pressure increases and, in turn, the antegrade systolic flow in the pulmonary veins diminishes. With severe regurgitation, systolic reversal of flow in the pulmonary veins may be present (Fig. 6.9B). The regurgitation is more severe when systolic reversal of flow is identified in pulmonary veins that are not in the direction of the regurgitant jet. These Doppler findings are subject to variations in hemodynamic state.

### Continuous Wave Doppler

CW Doppler is helpful in the assessment of MR. The density of the CW Doppler signal provides a gross reflection of the degree of

MR because it is determined by the number of red blood cells within the range of the ultrasound beam. In addition, the shape of the velocity curve reflects the shape of the pressure difference between the LV and LA. From an apical position, with the transducer angulated such that a M-shaped diastolic mitral inflow pattern is identified, MR is characterized by a holosystolic, high-velocity (5 to 6 m/s) signal directed away from the transducer. The regurgitant velocity profile peaks early in systole and then gradually decreases through the latter two thirds of systole. The CW recording demonstrates a smooth curve throughout the regurgitant cycle. In the setting of acute MR, a rise in LA pressure late in systole (the LA V wave) may be seen due to a steep pressure-volume relationship of the nondilated LA. The CW Doppler recording in acute MR reveals a notch (V wave) along the velocity curve as the LA pressure rises, LV–LA pressures equalize, and transmitral systolic pressure gradient falls abruptly. This correlates with a late systolic decline in the auscultatory intensity of the MR murmur in patients with acute severe MR.

### *Mitral Regurgitation Index*

An MR index has been described to determine MR severity (18). The index is derived from six variables: jet penetration, PISA, CW Doppler jet density, pulmonary veins flow, and LA size. Each variable is given a score between 0 and 3, and an averaged global score is obtained. Using an MR index ≥2, patients with a regurgitant fraction >40% were identified with a sensitivity of 100%, specificity of 95%, and positive predictive value of 91% (18). Therefore, the MR index appears to be an objective parameter for clinical evaluation of MR.

## SUMMARY

### Diagnostic Value of the History and Physical Examination

Tables 6.2 and 6.3 describe features of the physical examination that aid in the characterization and stratification of MR.

### Limitations of the History and Physical Examination

In the average patient, the audibility of mild MR is ≤20% and that of moderate or worse MR is uncertain. The audibility of a murmur is decreased in patients with depressed LV function despite the presence of moderate MR. In addition, cardiac tones may be diminished or inaudible, and palpable physical findings may be underappreciated in obese patients or patients with severe lung disease.

Many patients with overt congestive heart failure have severe MR despite a soft murmur. With appropriate medical therapy, LV function may improve; end-diastolic volume decreases, ejection fraction increases, and the murmur becomes louder. When there is profound pump failure and end-stage MR, the systolic murmur may be virtually inaudible.

In acute MR, as occurs in the setting of severe papillary muscle dysfunction or rupture, the murmur of MR may be inaudible. In papillary muscle dysfunction, the relationship between murmur intensity and severity of MR typically is poor due to the coexistence of serious abnormalities of LV contraction.

Eccentric MR jets may produce misleading physical findings. For example, posterior mitral leaflet prolapse may produce an anteriorly directed murmur as opposed to the typical apical murmur that radiates to the left axilla.

### Diagnostic Value of Echocardiography

Both TTE and TEE provide significant information regarding the etiology and degree of MR (Table 6.5), as well as the cardiovascular sequelae of MR.

### Limitations of Echocardiography

There are several limitations that must be recognized in order to ascertain the diagnostic value of echocardiography in the diagnosis and management of MR.

Unfortunately, a patient's body habitus as well as the presence of lung disease may limit image quality.

**TABLE 6.5.** *Assessment of mitral regurgitation severity*

| Method | Mild | Moderate | Moderate to severe | Severe |
|---|---|---|---|---|
| Jet length (cm) | <1.5 | 1.5–2.9 | 3.0–4.4 | >4.4 |
| Jet area (cm²) | <3 | 3–6 | — | >6 |
| Jet area/left atrial area ratio[a] | <20 | 20–40 | — | >40 |
| Vena contracta width (cm) | <0.3 | — | — | >0.5 |
| Regurgitant fraction (%) | <20 | 20–40 | 40–60 | >60 |
| Regurgitant orifice area (cm²) | ≤0.1 | >0.1–0.3 | — | >0.3 |
| Pulmonary venous inflow | — | Diastolic filling predominates | — | Systolic flow reversal and predominant diastolic filling |
| MR index (mean ± SD) | 1.2 ± 0.4 | 1.7 ± 0.4 | — | 2.4 ± 0.3 |

[a]Only in central mitral regurgitation (MR) jets.

Color Doppler can both overestimate and underestimate the degree of MR. Color flow imaging of jet size and length is influenced by instrument settings (pulse repetition frequency, depth, Nyquist limit, gain, etc.), loading conditions, and jet direction. Unfortunately, the vena contracta method of MR analysis is unpredictably affected by changes in LV afterload that may limit its utility. There are other pitfalls associated with this method of analysis, including geometric constraints of the flow convergence zone (i.e., eccentric jets), multiple jets, and a nonspherical orifice.

Analysis of the PISA may be limited in some cases if the hemisphere is difficult to define or the radius is difficult to measure. Although this method is accurate, the time and labor necessary to perform this technique limit its routine applicability.

Clinical scenarios that lead to LA hypertension, such as LV systolic dysfunction and atrial fibrillation, also lead to blunting of pulmonary flow. Thus, in these situations, pulsed wave Doppler assessment of pulmonary flow is a less specific indicator of the severity of MR. Likewise, in conditions with reduced preload or afterload (i.e., hypovolemia or hypotension), the systolic reversal velocity will be decreased concomitant with the reduction in LA pressure.

Two-dimensional imaging is just that, two dimensional. It requires a mental reconstruc-tion of the three-dimensional saddle-shaped mitral valve.

Because neither the physical examination nor any one echocardiographic parameter is adequate alone, evaluation of a patient with MR must take into account the patient's history, physical examination findings, and an integrated echocardiographic analysis.

## REFERENCES

1. Braunwald E, ed. Heart disease: a textbook of cardiovascular medicine. Philadelphia: WB Saunders, 1997.
2. Bonow RO, Carabello B, De Leon AC, et al. ACC/AHA guidelines for the management of patients with valvular heart disease. J Am Coll Cardiol 1998; 32:1486–1588.
3. Smith MD, Cassidy JM, Gurley JC, et al. Echo Doppler evaluation of patients with acute mitral regurgitation: superiority of transesophageal echocardiography with color flow imaging. Am Heart J 1995;129:967–974.
4. Crawford MH, Roldan CA. Quantitative assessment of valve thickness in normal subjects by transesophageal echocardiography. Am J Cardiol 2001;87:1419–1423.
5. Schulter M, Hanrath P. Transesophageal 2-D echocardiographic feature of flail mitral leaflet due to ruptured chordae tendineae. Am Heart J 1984;108:609–610.
6. Roldan CA, Chai A, Coughlin C, et al. Mechanism of mitral regurgitation post myocardial infarction. J Am Coll Cardiol 1998;31:255C.
7. Vasan RS, Shrivastava S, Vijayakumar M, et al. Echocardiographic evaluation of patients with acute rheumatic fever and rheumatic carditis. Circulation 1996;94:73–82.
8. Mugge A, Daniel WG, Frank G, et al. Echocardiography in infective endocarditis: reassessment of prognostic implications of vegetation size determined by the transthoracic and the transesophageal approach. J Am Coll Cardiol 1989;14:631–638.

9. Shively BK, Gurule FT, Roldan CA, et al. Value of transesophageal and transthoracic echocardiography in endocarditis. J Am Coll Cardiol 1991;18:391.
10. Castello R, Lenzen P, Aguirre F, et al. Quantitation of mitral regurgitation by transesophageal echocardiography with Doppler color flow mapping: correlation with cardiac catheterization. J Am Coll Cardiol 1992;19:1516–1521.
11. Helmcke F, Nanda NC, Msiung MC, et al. Color Doppler assessment of mitral regurgitation with orthogonal planes. Circulation 1987;75:175–183.
12. Miyatake K, Izumi S, Okamoto M, et al. Semiquantitative grading of severity of mitral regurgitation by real-time two-dimensional Doppler flow imaging technique. J Am Coll Cardiol 1986;7:82.
13. Bargiggia GS, Tronconi L, Sahn DJ, et al. A new method for quantification of mitral regurgitation based on color flow Doppler imaging of flow convergence proximal to regurgitant orifice. Circulation 1991;84:1481–1489.
14. Enriquez-Sarano M, Miller FA Jr, Hayes SN, et al. Effective mitral regurgitant orifice area: clinical use and pitfalls of the proximal isovelocity surface area method. J Am Coll Cardiol 1995;25:703–709.
15. Pu M, Vandervoort PM, Griffin BP, et al. Quantification of mitral regurgitation by the proximal convergence method using transesophageal echocardiography: clinical validation of a geometric correction for proximal flow constraint. Circulation 1995;92:2169–2177.
16. Pearlman AS, Otto CM. Quantification of valvular regurgitation. Echocardiography 1987;4:271–340.
17. Heinle SK, Hall SA, Brickner ME, et al. Comparison of vena contracta width by transesophageal echocardiography with quantitative Doppler assessment of mitral regurgitation. Am J Cardiol 1998;81:175–179.
18. Thomas L, Foster E, Schiller NB. Mitral regurgitation index: a new semiquantitative guide to evaluate severity. Circulation 1997;96[85 Suppl]:I-541.

# 7

# The Patient with Mitral Stenosis

Edward A. Gill, *Carlos A. Roldan, and †Jonathan Abrams

*Department of Internal Medicine, University of Washington School of Medicine; and Cardiology Division, Harborview Medical Center, Seattle, Washington; *Department of Internal Medicine, University of New Mexico School of Medicine; and Department of Internal Medicine, Veterans Affairs Medical Center, Albuquerque, New Mexico; †Cardiology Division, University of New Mexico School of Medicine; and Department of Internal Medicine, University Hospital, Albuquerque, New Mexico*

## INTRODUCTION

Mitral stenosis is a diagnosis that has been declining in frequency due to near eradication of rheumatic fever. In fact, in 1995, the Centers for Disease for Control declared that rheumatic fever was one of ten diseases that had been removed from the list of nationally notifiable diseases. Despite this fact, in the mid-1980s, after more than a decade of the apparent absence of cases of rheumatic fever, numerous outbreaks occurred in a variety of geographic and socioeconomic settings across the United States, most notably in Utah (1). In addition, patients who had rheumatic fever 30 to 50 years ago are now presenting with mitral stenosis. These state-

ments apply to the demographics of mitral stenosis in the United States, but they are not true for other parts of the world, where rheumatic fever is still endemic.

Rheumatic fever is the most common cause of mitral stenosis. Other immune-mediated valvulitis, such as systemic lupus erythematosus, and congenital mitral stenosis are rare causes of mitral stenosis (2). Although mitral annular calcification usually causes mitral regurgitation (MR), rare cases result in nonclinically significant mitral stenosis.

Chronic rheumatic valvulitis culminating in mitral stenosis is a result of thickening, sclerosis, retraction, and distortion of the valve leaflets and chordae tendineae, along with commissural fusion. Commonly, the process begins with commissural fusion resulting in a narrowed valve. Typically, the leaflets are thickened and have blunted and rolled edges. The chordae are foreshortened and often matted together. The entire valve apparatus becomes altered into a funnel-like sleeve; when severe, the mitral valve takes on a "fish mouth" appearance and loses the ability to open during diastole. Dense calcification is a frequent late accompaniment.

Pure mitral stenosis occurs in 25% of patients, whereas 40% have combined mitral stenosis and MR.

The most characteristic symptoms of mitral stenosis are similar to those of heart failure, and may include dyspnea on exertion, orthopnea, paroxysmal nocturnal dyspnea, fatigue, and lower extremity edema. Dyspnea, although nonspecific, is the most common symptom in patients with mitral stenosis. Palpitations are a common complaint in patients with atrial fibrillation.

## PHYSICAL EXAMINATION

### General Appearance

There are no distinguishing features in most patients. The majority of subjects are women. In individuals with severe mitral stenosis, especially with major pulmonary hypertension, "mitral facies" may be observed, i.e., a patchy, pinkish-purple appearance of the cheeks resulting from dilated venules. Such subjects often manifest peripheral cyanosis as well. Patients with advanced mitral valve disease and right ventricular (RV) failure typically are thin and often have acrocyanosis and peripheral edema.

### Blood Pressure and Radial Pulse

Blood pressure in patients with mitral stenosis is normal. It may be reduced somewhat in severe disease due to low cardiac output. In this setting, the radial pulse is diminished and the carotid arterial pulse is of small volume. An irregularly irregular pulse due to atrial fibrillation is common in chronic mitral stenosis.

### Jugular Venous Pressure

In patients in sinus rhythm, a prominent A wave is often seen. In patients with atrial fibrillation, the A wave and X descent disappear and there is only one crest (V wave) in the jugular venous pulse, which can be quite prominent even in the absence of tricuspid regurgitation. As many subjects with mitral stenosis develop pulmonary hypertension over time, RV hypertrophy and enlargement are common. Associated tricuspid regurgitation, either functional or in part related to organic rheumatic involvement of the tricuspid leaflets, is extremely common; thus, a prominent jugular V wave often is seen, both in the presence or absence of tricuspid regurgitation. When right atrial pressure is elevated, due to RV hypertrophy or RV dysfunction, the mean jugular pressure will be elevated (see Chapter 1).

### Examination of the Precordium

Examination of the precordium typically reveals a small or unimpressive left ventricular (LV) apical impulse due to diminished filling of a small LV. A palpable presystolic A wave makes significant mitral stenosis quite unlikely. If there is moderate or greater associated MR, the LV impulse may be prominent; this can misdirect the clinician, as the experienced examiner anticipates that the LV impulse in pure mitral stenosis is diminutive.

Typically, the first heart sound ($S_1$) is felt at or inside the site of the LV apex beat. An increased pulmonic valve component ($P_2$) and, less commonly, a pulmonary artery lift may be felt at the second to third left interspace. The opening snap (OS) often is palpable in the region between the lower left sternal border and cardiac apex. A diastolic thrill at the apex, produced by a very loud mitral rumble, occasionally may be detected in the left decubitus position.

*Right ventricular impulse:* It is common to detect parasternal activity in pure mitral stenosis. *Practical Point: To detect parasternal motion, it is desirable to use firm pressure with the heel of the hand during held-expiration* (Fig. 1.12). An RV impulse often will be detected in mitral stenosis even when resting pulmonary pressure is high normal or only moderately elevated. In individuals with more severe pulmonary hypertension, the RV impulse can be very prominent. The parasternal heave or major RV enlargement often extends leftward; in severe degrees of RV enlargement, the apex may be formed by the RV. The typical rumble of mitral stenosis may not be heard unless auscultation occurs when one listens precisely over the LV impulse, which may be displaced laterally to the anterior or mid-axillary line by a huge RV.

### Heart Sounds

#### *First Heart Sound*

A loud $S_1$ is heard when the mitral valve is thickened and stenosed, but remains flexible and is not heavily calcified (Fig. 7.1). The mitral valve leaflets remain maximally open un-til ventricular systole begins, at which point the valve closes quickly and creates a loud sound, in part related to decreased compliance of the leaflets themselves. Conversely, if the valve is particularly thick and calcified, there may be relatively little movement of the valve leaflets with opening or closing; hence, $S_1$ (and the OS) may be soft. The loud $S_1$ of mitral stenosis often is palpable.

#### *Second Heart Sound*

The pulmonic component ($P_2$) of the second heart sound often is increased in amplitude due to pulmonary hypertension. $P_2$ may be palpable and often is associated with an RV lift.

#### *Opening Snap*

The OS is one of the classic findings in cardiac physical diagnosis (Fig. 7.1). *Practical Point: A loud OS indicates the diagnosis of mi-*

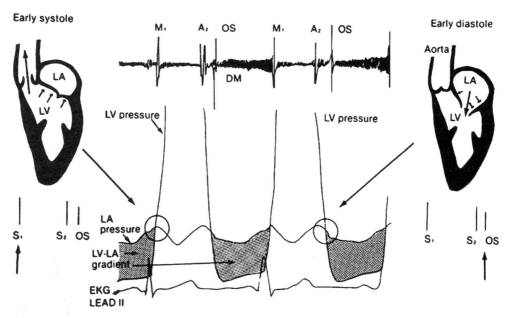

**FIG. 7.1.** Intracardiac pressure and sound relationships in mitral stenosis. Pressure crossover between the left atrium (LA) and left ventricle (LV) always precedes the cardiac sounds generated by mitral valve closure ($M_1$) and opening (opening snap [OS]). The persistence of a late diastolic gradient between the LA and LV in combination with the thickened mitral valve apparatus results in accentuated $S_1$. Similarly, the maximal opening excursion of the rigid and fibrotic valve generates an OS, which immediately precedes early diastolic filling of the LV and the resultant diastolic murmur (DM). (From Abrams J. Prim Cardiol 1983, with permission).

*tral stenosis.* The OS is the sound produced precisely when the stenotic mitral valve leaflets maximally open; as a loud $S_1$ in mitral stenosis requires the valve to be flexible and mobile, so does a prominent OS. The OS is due to sudden tensing of the valve leaflets just after the valve cusps have completed their opening excursion. (Figs. 7.1 and 7.2). Neither a loud $S_1$ nor an OS will be present with advanced deformity of the valve involving severe thickening and calcification. In fact, $S_1$ and the OS are reciprocal sounds caused by opposite movement of the valve. Paradoxically, although the absence of a loud $S_1$ and an OS predicts severe deformation of the valve, neither is a good indicator of the actual severity of the orifice stenosis.

The OS occurs earlier or closer to $S_2$ than the third heart sound ($S_3$). The unusual combination of an OS and an $S_3$ should make one think of combined mitral stenosis and MR.

An OS is classically a higher-pitched sound than an $S_3$. The shorter the duration from the aortic valve component ($A_2$) to the OS, the worse the severity of valvular stenosis. As left atrial (LA) pressure rises above LV pressure, the mitral valve opens. In severe mitral stenosis, the LA pressure is markedly elevated, LV pressure drops below the LA pressure very early in diastole and, hence, there is a short $A_2$–OS duration. Shortening of the $A_2$–OS interval over time suggests increasing mitral stenosis severity. *Dynamic auscultation* can affect the $A_2$–OS interval. For instance, standing will increase the $A_2$–OS interval, and sudden squatting will narrow the $A_2$–OS interval. The standing and squatting maneuvers may be helpful in distinguishing the $S_2$–OS complex in mitral stenosis from a split $S_2$, which will narrow on standing and widen on squatting (Table 7.1).

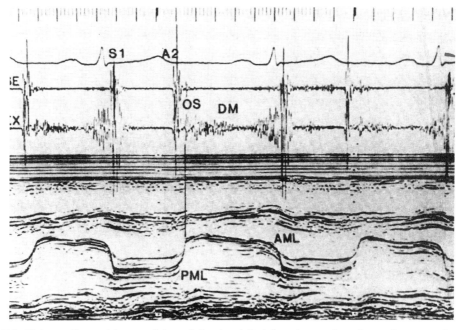

**FIG. 7.2.** Echocardiographic correlates of the loud first heart sound and opening snap in mitral stenosis. $S_1$ is produced by mitral valve closure and is accentuated and delayed due to elevation of left atrial pressure and the loss of valve compliance. A prominent presystolic diastolic murmur merges with $S_1$; this represents augmented transmitral flow with left atrial contraction. The opening snap (OS) times precisely with the maximum opening excursion of the anterior mitral leaflet of the mitral valve and is produced by tensing of the valve cusps during early diastole. Left ventricular filling and the resultant early to mid-diastolic murmur (DM) follows the OS. (From Reddy PS, Salerni R, Shaver JA. Normal and abnormal heart sounds in cardiac diagnosis. Part II. Diastolic sounds. Curr Prog Cardiol 1985;10:1, with permission.)

**TABLE 7.1.** *Dynamic cardiac auscultation and the murmur of mitral stenosis*

| Maneuver | Effect |
| --- | --- |
| Expiration | ↑ |
| Inspiration | ↓ |
| Isometric exercise | ↑ |
| Isotonic exercise | ↑ |
| Coughing | ↑ |
| Sudden squatting | ↑ |
| Sudden standing | ↓ |
| Valsalva maneuver | ↓ |
| Amyl nitrite | ↑ |

### Diastolic Murmur

The most notable finding on examination of patients with mitral stenosis, in addition to the OS, is a diastolic rumbling murmur (Fig. 7.3). It often is missed and can be difficult to hear, especially if one is not listening specifically for this murmur. Several clues usually are present that should influence the examiner

to suspect mitral stenosis, for instance, the loud $S_1$, which often is palpable. In addition, a parasternal heave or lift is common in mitral stenosis. Furthermore, the diastolic murmur may be palpable (thrill at the apex with the patient in the left lateral decubitus position). The

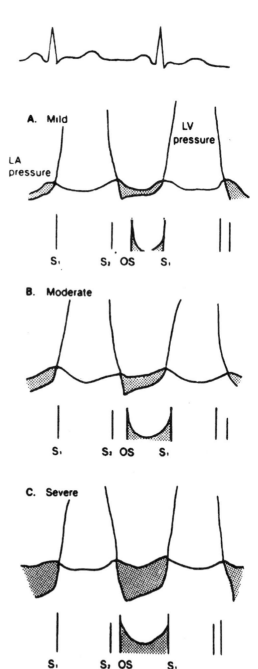

**FIG. 7.3.** Relationship of severity of mitral stenosis to timing of the diastolic murmur and opening snap (OS). There are two separate components to the murmur of mitral stenosis. The first occurs in early diastole during the rapid filling phase and immediately follows the opening snap. The second sound follows atrial contraction and represents late diastolic augmentation of blood flow across the mitral valve. **A:** Mild mitral stenosis. A murmur may be heard in early diastole, late diastole, or both. The OS is relatively late. **B:** Moderately severe mitral stenosis. There is a pressure gradient across the mitral valve that persists into late diastole. The mitral murmur typically begins with a loud rush, tapers in mid-diastole, and becomes louder in late diastole as it crescendos into the loud $S_1$ (presystolic accentuation). The OS occurs closer to $S_2$. **C:** Severe mitral stenosis. The large holodiastolic gradient and markedly elevated left atrial pressure produces blood flow across the mitral valve that is accompanied by considerable turbulence. A prominent holodiastolic murmur follows an early OS and extends to $S_1$. There may or may not be presystolic accentuation, depending upon whether the patient remains in sinus rhythm. When the murmur has dominant medium-frequency vibrations and is heard throughout diastole, it can mimic the murmur of aortic regurgitation (From Abrams J. Prim Cardiol 1983, with permission.)

**TABLE 7.2.** *Cardiac conditions that imitate the diastolic murmur of mitral stenosis*

1. Austin Flint murmur of aortic regurgitation
2. Diastolic flow murmur caused by excessive flow across the mitral valve, such as in a large ventricular septal defect or with severe mitral regurgitation
3. Medially located diastolic murmur caused by a large atrial septal defect with increased flow across the tricuspid valve
4. Carey Coombs murmur is the murmur of mitral valvulitis heard during acute rheumatic fever. It typically differs from the classic mitral stenosis murmur in that it is a soft, early diastolic murmur that is higher pitched and varies from day to day. In particular, the Carey Coombs murmur would be expected to resolve after treatment of acute rheumatic fever.
5. Atrial myxoma that causes partial obstruction of the mitral valve

diastolic murmur is characteristically low frequency and "rumbling" in character. It immediately follows the OS and may taper off in late diastole. It also may increase in loudness late in diastole after atrial contraction. This is known as presystolic accentuation (Figs. 7.1–7.2). In mild mitral stenosis, the late or presystolic component may be the only murmur heard. With severe mitral stenosis, the diastolic murmur extends from the OS to the loud S$_1$. When high-frequency vibrations predominates, a long murmur may be mistaken for that of aortic regurgitation. Table 7.2 lists cardiovascular conditions that can be confused with mitral stenosis.

*Listen at the apex:* The mitral diastolic rumble typically is best (or only) heard at the LV apex, using light pressure with the bell of the stethoscope, with the patient in the left lateral position. This murmur may be heard more easily after several coughs, handgrip, or turning to the left decubitus position. The inexperienced examiner may have difficulty identifying systole and diastole in the presence of the mitral diastolic murmur and a prominent OS. Careful attention to assessment of systole and diastole is critical.

**Assessment of Severity**

Several findings on the physical examination may help to define the severity of mitral stenosis (Table 7.3).

**TABLE 7.3.** *Assessment of mitral stenosis severity by physical examination*

| Physical finding | Mild | Moderate | Severe |
|---|---|---|---|
| General appearance | Normal | Normal | May have overt signs of congestive heart failure. Cachexia if very advanced. |
| Carotid and arterial pulses | Normal | Normal or atrial fibrillation | Small volume. Atrial fibrillation common. |
| Jugular venous pressure | Normal | Normal | Elevated mean pressure common. Big V waves if tricuspid regurgitation. Loss of A wave if atrial fibrillation. |
| Apical impulse | Normal. Palpable S$_1$ and OS. | RV lift. Palpable S$_1$, OS, apical diastolic thrill. LV impulse small unless associated MR. | RV lift prominent. Palpable S$_1$, OS, P2, diastolic apical thrill. LV impulse small unless associated MR. |
| Heart sounds | Increased S$_1$, OS | Increased S$_1$, OS, increased P2 | Increased S$_1$, OS, P2. |
| Diastolic murmur (use left lateral position, bell of stethoscope) | May only be early diastolic or presystolic. Sound gap between two murmurs | Holodiastolic murmur after OS, accentuated in mid and late diastole; may have a thrill. Occasionally medium–high frequency | Holodiastolic, even with long cycle lengths. Can be quite loud (with thrill) at apex. |

LV, left ventricle; MR, mitral regurgitation; OS, opening snap; RV, right ventricle.

### Mild Mitral Stenosis

In patients with a small resting LA–LV gradient, there may be either a short early diastolic murmur or, on occasion, only a presystolic crescendo murmur.

### Mild to Moderate Mitral Stenosis

Both the early and late murmurs are heard.

### Moderate to Severe Stenosis

In patients with a substantial and persistent LA–LV gradient, the diastolic rumble truly is *pandiastolic*; sound vibrations start with the OS and extend to $S_1$, typically with an increase in intensity at end-diastole. In subjects with slow heart rates or variable cycle lengths during atrial fibrillation, it is important to carefully assess the length of the murmur. *Practical Point: A holodiastolic murmur following the OS during long R-R intervals in sinus rhythm or atrial fibrillation is consistent with major obstruction at the mitral valve level.*

### Silent Mitral Stenosis

It is uncommon for mitral stenosis to be truly undetectable or silent, but this situation does occur. In very mild mitral stenosis with a large mitral valve orifice and a small gradient, the murmur may be absent. The most common cause of silent mitral stenosis is poor auscultatory technique, such as improper application of the stethoscope (failure to use the left decubitus position, failure to use light pressure with the bell), erroneous identification of the cardiac apex, lack of the use of murmur enhancement techniques, or misinterpretation of cardiac findings. Very severe mitral stenosis, associated pulmonary hypertension, and combination lesions (e.g., aortic valve disease) commonly result in silent mitral stenosis on auscultation.

## ECHOCARDIOGRAPHY

### Introduction

Transthoracic (TTE) and transesophageal (TEE) M-mode, two-dimensional (2-D), pulse, continuous wave, and color Doppler echocardiography play essential roles in the diagnosis and assessment of severity of mitral stenosis. These techniques are important in defining the timing and most appropriate type of therapy for mitral stenosis. TTE or TEE M-mode, especially 2-D, and recently three-dimensional echocardiography accurately characterize the morphology of the mitral valve and subvalvular apparatus (thickening, sclerosis, calcification, and mobility), identify patients who are candidates for mitral valvuloplasty, and predict patient prognosis. TEE is helpful in detecting LA thrombi and can be used to guide and assess outcome of mitral valve balloon valvuloplasty. Pulse, continuous wave, and color Doppler echocardiography allow for accurate assessment of the severity of mitral stenosis and associated regurgitation.

### Transthoracic M-Mode and Two-Dimensional Echocardiography

Mitral stenosis is one of the most important contributions of M-mode echocardiography in the diagnosis of cardiovascular diseases. In fact, mitral stenosis on M-mode images has unique or specific characteristics. The mitral leaflets are thickened, have markedly decreased mobility with blunting to disappearance of the E to F slope, and parallel anterior motion of both leaflets due to commissural fusion and subvalvular/chordal thickening and fusion (Figs. 7.2 and 7.4)

Two-dimensional echocardiography is more accurate than M-mode echocardiography in the diagnosis of mitral stenosis. Typical findings include thickening predominantly of the leaflet tips. Restricted leaflet mobility with a characteristic diastolic doming pattern, especially of the anterior leaflet (called *hockey stick*), is easily defined (Fig. 7.5). This characteristic leaflet mobility pattern is due to tethering of the leaflets by retracted and fused chordae tendineae and in part due to commissural fusion. The extent of subvalvular apparatus thickening and calcification also is determined.

TTE 2-D echocardiography has been used to measure the actual orifice area. This method

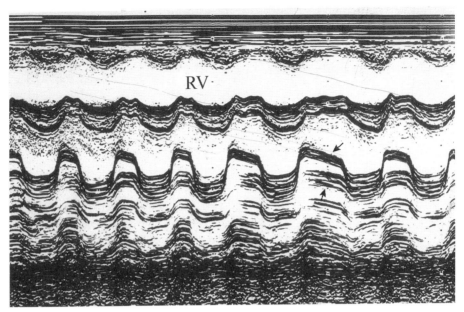

**FIG. 7.4.** M-mode echocardiogram of a severely stenotic mitral valve. Note the marked thickening, decreased mobility, and parallel anterior motion of both anterior and posterior mitral leaflets *(arrows)*. (Courtesy of Albuquerque New Mexico Veterans Affairs Medical Center Echocardiography Laboratory.)

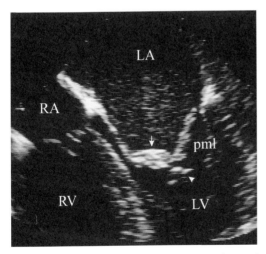

**FIG. 7.5.** Two-dimensional transesophageal echocardiogram of severe mitral stenosis. Note the severe thickening predominantly of the anterior mitral leaflet tip *(arrow)*. Tethering of the anterior mitral leaflet results in doming mobility of the leaflet and its characteristic hockey stick appearance *(arrow)*. The posterior leaflet (pml) appears diffusely thickened and is fixed. Note involvement of the subvalvular apparatus *(arrowhead)*. Left atrial (LA) spontaneous echo contrast is noted. RA, right atrium; RV, right ventricle; LV, left ventricle. (Courtesy of the Albuquerque New Mexico Veterans Affairs Medical Center Echocardiography Laboratory.)

correlates well with other echocardiographic parameters of assessing valve area and moderately when tested against the Gorlin formula, and has demonstrated up to 0.95 correlation when compared with a true anatomic orifice (3,4). The accuracy of this method is dependent of the ability to define the true valve orifice at the level of the leaflet tips.

By 2-D echocardiography, a scoring system has been developed to assess the extent of mitral leaflet and submitral valve apparatus involvement. This score determines the feasibility of balloon or surgical valvuloplasty; predict its short- and long-term success; and predicts development of complications (Table 7.4) . Thickening, mobility, and calcification of the mitral leaflets as well as of the chordae tendineae are scored from 1 (mild involvement) to 4 (severe) (5). Therefore, the lowest score is 4 and the highest is 16. A score <8 predicts short- and long-term success of mitral balloon valvuloplasty. Parameters of a successful balloon valvuloplasty include an increase in valve area of >50%, valve area >1.5 cm², and ≤2+ MR. Patients with a successful procedure have an event-free survival (death, repeat valvuloplasty, or valve replacement) of

**TABLE 7.4.** *Grading of mitral valve characteristics from the echocardiographic examination*

| Grade | Mobility | Subvalvar thickening | Thickening | Calcification |
|-------|----------|---------------------|------------|---------------|
| 1 | Highly mobile valve with only leaflet tips restricted | Minimal thickening just below the mitral leaflets | Leaflets near normal in thickness (4–5 mm) | Single area of increased echo brightness |
| 2 | Leaflet mid and basal portions have normal mobility | Thickening of chordal structures extending up to one third of the chordal length | Mid leaflets normal, considerable thickening of margins (5–8 mm) | Scattered areas of brightness confined to leaflet margins |
| 3 | Valve continues to move forward in diastole, mainly from the base | Thickening extending to the distal third of the chords | Thickening extending through the entire leaflet (6–8 mm) | Brightness extending into the mid portion of the leaflets |
| 4 | No or minimal forward movement of the leaflets in diastole | Extensive thickening and shortening of all chordal structures extending down to the papillary muscles | Considerable thickening of all leaflet tissue (>8–10 mm) | Extensive brightness throughout much of the leaflet tissue |

80% to 96% at 1 year, >60% at 4 years, and >55% at 6 years (6,7). Furthermore, valve scores >10 and commissural calcification have been associated with a 9% to 13% incidence of moderate to severe MR after single balloon valvuloplasty (8). The mechanism of moderate MR is excessive commissural tear (60% to 65%) and leaflet or chordal rupture or perforation (35% to 40%). However, severe MR is more commonly caused by leaflet rupture (73%), chordal rupture (18%), and excessive commisural tear (9%) (9).

With the recent advent of harmonic imaging, TTE can detect LA spontaneous echo contrast or pseudocontrast in >80% of patients with pseudocontrast on TEE (10). This finding contrasts with a detection rate of <10% by fundamental imaging.

### Pulse and Continuous Wave Doppler Echocardiography

Pulse and continuous wave Doppler echocardiography are the most important imaging techniques in assessing the severity of mitral stenosis. These techniques allow accurate estimation of mitral valve area as well as valve peak and mean gradients by using the continuity equation and pressure half-time ($P_{1/2}$).

### *Continuity Equation*

The continuity equation is used almost routinely to determine mitral valve area (11). The principle of this equation is that the flow rate through a stenotic valve is the same as that of a nonstenotic valve. This equation commonly uses the estimated flow rate or stroke volume at the aortic and mitral valves.

The equation includes both pulse and continuous wave Doppler parameters as follows: Mitral valve area = LV outflow tract area ($cm^2$) × pulse Doppler velocity time integral of the LV outflow tract (cm/s) divided by the continuous wave Doppler velocity time integral across the mitral valve (cm/s). The outflow tract area is derived from the LV outflow tract diameter obtained from the TTE parasternal or TEE long-axis view as $r^2 \times \pi$. *Mitral stenosis is mild if the calculated valve area is >1.5 $cm^2$, moderate if 1.0 to 1.5 $cm^2$, and severe if <1$cm^2$.*

The continuous wave velocity time integral across the stenotic mitral valve orifice also determines the peak and mean valve gradients (12). *Mitral stenosis is mild if the mean gradient is <5 mm Hg, moderate if 5 to 10 mm Hg, and severe if >10 mm Hg* (Fig. 7.6A).

### *Pressure Half-Time*

$P_{1/2}$ measures the time (in milliseconds) it takes for the peak mitral valve gradient, as determined by continuous wave Doppler, to decrease by 50%. The longer the $P_{1/2}$, the worse is the mitral stenosis. *Mitral valve area is calculated then as the constant 220 divided by $P_{1/2}$* (Fig. 7.6B). *Mitral stenosis is mild if $P_{1/2}$ is <130 ms, moderate if 130 to 220 ms, and severe if >220 ms.* The Doppler $P_{1/2}$ has been validated against catheterization data (13,14).

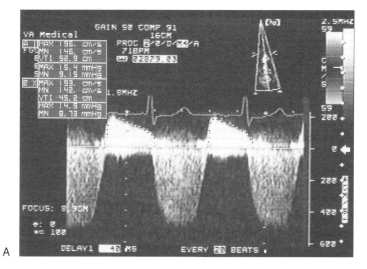

A

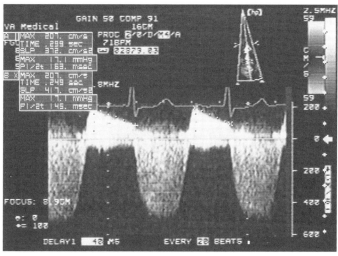

B

**FIG. 7.6.** Mitral stenosis and regurgitation. **A:** Continuous wave Doppler velocity time integrals of the transmitral flow demonstrate mean gradients of 8 to 9 mm Hg. **B:** Pressure half-time of the transmitral flow ranged from 145 to 163 ms. These values are consistent with moderate mitral stenosis and correlated well with a mitral valve area of 1.3 cm² calculated by the continuity equation. Associated mitral regurgitation also was detected. (Courtesy of the Albuquerque New Mexico Veterans Affairs Medical Center Echocardiography Laboratory.)

The correlation coefficient of this method when compared with direct measurement of an anatomic valve orifices is at least 0.80.

### Color Doppler Echocardiography

With this technique, high-velocity flow can be demonstrated at the valve orifice (vena contracta) as well as proximal to the stenotic area in the LA side. Proximal to the stenotic orifice, an acceleration zone, flow convergence zone, or proximal isovelocity surface area (PISA) is generally seen. The PISA can be used to calculate the mitral valve area (14). To define the PISA, the color Doppler settings must be adjusted to define a hemispheric aliasing surface area (Fig. 7.7). The velocity at the outer shells of the PISA equals

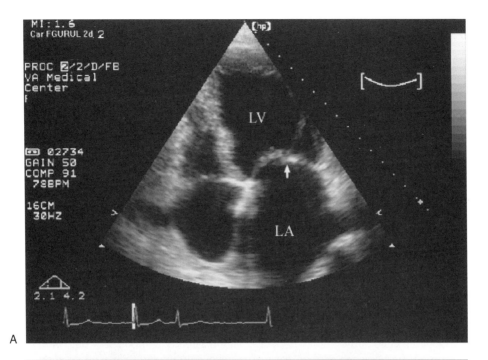

A

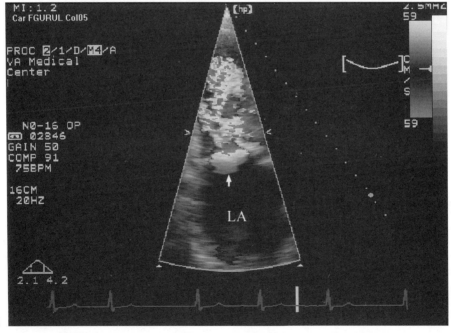

B

**FIG. 7.7.** Color Doppler assessment of mitral stenosis. **A:** Four-chamber transthoracic echocardio-gram shows marked thickening and decreased and doming mobility of both anterior and posterior mitral leaflets *(arrow)*. **B:** Large flow convergence zone *(arrow)* is noted proximal to the mitral orifice. The mitral valve area calculated with the proximal isovelocity area was 0.9 cm$^2$ and correlated well with that calculated by the pressure half-time and continuity equation. Abbreviations as in Fig. 7.5. (Courtesy of the Albuquerque New Mexico Veterans Affairs Medical Center Echocardiography Lab-oratory.) (See Color Figure 7.7B.)

that of the Nyquist limit. The PISA length allows for calculation of the flow rate proximal to the valve orifice, which equals the flow rate across the stenotic orifice (principle of the continuity equation).

*Therefore, flow rate (cm³/s) proximal to the stenotic orifice is calculated using the formula for a hemispheric or hemielliptic model as $2 \times \pi \times r^2 \times Vr$, where r is the radius or length of the PISA and Vr is the corresponding color Doppler aliasing velocity (cm/s). This value can be multiplied by a factor that corrects for the mitral inflow angle ($\theta/180$). The proximal flow rate then is divided by the continuous wave Doppler peak velocity time integral across the mitral valve to obtain the mitral valve area* (4,14) (Fig. 7.7). This method has demonstrated a correlation coefficient of 0.87 when compared with direct measurement of an anatomic valve orifice.

Color Doppler echocardiography is accurate in defining the presence and severity of associated MR. This is especially important, because ≥mild MR is a contraindication to perform balloon valvuloplasty. Also, this technique can assess the development and severity of MR during or following balloon valvuloplasty.

### Exercise or Dobutamine Echocardiography

In some patients, echocardiography may reveal resting hemodynamics (valve area, peak and mean gradients, or pulmonary artery pressure) that are disproportional to patients' symptoms. In these patients, exercise or dobutamine echocardiography are of complementary diagnostic value. During stress, a significant increase in peak and mean gradients as well as pulmonary artery pressure can be demonstrated. These data are important in the decision to recommend balloon valvuloplasty or valve replacement (15–17).

### Transesophageal Echocardiography

Adequate TTE studies generally provide most of the information needed to define the presence and severity of mitral stenosis and its hemodynamic impact on LA size; LA and pulmonary artery pressures; presence and severity of associated MR; and assessment of LV size and function. This technique also allows adequate evaluation of valve morphology, including commissural fusion.

However, because of the proximity of the transducer to the mitral valve, LA, and interatrial septum, TEE provides complementary and additive information to TTE about the morphology and function of these structures. Using TEE M-mode or 2-D images, mitral leaflet thickness can be quantitatively assessed (18). TEE can accurately assess the extent of leaflet calcification and decreased mobility; severity of associated MR; and extent of subvalvular apparatus involvement. This technique also can determine the extent of commissural fusion. These data are especially important in predicting feasibility and potential outcome of percutaneous mitral valvuloplasty.

The presence of LA thrombus is a contraindication to balloon valvuloplasty. TEE has a sensitivity, specificity, and predictive accuracy of 95% to 100% for detecting LA thrombi (19). Spontaneous echo contrast or pseudocontrast in the LA (a predictor of LA thrombi formation and future cardioembolism) also is detected better by TEE than TTE. The prevalence of LA thrombi (more common in the appendage and LA posterior wall) and pseudocontrast in patients with mitral stenosis is 7% to 15% and >60%, respectively. LA thrombi and pseudocontrast are related to the severity of mitral stenosis, LA size, and atrial fibrillation (20). However, pseudocontrast can be detected by TEE in about 25% of patients in normal sinus rhythm (21).

The prevalence of LA thrombi and pseudocontrast is lower in patients with moderate or worse MR (17%) compared to patients without significant MR (94%) (22).

On-line TEE is a feasible, safe, and well-tolerated alternative to fluoroscopy-guided percutaneous balloon valvuloplasty (23,24). This technique can guide transseptal catheterization and balloon placement; detect LA thrombi; and assess postvalvuloplasty valve area, gradient, and degree of MR. Using TEE, the fluoroscopy time can be reduced by at least 50%. This advantage is of most importance in pregnant patients in need of an emergent valvuloplasty (25).

### Three-Dimensional Echocardiography

This technique currently is used to evaluate commissural fusion as an important predictor of outcome in patients considered for percutaneous mitral valvuloplasty (Fig. 7.8) (26). The planimetered valve area before and after valvuloplasty by this technique correlate well with that measured by $P_{1/2}$ and the continuity equation. Complete and partial commissural split is the main determinant of postprocedure valve area. This technique also allows detection of tears in the mitral leaflets leading to postprocedure MR (26).

### Other Echocardiographic Findings

In addition to evaluation of mitral valve area and gradients, other structural and hemodynamic parameters reflective of mitral stenosis severity need to be evaluated.

LA size and pressure increase in proportion to the severity of mitral stenosis. The more se-

vere the stenosis is, the larger the LA size and the more likely atrial fibrillation will occur.

Pulmonary venous Doppler flow patterns have been assessed in patients with mitral stenosis and have demonstrated decreases in systolic, diastolic, and atrial reversal velocities. These velocities increase significantly after mitral valvuloplasty (27), but these data are of uncertain clinical value.

Pulmonary hypertension develops because of elevated LA pressure and corresponding elevated pulmonary capillary wedge pressure. Consequently, RV dilation and hypertrophy and tricuspid regurgitation develop.

Because rheumatic heart disease can affect all heart valves, it is important to carefully evaluate other valves for the presence and severity of regurgitation or stenosis.

### SUMMARY

### Diagnostic Value of the Physical Examination

A careful and complete physical examination should allow for diagnosis of mitral stenosis, especially if the stenosis is of moderate or worse degree. The physical examination also is important in the selection of patients for balloon valvotomy. Presence of an

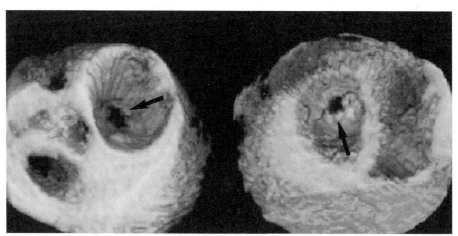

A                                                                                                B

**FIG. 7.8.** Three-dimensional echocardiogram in mitral stenosis. **A:** Three-dimensional echocardiogram showing a stenotic mitral valve viewed from above the valve (*arrow*). **B:** Three-dimensional echocardiogram showing a stenotic mitral valve viewed from below the valve (*arrow*).

**TABLE 7.5.** *Echocardiographic assessment of mitral stenosis severity*

| Severity | Valve area (cm$^2$) | Mean gradient (mm Hg) | P$_{1/2}$ time (ms) |
|---|---|---|---|
| **Mild** | 1.6–2.0 | <5 | ≤130 |
| **Moderate** | 1.1–1.5 | 6–10 | 130–220 |
| **Severe** | ≤1.0 | >10 | >220 |

OS and a loud S$_1$ indicates a flexible valve that is likely to respond favorably to percutaneous mitral valvotomy. Also, clinically detectable MR suggest more than mild MR. Although several components of the cardiovascular physical examination can help in determining the extent of mitral stenosis (Table 7.3), echocardiography is necessary to reliably assess the severity of the disease and determine its appropriate therapy.

### Diagnostic Value of Echocardiography

M-mode, 2-D, color Doppler, and, in specific situations, TEE or stress echocardiography are highly accurate in the diagnosis and assessment of the severity of mitral stenosis (Table 7.5). In addition, echocardiography is important and necessary in determining the time and most appropriate type of therapy (i.e., careful and serial clinical and/or echocardiographic follow-up vs. percutaneous balloon valvuloplasty or valve replacement). Finally, on-line TEE can be used to exclude atrial thrombi; guide balloon valvuloplasty; and determine postprocedure mitral valve area, gradient, and degree of MR.

In patients with suspected or known to have mitral stenosis, use of echocardiography needs to be judicious and should follow specific clinical criteria as suggested by the American College of Cardiology/American Heart Association (ACC/AHA) guidelines for the application of echocardiography and guidelines for the management of patients with valvular heart disease (Table 7.6) (28,29).

### Limitations of Echocardiography

Although echocardiography is highly accurate in the assessment of the severity of mitral stenosis, a few limitations of the technique need to be emphasized to prevent misdiagnoses.

1. A reduced E to F slope is relatively nonspecific for diagnosis of mitral stenosis and can be influenced by reduced LV preload, compliance and contractility. Therefore, a reduced E to F slope can be observed in patients with LV systolic dysfunction, elevated LV end-diastolic pressure, or aortic regurgitation (regurgitant jet does not allow normal opening of the anterior leaflet).

**TABLE 7.6.** *Class I indications for echocardiography in patients with mitral stenosis*

1. Diagnosis of mitral stenosis, assessment of hemodynamic severity (mean gradient, mitral valve area, pulmonary artery pressure), and assessment of right ventricular size and function
2. Assessment of valve morphology to determine suitability for percutaneous mitral balloon valvotomy
3. Diagnosis and assessment of concomitant valvular lesions
4. Reevaluation of patients with known mitral stenosis with changing symptoms or signs
5. Assessment of changes in hemodynamic severity and ventricular compensation in patients with known mitral stenosis during pregnancy
6. Assessment of left ventricular and right ventricular size, function, and/or hemodynamics
7. Postintervention (percutaneous valvotomy) baseline studies for valve function (early) and ventricular remodeling (late)
8. Use of transesophageal echocardiography to perform percutaneous balloon valvotomy
9. Assessment for atrial thrombus prior to mitral balloon valvotomy or cadioversion[a]

[a]This is a class IIa indication.

2. The continuity equation is less accurate in patients with associated aortic regurgitation or MR, unless the degree of regurgitation of both valves is equal or of trivial to mild degree.

3. Several factors decrease the accuracy of the calculation of mitral valve area when using $P_{1/2}$. Any condition that leads to elevation of LV end-diastolic pressure will shorten the time it takes for the LA and LV pressures to equilibrate, shorten $P_{1/2}$, and therefore overestimate the mitral valve area. Aortic regurgitation and increased LV end-diastolic pressure due to other valvular or myocardial disease will shorten $P_{1/2}$ and lead to overestimation of mitral valve area. An abnormally decreased LV relaxation (especially in the elderly) can result in prolongation of $P_{1/2}$ and underestimation of mitral valve area.

4. Doppler $P_{1/2}$ has been shown to be an unreliable method to evaluate stenosis severity immediately after valvotomy because of worsening of LA compliance (30).

5. During tachycardia, fusion of the initial and late velocities of the mitral inflow precludes assessment of $P_{1/2}$.

## REFERENCES

1. Bisno AL. Group A streptococcal infections and acute rheumatic fever. N Engl J Med 1991;325:783–793.
2. Roldan CA, Shively BK, Crawford MH. An echocardiographic study of valvular heart disease associated with systemic lupus erythematosus. New Engl J Med 1996;335:1424–1430.
3. Shiran A, Goldstein SA, Ellahham S, et al. Accuracy of two-dimensional echocardiographic planimetry of the mitral valve area before and after balloon valvuloplasty. Cardiology 1998;90:227–230.
4. Faletra F, Pezzano A Jr, Fusco R, et al. Measurement of mitral valve area in mitral stenosis: four echocardiographic methods compared with direct measurement of anatomic orifices. J Am Coll Cardiol 1996;28:1190–1197.
5. Wilkins GT, Wehman AE, Abascal VM. Percutaneous mitral valvotomy: an analysis of echocardiographic variables related to outcome and the mechanism of dilatation. Br Heart J 1988;60:299.
6. Dean LS, Mickel M, Bonan R, et al. Four-year follow up of patients undergoing percutaneous valvuloplasty. A report from the National Heart, Lung, and Blood Institute Balloon Valvuloplasty Registry. J Am Coll Cardiol 1996;28:1452–1457.
7. Hildick-Smith DJ, Taylor GJ, Shapiro LM. Inoue balloon mitral valvuloplasty: long term clinical and echocardiographic follow-up of a predominantly unfavorable population. Eur Heart J 2000;21:1690–1697.
8. Padial LR, Abascal VM, Moreno PR, et al. Echocardiography can predict the development of severe mitral regurgitation after percutaneous mitral valvuloplasty by the Inoue technique. Am J Cardiol 1999;83:1210–1213.
9. Kaul UA, Singh S, Kalra GS, et al. Mitral regurgitation following percutaneous mitral commissurotomy: a single center experience. J Heart Valve Dis 2000;9:262–266.
10. Ha JW, Chung N, Kang SM, et al. Enhanced detection of left atrial spontaneous echo contrast by transthoracic harmonic imaging in mitral stenosis. J Am Soc Echocardiogr 2000;13:849–854.
11. Bargiggia GS, Scopelliti P, Bertucci C, et al. Doppler estimation of the stenotic mitral valve area. Direct application of the continuity equation to the flow convergence region. G Ital Cardiol 1991;8:815–823.
12. Nishimura RA, Rihal CS, Tajik AJ, et al. Accurate measurement of the transmitral gradient in patients with mitral stenosis: a simultaneous catheterization and Doppler echocardiographic study. J Am Coll Cardiol 1994;24:152–158.
13. Thomas JD, Weyman AE. Doppler mitral pressure half-time: a clinical tool in search of theoretical justification. J Am Coll Cardiol 1987;10:923.
14. Oku K, Utsunomiva T, Mori H, et al. Calculation of mitral valve area in mitral stenosis using the proximal isovelocity surface area method. Comparison with two-dimensional planimetry and Doppler pressure half-time method. Jpn Heart J 1997;38:811–819.
15. Aviles RJ, Nishimura RA, Pellika PA, et al. Utility of stress Doppler echocardiography in patients undergoing percutaneous mitral valvotomy. J Am Soc Echocardiogr 2001;14:676–681.
16. Leavitt JI, Coats MH, Falk RH. Effects of exercise on transmitral gradient and pulmonary artery pressure in patients with mitral stenosis or a prosthetic valve: a Doppler echocardiographic study. J Am Coll Cardiol 1991;17:1520–1526.
17. Decena BF 3rd, Tischler MD. Stress echocardiography in valvular heart disease. Cardiol Clin 1999;17:555–572.
18. Crawford MH, Roldan CA. Quantitative assessment of valve thickness in normal subjects by transesophageal echocardiography. Am J Cardiol 2001;87:1419–1423.
19. Koca V, Bozat T, Akkaya V, et al. Left atrial thrombus detection with multiplane transesophageal echocardiography: an echocardiographic study with surgical verification. J Heart Valve Dis 1999;8:63–66.
20. Goswami KC, Yadav R, Rao MB, et al. Clinical and echocardiographic predictors of left atrial clot and spontaneous echo contrast in patients with severe rheumatic mitral stenosis: a prospective study in 200 patients by transesophageal echocardiography. Int J Cardiol 2000;73:273–279.
21. Agarwal AK, Venugopalan P. Left atrial spontaneous echo contrast in patients with rheumatic mitral valve stenosis in normal sinus rhythm: relationship to mitral valve and left atrial measurements. Int J Cardiol 2001;77:63–68.
22. Kranidis A, Koulouris S, Filippatos G. Mitral regurgitation protects from left atrial thrombogenesis in patients with mitral valve disease and atrial fibrillation. Pacing Clin Electrophysiol 2000;23:1863–1866.

23. Goldstein SA, Campbell A, Mintz GS, et al. Feasibility of on-line transesophageal echocardiography during balloon mitral valvulotomy: experience with 93 patients. J Heart Valve Dis 1994;3:136–148.

24. Park SH, Kim MA, Hyon MS. The advantages of on-line transesophageal echocardiography guide during percutaneous balloon mitral valvuloplasty. J Am Soc Echocardiogr 2000;13:26–34.

25. Martinez-Reding J, Cordero A, Kuri J, et al. Treatment of severe mitral stenosis with percutaneous balloon valvotomy in pregnant patients. Clin Cardiol 1998;21:659–663.

26. Applebaum RM, Kasliwal RR, Kanojia A, et al. Utility of three-dimensional echocardiography during balloon mitral valvuloplasty. J Am Coll Cardiol 1998;32:1405–1409.

27. Srinivasa KH, Manjunath CN, Dhanalakshmi C, et al. Transesophageal Doppler echocardiographic study of pulmonary venous flow pattern in severe mitral stenosis and the changes following balloon mitral valvuloplasty. Echocardiography 2000;17:151–157.

28. Cheitlin MD, Alpert JS, Armstrong WF, et al. ACC/AHA guidelines for the clinical application of echocardiography. Circulation 1997;95:1686–1744.

29. Bonow RO, Carabello B, De Leon AC, et al. ACC/AHA guidelines for the management of patients with valvular heart disease. J Am Coll Cardiol 1998;32:1486–1588.

30. Thomas JD, et al. Inaccuracy of mitral pressure half-time immediately after percutaneous mitral valvotomy. Circulation 1988;78:980.

# 8

# The Patient with Aortic Valve Sclerosis or Stenosis

Kirsten Tolstrup,*Carlos A. Roldan, and †Jonathan Abrams

*Department of Internal Medicine, University of California Los Angeles; and Department of Internal Medicine, Cedars-Sinai Medical Center, Los Angeles, California; *Department of Internal Medicine, University of New Mexico School of Medicine; and Department of Internal Medicine, Veterans Affairs Medical Center, Albuquerque, New Mexico; †Cardiology Division, University of New Mexico School of Medicine; and Department of Internal Medicine, University Hospital, Albuquerque, New Mexico*

## INTRODUCTION

### Definition

Aortic valve sclerosis is present when the aortic valve cusps are thickened and hyperreflectant, but there is no obstruction to left ventricular (LV) outflow. Aortic stenosis is defined as an obstruction to LV outflow. The obstruction can be valvular (most common), subvalvular, or supravalvular. This chapter focuses mainly on valvular aortic stenosis.

### Etiology

Aortic valve sclerosis represents a degenerative process that occurs mainly in the elderly. As is the case with degenerative aortic valve stenosis, it may be the result of valvular stress, a primary degenerative process, or an expression of more generalized atherosclerosis (1). Recently, an atherosclerotic pathogenesis has been suggested by its association with atherogenic risk factors; coronary, carotid, and peripheral vascular disease; and cardiovascular events and cardiac death (2–6). In addition, on histopathology, aortic valve sclerotic lesions are similar to coronary atherosclerotic lesions.

Aortic valve stenosis has three major causes: degenerative, congenital, and rheumatic. In older patients, the most common etiology is degeneration of an inherently normal trileaflet aortic valve. Congenital aortic valve stenosis may be due to a unicuspid, bicuspid, or tricuspid valve. In addition, a dome-shaped diaphragm may be present. Cases of isolated aortic stenosis in patients <50 years of age most commonly are due to congenital defects, usually a bicuspid aortic valve. In infants, congenital aortic stenosis can be part of a generalized hypoplasia of the aorta and/or left heart. Rheumatic heart disease is more likely to be the cause if rheumatic mitral valve disease coexists.

## Prevalence and Incidence

Aortic valve sclerosis affects 21% to 29% of the general population >65 years of age and has a prevalence of 55% in the ninth to tenth decade (2,5). The prevalence in a veteran hospital population >50 years of age (mean age 67 years) has been found to be 42% (6).

Degenerative aortic valve stenosis has a prevalence of 2% to 4% in men and women >65 years of age. Aortic valve stenosis without accompanying mitral valve disease is more common in men and usually is congenital (younger subjects) or degenerative (older subjects) in origin. A bicuspid aortic valve is seen in 1% to 2% of the general population. Rheumatic heart disease has become less common in the United States with the decline of acute rheumatic fever.

## Natural History/Prognosis

### *Aortic Valve Sclerosis*

A recent study has suggested that asymptomatic subjects >65 years of age with aortic

valve sclerosis may have a 50% increased risk for myocardial infarction, angina, congestive heart failure, stroke, and death (3). Aortic valve sclerosis also has been found to be highly associated with aortic atheromatous disease in male patients >50 years of age (6). Also, some studies indicate that aortic valve sclerosis may progress to significant aortic valve stenosis.

### *Degenerative Aortic Valve Stenosis*

Degenerative aortic valve stenosis is now the most frequent cause of aortic stenosis requiring valve replacement. Sclerosis and calcifications are present at the bases and margins of the cusps and may extend to the tip portions, but no commissural fusion is present. The condition typically is not accompanied by significant aortic regurgitation. A prolonged asymptomatic period and very low morbidity and mortality usually are the case. The average rate of change in aortic valve area in patients with aortic valve stenosis is 0.12 cm$^2$ per year. However, it is impossible with the methods currently available to predict the rate of progression in the individual patient. More than half of patients will show little or no progression over a 3- to 9- year period, whereas others will have rapid progression with increases in pressure gradients of 15 to 19 mm Hg per year and a decrease of aortic valve area of 0.1 to 0.3 cm$^2$ per year (7,8). For these reasons, careful clinical and echocardiographic follow-up is mandatory in patients with moderate to severe aortic valve stenosis. Several studies have indicated the relationship of atherosclerotic risk factors with aortic valve stenosis, and a recent study found that lipid-lowering therapy with hydroxy methyl glutaryl coenzyme A (HMG-CoA) inhibitors may halt the progression of stenosis (2,9–11).

### *Congenital Aortic Valve Stenosis*

Unicuspid aortic valves cause severe outflow obstruction in infancy and are the most frequent malformations found in fatal aortic valve stenosis in children <1 year of age. Bicuspid aortic valves usually are not responsible for serious outflow obstruction during childhood. The changes causing stenosis resemble those occurring in adult-onset, trileaflet, degenerative aortic valve stenosis, except that the congenitally bicuspid valve becomes stenotic several decades earlier. Rarely, a congenitally bicuspid aortic valve is purely or predominantly regurgitant in the absence of a preceding infection. The congenitally malformed tricuspid valve has cusps of unequal size and some commissural fusion, and many of these valves retain normal function throughout life, as do a number of bicuspid valves.

### *Rheumatic Aortic Valve Stenosis*

Adhesion and fusion of the commissures, thickening predominantly at the tip portions of the cusps, and retraction and stiffening of the free borders of the cusps lead to aortic stenosis. Consequently, concomitant aortic regurgitation and stenosis often are present.

## HISTORY

Patients with aortic valve sclerosis are asymptomatic. However, these patients appear to have an increased incidence of cardiovascular morbidity and mortality.

In adults with aortic valve stenosis, the outflow obstruction increases gradually over a prolonged period. Cardiac output is maintained by the development of LV hypertrophy, which may sustain cardiac performance for many years without any symptoms despite a large pressure gradient across the aortic valve. The cardinal clinical manifestations of severe aortic valve stenosis are angina pectoris, syncope, dyspnea, and heart failure. Without relief of the obstruction, the time from onset of symptoms to death is approximately 5 years for angina, 3 years for syncope, and 2 years for heart failure. Up to two thirds of patients with critical aortic valve stenosis have classic angina pectoris, only half of whom have obstructive

coronary artery disease. Syncope usually is exertional and related to reduced cerebral blood flow due to a fixed cardiac output and systemic vasodilation. Warning symptoms may occur, and exertional dizzy spells and near fainting are common. Syncope at rest can be due to ventricular fibrillation, atrial fibrillation, or atrioventricular block due to calcific extension into the conduction system. Loss of atrial contraction, as occurs in atrial fibrillation or atrioventricular dissociation, may result in rapid clinical deterioration in patients with severe aortic stenosis. Left heart failure symptoms and manifestation of low cardiac output usually are late symptoms. Sudden death usually occurs in patients who have manifested symptoms related to aortic stenosis.

Gastrointestinal bleeding may occur in patients with calcific aortic valve stenosis; its etiologies are idiopathic, angiodysplasia, or other vascular malformations. The bleeding episodes may stop after valve replacement. Infective endocarditis is more common in younger patients with milder valvular deformities. Rarely, microthrombi and calcific emboli may cause embolization to various organs, including the brain, eye, kidneys, and heart.

Therapeutic decisions are based largely on the presence or absence of symptoms. Thus, the absolute valve area usually is not the primary determinant of the need for valve replacement.

Recent studies confirm the value of serial echocardiography in older individuals to identify those in whom the disease progresses to severe aortic valve stenosis.

## PHYSICAL EXAMINATION

### Blood Pressure and Arterial Pulse

In the absence of hypertension or associated aortic regurgitation, systolic blood pressure is normal in aortic valve sclerosis and aortic stenosis. With advanced degrees of outflow obstruction, the pulse pressure narrows as systolic arterial pressure decreases. Even in severe aortic stenosis, only a minority of patients will have a systolic blood pressure ≤100 mm Hg.

Contrary to popular belief, systemic arterial hypertension can be associated with significant aortic valve stenosis, particularly in the older population. When substantial aortic regurgitation also is present, systolic arterial pressure will increase and diastolic pressure decrease.

In detecting aortic stenosis, the focus of the examination of the arterial system should be on the carotid arteries and not on the peripheral pulses. The normal alteration of increased amplitude and rate of rise of the arterial wave contour in the peripheral circulation (see Chapter 1, Arterial Pulse) reduces the diagnostic usefulness obtainable from palpation of the brachial or radial arteries.

The hallmark of aortic stenosis is the typical slow-rising, small-volume carotid arterial pulse, also labeled pulsus parvus et tardus (slow and late). There can be an associated systolic thrill or shudder on the upstroke of the carotid pulse. *Practical Point: The classic carotid pulse in aortic stenosis has a slow upstroke, reduced amplitude, and sustained contour, with or without an accompanying thrill (Fig. 8.1).*

The severity of valvular obstruction is roughly proportional to the degree of abnormality of the carotid pulse. However, it is not uncommon to seriously underestimate or overestimate the severity of aortic stenosis by carotid artery palpation. *Practical Point: In an adult <55 to 60 years of age with clinically*

*normal LV function, a completely normal carotid pulse contour and arterial pulse pressure generally excludes moderate to severe aortic stenosis. A distinctly delayed carotid upstroke in the same setting is consistent with moderate to severe obstruction.*

In patients with LV dysfunction, alteration of peak systolic pressure and rate of rise is common; therefore, the carotid pulse may not be helpful to assess the severity of stenosis.

## Jugular Veins

The venous pulse configuration and pressure are unremarkable in aortic valve sclerosis and stenosis. Occasionally, in aortic stenosis, the jugular A wave will be prominent in the absence of an elevation in mean jugular pressure. Rarely, the mean jugular pressure will be elevated. This may be caused by the Bernheim effect, where the hypertrophied LV septum bulges into the right ventricular cavity and thereby impairs right ventricular filling.

## Precordial Percussion and Palpation

In hemodynamically important, compensated aortic stenosis, the apex impulse typically is a sustained LV lift with little or no leftward displacement of the point of maximal impulse. The duration and force of the LV impulse is increased due to increased LV mass, high intraventricular pressure, and obstruction to ventricular outflow. During precordial palpation, pay close attention to the duration of the apex impulse, which may be sustained into the second half of systole in significant aortic valve obstruction.

A normal LV impulse is characteristic of aortic valve sclerosis and mild aortic stenosis. In subjects with lung disease, obesity, deep chests, or large breasts, the apex beat may be diminutive or impalpable even in the presence of severe aortic stenosis. The presence of a sustained but otherwise unimpressive LV impulse in an older subject with a large chest and a long systolic murmur suggests important obstruction. *Practical Point: The concentrically hypertrophied LV of isolated aortic stenosis does not produce significant lateral*

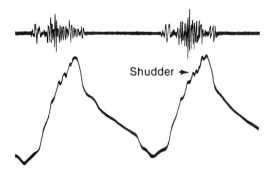

**FIG. 8.1.** Carotid arterial pulse in aortic stenosis. Note the delayed upstroke and the jagged contour representing a palpable shudder or transmitted thrill. Pulse volume usually is decreased as well (pulsus parvus et tardus).

*or downward displacement unless cardiac dilation has occurred or there is associated aortic regurgitation.*

A palpable A wave (presystolic distension of the LV) in the supine or left lateral position is a most valuable observation (Figs. 1.11 and 1.15). This finding indicates elevation of LV end-diastolic pressure and suggests a thick, noncompliant chamber. The murmur of aortic stenosis often is accompanied by a systolic thrill, which most commonly is located to the first or second right intercostal space with radiation upward and rightward toward the neck and right shoulder. *Practical Point: For optimal detection of the systolic thrill, have the subject sit up and lean forward while holding the breath in expiration.* A systolic thrill is the rule, not the exception, in aortic stenosis. Detection of a thrill indicates that aortic stenosis is present, but it does not necessarily indicate severe obstruction.

## Auscultation

### *First and Second Heart Sounds*

The first heart sound ($S_1$) usually is unaltered in aortic valve sclerosis and isolated aortic stenosis. It may be decreased in intensity, but never accentuated. A loud "$S_1$" in a patient with suspected or proven aortic stenosis suggests the presence of an aortic ejection sound or associated mitral stenosis. Abnormalities in the amplitude of the aortic valve component ($A_2$) and in the inspiratory behavior of the second heart sound ($S_2$) are common in aortic stenosis. $A_2$ may be normal or even increased in amplitude in patients with pliable and relatively thin aortic leaflets. This is typical for bicuspid aortic valve stenosis without calcification and occasionally may be found in young subjects with severe aortic obstruction. However, as thickening and rigidity of the aortic valve ensues, the amplitude of $A_2$ decreases. Calcification of the valve usually contributes to the diminished loudness of $A_2$. In severe aortic stenosis, $A_2$ may be totally inaudible. *Practical Point: The amplitudes of the aortic ejection click and $A_2$ are closely related.*

*Both are prominent in subjects with a pliable, noncalcified bicuspid valve. Both are decreased in intensity in the presence of calcium or significant valvular thickening.* Because $A_2$ commonly is soft or absent in aortic stenosis, a normal or increased pulmonic valve component ($P_2$) can readily be mistaken for $A_2$. Hemodynamically significant aortic stenosis causes abnormal splitting of $S_2$. The characteristic alteration of $S_2$ in aortic stenosis is an increase in the Q–$A_2$ interval with $A_2$ occurring later than usual (therefore moving closer to $P_2$), and a tendency for $S_2$ to become single. If LV ejection time is substantially delayed, reversed or paradoxic splitting of $S_2$ occurs. (Fig. 8.2) *Practical Point: Detection of paradoxic splitting of $S_2$ in aortic stenosis in the absence of left bundle branch block or impaired LV function is an important observation, which implies that the LV–aortic gradient is ≥75 mm Hg, e.g. severe aortic stenosis is present.*

Normal splitting of $S_2$ generally is found in aortic valve sclerosis, mild aortic stenosis in adults, and commonly in congenital aortic stenosis, even when severe. A single $S_2$ also may result from a decreased intensity of $A_2$ due to fibrocalcific changes. *Practical Point: In approximately two thirds of older patients with moderate to severe aortic stenosis, $S_2$ will be single. $S_2$ will be reversed or paradoxic in another 20% to 25%, and it will be completely normal in a small number of patients.*

A prominent, long systolic murmur can mask audible splitting of $S_2$; therefore, one must listen carefully for the characteristics of splitting at the apex, second right, and second left intercostal space. Typically, $P_2$ is not audible at the apex unless there is pulmonary hypertension. If the systolic murmur of aortic stenosis is loud and prolonged, $A_2$ and $P_2$ may be obscured within the murmur and be inaudible.

### *Third and Fourth Heart Sounds*

A third heart sound ($S_3$) is not a normal or expected finding in adults with aortic valve sclerosis or aortic stenosis. Its presence suggests significant LV dysfunction or decompen-

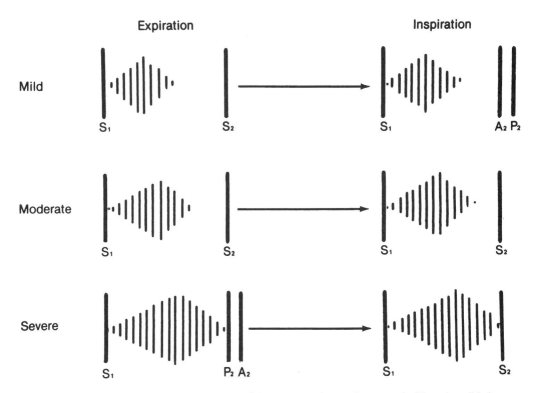

**FIG. 8.2.** Patterns of $S_2$ splitting and shape of the murmur in aortic stenosis. **Top:** In mild degrees of left ventricular (LV) obstruction, splitting of $S_2$ remains physiologic. **Middle:** Frequently, a single $S_2$ is heard in aortic stenosis, reflecting moderate obstruction. The delayed $A_2$ results in fusion of the two components of $S_2$. Marked attenuation in the intensity of $A_2$ from severe fibrocalcific changes may cause $A_2$ to be inaudible and result in a single $S_2$ (which is actually $P_2$). **Bottom:** With advanced aortic stenosis, LV ejection time is prolonged sufficiently such that, in expiration, aortic valve closure follows pulmonic closure. During inspiration, $P_2$ moves away from $S_1$ and may become synchronous with $A_2$, resulting in paradoxic or reversed splitting of $S_2$. The figure also illustrates the relationship of the shape of the systolic murmur to severity of the underlying aortic stenosis. As obstruction to LV outflow becomes more severe, the murmur becomes longer and the time to peak intensity is delayed. Note the lack of respiratory variation in timing and intensity of the murmur.

sated heart failure. A fourth heart sound ($S_4$) is a valuable clue to the presence of LV hypertrophy and decreased LV compliance associated with severe aortic stenosis, especially in younger patients (<40 to 50 years old). An audible or palpable $S_4$ in such individuals correlates with an LV–aortic gradient (>70 mm Hg) and an abnormally elevated LV end-diastolic pressure. Because an $S_4$ is normal in young children and commonly is found in older patients with coexisting atherosclerotic heart disease or hypertension, its prognostic significance is considerably reduced in these age groups. *Practical Point: The presence of an au-*

*dible $S_4$ in an older patient does not necessarily mean the aortic stenosis is severe.* However, the finding of a *palpable* $S_4$ in a patient with aortic stenosis implies that the valve obstruction is of major hemodynamic importance.

### *Aortic Ejection Click*

The ejection click is a high-frequency, crisp sound. It occurs 40 to 80 ms after $S_1$ [longer interval than that separating the closure of the mitral valve ($M_1$) and tricuspid valve ($T_1$)] (Fig. 8.3). The ejection click usually is heard best at the cardiac apex, where it often is

**Aortic Ejection Click of Aortic Stenosis**

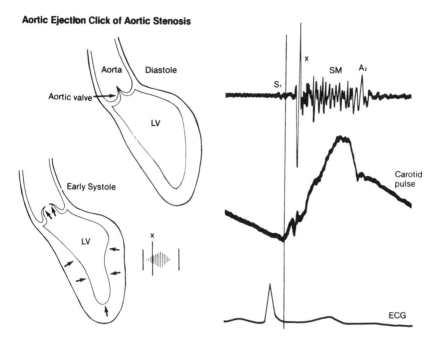

**FIG. 8.3.** Aortic ejection click associated with aortic stenosis due to a congenitally bicuspid valve. Note the high-frequency, high-amplitude sound (x) that follows $S_1$ and is coincident with the onset of ejection into the aorta. The aortic ejection sound is formed by sudden cessation of the opening motion of the abnormal valve leaflets (doming). Note also the delayed carotid upstroke and long systolic murmur.

louder than both $S_1$ and $S_2$. A typical click has a "snappy" quality and is heard throughout the precordium. It is readily mistaken for $S_1$, particularly at the base of the heart. One should remember that a "split" $S_1$ at the apex and left sternal border may represent an $S_1$–ejection click complex. The aortic ejection click does not vary with inspiration and, therefore, is distinguishable from a pulmonary ejection sound. The detection of an aortic ejection click or sound is an important observation. It confirms the diagnosis of structural heart disease in a patient with a systolic ejection murmur. It localizes the abnormality to the aortic valve (in the absence of a dilated aorta or chronic hypertension). It suggests that the etiology of the valve abnormality is a congenitally deformed aortic valve, usually a bicuspid valve. *Practical Point: Although an ejection click indicates that the deformity is at aortic valve level, its presence does not correlate with the severity of the lesion.* With increasing calcification and thick-

ening, the valve cusps lose mobility and their excursion lessens; the click softens and ultimately may disappear.

An ejection sound is found less commonly in acquired trileaflet aortic stenosis. *Practical Point: Systolic ejection clicks are present in less than one third of older patients with aortic valve stenosis (>50 years old), but they are the rule in congenital aortic valve stenosis. Clicks are heard less commonly in severe congenital aortic stenosis.*

### Heart Murmurs

Aortic valve sclerosis produces a less than grade 3/6 systolic ejection murmur best heard at the second right intercostal space. It has an early to mid-systolic peak, may be somewhat harsh in character, and ends well before a normal $A_2$. It may be transmitted to the carotid arteries, which will have a normal upstroke.

Aortic stenosis produces the prototype of the classic systolic ejection murmur: a crescendo-decrescendo murmur that begins after $S_1$ and ends before $S_2$ (Fig. 8.2). The murmur typically is harsh, rough, or grunting and maximal at the second right intercostal space, the so-called aortic area. However, it is not uncommon for the murmur to be maximal at the second or third left intercostal space (Erb point). In older patients with large chests or obstructive lung disease, the murmur may be loudest at the apex. The murmur at the cardiac base typically radiates upward and to the right and often is well heard over both carotid arteries. In general, the length of the murmur is proportional to the severity of the valvular obstruction in the absence of other factors that modify stroke volume or the rate of ejection. In the presence of decreased LV function or overt congestive heart failure, the murmur of aortic stenosis may shorten or completely disappear. Some studies have shown that the time to peak intensity of the murmur is a better predictor of severity of aortic stenosis than its overall length (Fig. 8.2). *Practical Point: It is important to assess the duration to the maximal murmur intensity in the evaluation of the severity of aortic stenosis. A murmur that peaks within the first third or half of systole suggests mild aortic stenosis. A murmur that peaks within the second half of systole indicates severe disease.*

In adults with acquired aortic stenosis, the systolic murmur at the apex can be quite musical in its pure frequency and high-pitched sound (the Gallavardin murmur). This murmur typically is confused with mitral regurgitation. Thus, it is important to recognize that, in older patients, particularly those with an increased chest diameter, the systolic murmur of aortic stenosis may be markedly different in tone at the base and apex, although the shape and length of the murmur are similar (ejection murmur).

In general, the louder the murmur of aortic stenosis, the more severe the valve obstruction. This relationship is less reliable in adults, as evidenced by the soft and unimpressive murmur that occasionally is found in patients with severe aortic stenosis. In the presence of chronic obstructive lung disease, obesity, or a big chest, it is important to auscultate at the base of the heart with the patient upright and

leaning forward. The murmur of aortic stenosis in such individuals often is heard very well over and above the clavicles and in the neck. Conversely, in such patients or in the presence of congestive heart failure or in those with co-existing mitral stenosis, the finding of a prominent grade 3-4/6 murmur of aortic stenosis is a most important observation that suggests severe valvular obstruction. The systolic murmur usually is quite soft and unimpressive in these situations, giving the false impression that the aortic stenosis is mild or absent. Many patients, especially those with rheumatic aortic valve stenosis, have some degree of aortic regurgitation, even in the presence of severe stenosis. The rigid, contracted, and often calcified valve may be truly immobile, unable to adequately open or close. It is common for some degree of aortic regurgitation to coexist with severe aortic stenosis, resulting in a grade 1 to 2/6 high-frequency aortic regurgitation blow. *Practical Point: While using firm pressure with the diaphragm of the stethoscope, specifically listen for a blowing diastolic murmur in all patients with suspected aortic stenosis by having the subject sit up and lean forward with the breath held in expiration.* The presence of aortic regurgitation of any magnitude will tend to augment the stroke volume and, thus, the intensity and length of the systolic murmur for any degree of valve obstruction. The murmur of aortic valve stenosis is augmented by amyl nitrite and by squatting, which increases stroke volume. It is decreased in intensity by Valsalva strain, vasopressors, moderate isometric exercise, or standing.

### Differential Diagnosis

When an aortic stenosis murmur radiates to the apex or is louder at the apex, the differential diagnosis should include mitral regurgitation. This is a particular problem in the older patient or in the subject with a large chest in whom the apical aortic murmur is likely to be of a higher frequency and have a more musical tone. To make the distinction between a murmur of aortic and mitral origin, it is critical to assess the length of the murmur and pay close attention to late systole. The murmur of aortic

stenosis is often heard above the clavicles; the murmur of mitral regurgitation usually radiates well into the axilla. A normal carotid pulse favors mitral regurgitation. The intensity of the aortic stenosis murmur varies directly with the magnitude of the LV stroke volume, whereas a mitral regurgitation murmur tends to be equally loud independently of LV volume changes on a beat to beat basis. Thus, in a postpremature ventricular beat or following a long R-R cycle in atrial fibrillation, the murmur of aortic stenosis will increase in loudness, but there will be no change in intensity of the mitral regurgitation murmur.

### Other Peripheral Manifestations

Patients may rarely manifest symptoms of peripheral embolization from microthrombi or calcific embolization. Aortic valve sclerosis and degenerative aortic valve stenosis are associated with atherosclerosis, and these patients may clinically manifest or have occult but significant peripheral vascular disease or coronary artery disease.

### ECHOCARDIOGRAPHY

Patients with physical findings suggestive of aortic valve stenosis should have an electrocardiogram, chest x-ray film, and echocardiogram. The echocardiographic evaluation of a patient with suspected aortic valve stenosis should focus on defining the presence and severity of the stenosis, and should include assessment of LV systolic and diastolic function, and LV wall thickness and chamber size. The evaluation also should include quantification of associated regurgitant lesions (mitral and aortic regurgitation), estimation of pulmonary artery pressure, measurement of aortic root diameter, and assessment of the severity of associated root sclerosis.

Echocardiographically, aortic valve sclerosis is defined as increased reflectance and thickness of the aortic valve cusps, but without significant outflow tract obstruction (gradient <16 mm Hg or peak velocity <2.0 m/s). On the other hand, aortic valve stenosis is defined as any abnormality of the aortic valve in which the cusps

physically encroach on the lumen of the outflow tract. Depending on its severity, such anatomic deformity may produce hemodynamically significant obstruction. Obstruction is defined by an abnormal transvalvular pressure gradient ($\geq$16 mm Hg). All echocardiographic techniques [M-mode, two-dimensional (2-D), and color Doppler] play an important role in diagnosing and assessing the severity of aortic stenosis; assessing the hemodynamic consequences of the obstruction on LV structure and function; and defining its etiology. The contributions of each of the modalities are outlined in the subsequent sections.

### M-Mode Echocardiography

M-mode echocardiography currently plays a lesser role in the assessment of aortic valve sclerosis or stenosis. Thickness and mobility of the aortic valve leaflets can be assessed as accurately as by 2-D echocardiography. Although the technique is not accurate for defining the severity of aortic stenosis, aortic cusp separation of $\geq$1cm indicates noncritical aortic valve stenosis. However, this criterion may lack specificity in bicuspid and rheumatic aortic valve stenosis. Although it is difficult to accurately determine the etiology of aortic stenosis (degenerative vs. congenital vs. rheumatic) by M-mode echocardiography, eccentric valve closure in relation to the aortic root walls has been related to the presence of a bicuspid aortic valve (Fig. 8.6C). Also, M-mode echocardiography suggests the presence of a membranous form of subaortic stenosis by a characteristic coarse systolic flutter of the aortic cusps and a mid-systolic partial closure of the valve. However, this finding is nonspecific for significant subvalvular outflow obstruction and is also seen in patients with hypertrophic obstructive cardiomyopathy.

### Two-Dimensional Echocardiography

Two-dimensional echocardiography provides excellent morphologic characterization of the sclerotic or stenotic aortic valve cusps, and it can identify the subvalvular and

supravalvular causes of outflow tract obstruction. The normal aortic valve appears as two
thin parallel lines that lie close to the aortic
walls in systole in the parasternal long-axis
view. During diastole, the leaflets come together. Because most of the valve is parallel to
the beam, it is visualized only faintly, if at all.
The point of coaptation is seen as a small linear echo in the middle of the aorta. With aortic
valve sclerosis and all forms of aortic valve
stenosis, the valve cusps become thickened and
frequently are visualized in diastole. The short-
axis view provides semiquantitative assessment of the aortic valve sclerosis or stenosis
with assessment of cusp morphology, mobility,
and their degree of opening. Unsuccessful attempts have been made to quantitate aortic
stenosis by measuring the cross-sectional area
of the valve in the parasternal short-axis view.

### Aortic Valve Sclerosis

Aortic valve sclerosis is demonstrated
when one or more of the aortic cusps are hyperreflectant and thickened. Mobility usually
is normal, but it can be mildly or moderately
decreased. Valve thickening can be diffuse,

localized, or nodular. It may affect all areas of
the cusps, but most frequently it is seen involving the margins and basal portions of the
cusps (Fig. 8.4). The sclerosis is mild when
cusp mobility is normal or minimally reduced
and cusp thickening is <4 mm; moderate
when cusp sclerosis is 4 to 6 mm and associated with decreased mobility; and severe
when, in addition to decreased mobility and
increased thickness, velocity across the valve
is increased but <2 m/s (6,12).

### Degenerative Aortic Valve Stenosis

Degenerative aortic valve stenosis most often is evidenced by immobility and decreased
separation of the valve cusps with a decrease in
orifice area. The cusps are hyperreflectant,
thickened, and calcified. The fibrosis, nodular
deposits, and calcification usually begin and
are more severe at the base of the cusps, extend
to the cusp margins and commissural regions,
and then progress to the free edge (Fig.
8.5A–B). The base of the leaflets may become
fixed and immobile. Commissural fusion may
occur rarely. Associated aortic annular and root
sclerosis and calcification are common.

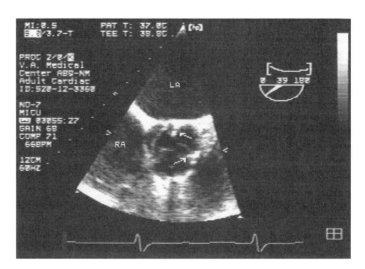

**FIG. 8.4.** Aortic valve sclerosis. Transesophageal echocardiographic short-axis view during systole
of the aortic valve in a 75-year-old man demonstrates moderate nodular valve sclerosis predominantly at the commissural portions of the left and right coronary cusps *(arrows)*. Note the decreased
mobility of the left and right coronary cusps. Doppler tracings revealed a peak gradient of only 12
mm Hg. LA, left atrium; RA, right atrium.

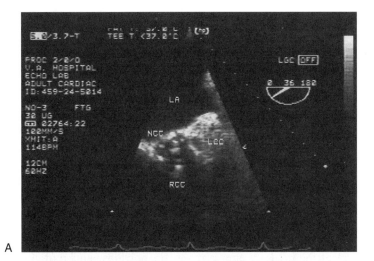

A

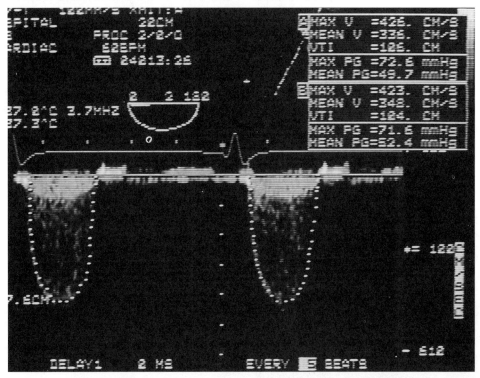

B

**FIG. 8.5.** Degenerative aortic valve stenosis. **A:** Transesophageal echocardiographic short-axis view during systole in a 70-year-old man with degenerative calcific aortic valve stenosis demonstrates a distorted valve with nodular deposits and calcifications predominantly at the bases and margins of the cusps. Systolic opening is barely discernible. **B:** Corresponding continuous wave Doppler tracing measuring peak velocity across the valve of 4.23 m/s and mean pressure gradient of 52.4 mm Hg consistent with severe stenosis. The tracing illustrates the typical envelope of flow beginning at aortic valve opening and terminating at valve closure click. LA, left atrium; LCC, left coronary cusp; NCC, noncoronary cusp; RCC, right coronary cusp.

### Congenital Aortic Valve Stenosis

In congenital aortic valve stenosis, there is increased echogenicity of the cusps due to thickening, sclerosis, and calcification. It usually is possible to directly visualize the cusps in the parasternal short-axis view. In this view, during diastole, the commissures of the cusps of a normal trileaflet valve appear as a "Y" (or an inverted Mercedes Benz sign). A bicuspid valve has two cusps of nearly equal size and a single linear commissure. If a raphe is present, the bicuspid valve may appear tricuspid-like. However, the number of cusps will become apparent in systole. In the long axis-view, the eccentric closure of the bicuspid valve will become apparent (Fig. 8.6A–C). High-resolution images are required for adequate visualization of the bicuspid valve, but this is not possible in all patients. A more important early sign of this type of valve stenosis is systolic doming of the cusps, where the edges of the leaflets are no longer parallel to the aorta, but are curved toward the center of the aorta. This finding suggests pliable cusps, but with restricted mobility of the tips relative to the bodies of the cusps. Occasionally, only one of the aortic cusps is visualized well in systole (usually the one normally corresponding to the right coronary cusp). A domed but thickened and sclerotic aortic cusp usually indicates the presence of aortic stenosis (Fig. 8.7). Doming is probably the most important 2-D echocardiographic finding for congenital, but also for rheumatic, valvular stenosis.

### Rheumatic Aortic Valve Stenosis

The usual pattern of rheumatic aortic valve stenosis is commissural fusion, thickening of the tip portions, and retraction of the cusps, with focal thickening of the edges (Fig. 8.7). Often all commissures are affected, and the severity of stenosis depends on the extent and numbers of cusps affected. Secondary calcification is common; at the extreme, it is impossible to discern between a late and chronically healed rheumatic stenosis and the degenerative form (associated mitral stenosis helps in diagnosing the stenosis as rheumatic).

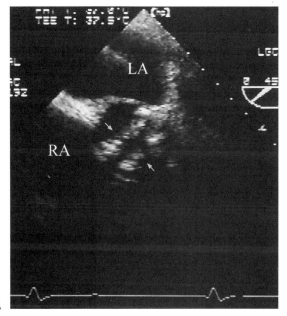

A

**FIG. 8.6.** Bicuspid aortic valve. **A:** Transesophageal echocardiographic short-axis view during systole demonstrates thickened and calcified bicuspid aortic valve leaflets *(arrows)* in a 57-year-old man with aortic valve stenosis.

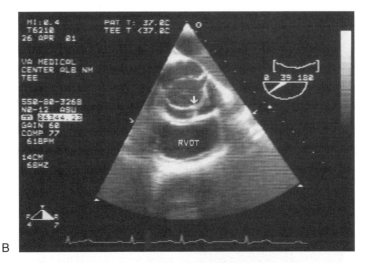

B

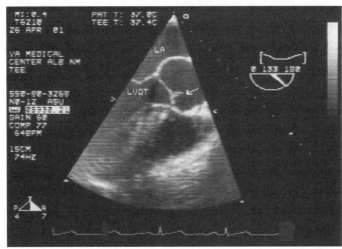

C

**FIG. 8.6.** *Continued.* **B:** For comparison, transesophageal echocardiographic short-axis view illustrates a non-stenotic bicuspid aortic valve in a 51-year-old man. The leaflets are thin and mobile and a raphe is present *(arrow)*, creating the illusion of a tricuspid valve. **C:** Same patient as shown in **B**, but long-axis view image obtained during diastole demonstrates eccentric closure of the valve *(arrow)*. LA, left atrium; LVOT, left ventricular outflow tract; RA, right atrium; RVOT, right ventricular outflow tract.

The extent of valve calcification has been shown to be a strong predictor of subsequent events in asymptomatic patients with severe aortic valve stenosis (13). Event-free survival (endpoints are death and aortic valve replacement) in patients with no or mild calcification was 92% ± 5% at 1 year compared with 60% ± 6% for those with moderate or severe calcifications. The 4-year event-free survival in these two groups was 75% ± 9% and 20% ± 5%, respectively. Therefore, characterization of valve morphology by 2-D echocardiography in patients with aortic valve stenosis has diagnostic and prognostic implications.

Two types of subvalvular outflow tract obstruction are known, in addition to hypertrophic cardiomyopathy. One is a discrete

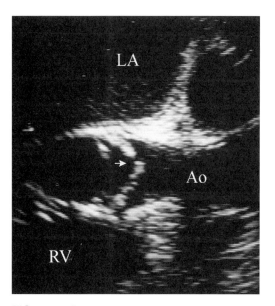

**FIG. 8.7.** Rheumatic aortic valve stenosis. Transesophageal echocardiographic long-axis view in a 45-year-old woman demonstrates eccentric closure, leaflet tip thickening, retraction of the noncoronary cusp, and systolic doming *(arrow)*. Severe aortic stenosis was demonstrated by Doppler data. Ao, ascending aorta; LA, left atrium; RV, right ventricle.

ally is associated with other congenital abnormalities, such as accessory mitral valve chordae, anomalous papillary muscle insertion, and abnormal insertion of the anterior mitral leaflet, all of which are detectable by 2-D echocardiography.

The least common site for congenital aortic stenosis is in the supravalvular area. Three morphologic types exist: fibromuscular thickening above the sinuses causing an hourglass-shaped narrowing; discrete fibrous membrane in a normal sized aorta, usually near the sinotubular junction (Fig. 8.8A–B); and diffuse hypoplasia of the ascending aorta. Two features often accompany the supravalvular aortic stenosis: dilation of the coronary arteries and thickening of the aortic valve cusps. The supravalvular lesions are recognized most easily from the parasternal long-axis and high right parasternal views. The parasternal short-axis view is useful for evaluation of the associated proximal coronary artery dilation.

**Pulse and Continuous Wave Doppler**

Doppler echocardiography provides the principal means of establishing the presence and quantitating the severity of aortic valve stenosis, and it serves to prove the lack of significant outflow tract obstruction in aortic valve sclerosis. Because valvular stenosis narrows the outflow tract, flow velocity through the restricted area must increase to maintain a constant flow volume. The increased flow velocity starts just proximal to the obstruction (flow acceleration) and reaches its maximum at a point just distal to the obstruction where the flow jet is narrowest, called the vena contracta. Detection of this local increase in velocity is the basis for Doppler diagnosis of aortic valve stenosis. The degree of increase in velocity is related to the severity of aortic stenosis and the systolic pressure difference between the LV and aorta across the valve as described by the Bernoulli equation. The simplified Bernoulli equation ($\Delta P = 4v^2$) has proven accurate

form of subaortic stenosis resulting from a crescent-shaped, thin and fibrous membrane located just below the aortic valve. It usually extends from the anterior septum to the anterior mitral leaflet and is seen as a discrete linear echo in the LV outflow tract (LVOT) perpendicular to the interventricular septum. Multiple transducer positions may be needed to record the structure, which is parallel to the ultrasound beam in the parasternal long-axis view. The membrane is recognized more easily in the apical view, where the beam is perpendicular to the membrane. The second form of subvalvular aortic stenosis is a fibromuscular ridge or tunnel. The tunnel type is very rare in adults and is characterized by diffuse thickening and narrowing of the outflow tract below the valve. The fibromuscular ridge appears as the membranous type, but thicker and less discrete. Subvalvular aortic stenosis occasion-

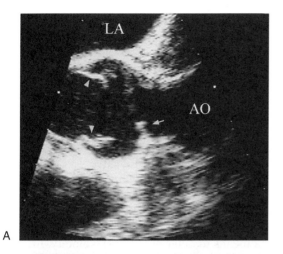

A

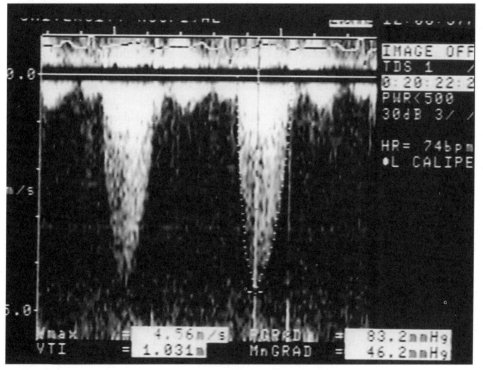

B

**FIG. 8.8.** Supravalvular aortic stenosis. **A:** Transesophageal echocardiographic long-axis view in a 32-year-old woman with membranous supravalvular aortic stenosis localized to the sinotubular junction *(arrow)*. A mildly sclerotic aortic valve is demonstrated *(arrowheads)*. **B:** Corresponding continuous wave Doppler tracings reveals a peak velocity of 4.56 m/s across the membrane. There was no gradient across the valve. AO, ascending aorta; LA, left atrium.

compared with simultaneous pressure gradient measurements by cardiac catheterization (14,15). For native aortic valve stenosis, the mean and maximum transaortic pressure gradients are linearly related. Therefore, because maximum jet velocity is related to maximum pressure gradient as described by the simplified Bernoulli equation, a given maximum jet velocity consistently and reliably corresponds to a given maximum and mean pressure gradient (Fig. 8.5B). The close relationship among maximum jet velocity and the maximum and mean gradients explains why maximum jet velocity data alone are useful for evaluation of the severity of aortic valve stenosis.

Most of the data discussed have been obtained by continuous wave Doppler, but high pulse repetition frequency Doppler can be used to make similar measurements. Multiple echocardiographic windows usually are necessary to find the highest peak velocity. These windows include the left parasternal, right parasternal, apical, suprasternal notch, and, especially in children, subcostal approach. *However, in at least 90% of patients, the highest velocity is obtained from the apical views.* A correctly sampled aortic stenosis jet has a distinctive high-velocity audible sound, and the spectral display usually shows a fine feathery appearance that is less dense than the more dominant lower-frequency velocity from the parajet. The jet starts after the isovolumetric phase (after Q of the QRS) and ends at the aortic valve closing click. The opening and closing valve clicks are inversely related to the severity of aortic stenosis (i.e., less noticeable in severe stenosis).

*Generally, in a patient with normal stroke volume, an aortic peak velocity ≥4 m/s or <2.5 m/s (but ≥2 m/s) determines the presence of severe or mild aortic stenosis, respectively.*

The combination of cusp calcification and a rapid increase in aortic jet velocity identifies a group of asymptomatic patients at high risk for adverse outcome. About 80% of patients with moderately or severely calcified valves with an increase in jet velocity ≥0.3 m/s per year will undergo valve replacement for symptoms or die within 2 years (13). A ratio of aortic valve area at mid acceleration and mid deceleration to valve area at peak velocity ≥1.25 predicted rapid progression of aortic stenosis with a sensitivity of 64%, specificity of 72%, and positive predictive value of 80% (16).

An important parameter in the assessment of the severity of aortic stenosis is the calculation of valve area or valve area index. A simple approach to calculate the aortic valve area using Doppler techniques relies on the continuity equation (17,18). Blood flow or stroke volume through the aortic valve is equal to the aortic valve velocity time integral (VTI) × cross-sectional valve area. Blood flow through the LVOT is derived from VTI at the LVOT × LVOT cross-sectional area. Blood flow in the LVOT must equal the flow through the aortic valve. Therefore, the aortic valve area can be calculated as area $_{LVOT}$ × VTI$_{LVOT}$ = area$_{AV}$ × VTI $_{AV}$, where AV = aortic valve. LVOT area can be calculated from a systolic diameter measured with 2-D echocardiography in the parasternal long-axis view within 1 cm from the aortic annulus. Pulsed Doppler provides the means to determine LVOT velocity. Ideally, the velocity time integrals of both LVOT and aortic valve should be measured. As an alternative to the velocity time integrals, the maximum velocities can be used. The largest source of variability in the calculation of aortic valve area using the continuity equation is the measurement of outflow tract diameter. However, outflow tract diameter remains relatively constant over time, so that a change in valve area >0.1 cm$^2$ most likely represents an actual interval change. Aortic valve area calculated by the Doppler continuity equation has the advantage of noninvasive data collection and the absence of an empiric constant, as in the Gorlin formula used in cardiac catheterization.

*Aortic valve stenosis severity is graded as mild when valve area is >1.5 cm$^2$, moderate when >1.0 to 1.5 cm$^2$, and severe when ≤1.0 cm$^2$* (19). Mean systolic pressure gradient >50 mm Hg in the presence of normal cardiac output or an effective aortic orifice <0.8 cm$^2$ in an average-sized adult (less than one fourth of the normal orifice) is generally considered to represent critical aortic stenosis. In contrast, mean gradient <20 mm Hg corresponds to mild aortic stenosis in the presence of normal LV systolic function.

Pulsed, continuous wave, and often high pulse repetition frequency Doppler studies are used in patients with subvalvular and supravalvular aortic stenosis. The Doppler-derived values correspond well with catheter-derived data, as long as there is no coexisting stenosis at other levels. In the event there are multiple serial stenoses or the stenosis is tubular, the Doppler measurements may overestimate the catheter-based gradient.

## Color Doppler

Color flow imaging can help identify the direction and location of the systolic jet in aortic stenosis to make certain that the ultrasonic beam is as parallel as possible to the vena contracta. It can detect the presence of concomitant subaortic valve obstruction in occasional patients. Color Doppler imaging also is useful for the evaluation of coexisting aortic and mitral regurgitation.

## Exercise and Dobutamine Echocardiography

In general, regular exercise testing should not be performed in symptomatic patients with moderate or severe aortic stenosis. However, in asymptomatic patients, exercise testing probably is safe and may provide added information to the initial evaluation by quantifying the functional capacity and symptoms, and providing information regarding hemodynamic severity of aortic stenosis.

A clinical and echocardiographically challenging subset of patients are those suspected of having aortic stenosis in the presence of significant LV systolic dysfunction (ejection fraction <35%). True aortic valve areas tend to be underestimated in patients with severely sclerotic and frequently calcified aortic cusps with decreased mobility suggestive of aortic stenosis, low transvalvular mean gradient (≤30 mm Hg), and calculated aortic valve area ≤1 cm² in the presence of decreased LV systolic function. Therefore, resting Doppler echocardiography cannot separate patients with LV dysfunction due to severe aortic valve stenosis from those with mild or moderate aortic stenosis and an unrelated cardiomyopathy. Dobutamine echocardiography has proven to be of important diagnostic and prognostic value in these patients. Before dobutamine is infused, a baseline wall-motion score and index is calculated and the ejection fraction estimated. Then, dobutamine is started at 5 μg/kg/min and increased by 5 μg every 3 to 5 minutes to a peak dose of 20 to 30 μg/kg/min. Patients with contractile reserve will demonstrate an improvement in wall-motion score or index of ≥20%, improvement in ejection fraction of ≥10%, or increase in stroke volume of >50%. In these patients, an increase in peak velocity of >0.6 m/sec, increase in peak gradient of ≥20 mm Hg or >25% from baseline, but no change or <20% change in valve area indicates underlying severe aortic stenosis (Fig. 8.9A–B). In contrast, patients with contractile reserve, but with an increase in peak gradient <20 mm Hg and >25% increase in valve area, have mild or moderate stenosis (20–22). Unfortunately, a small proportion of these patients show no contractile reserve and a separation will not be possible.

## Transesophageal Echocardiography

Transesophageal echocardiography (TEE) can accurately characterize the morphology of a sclerotic or stenotic aortic valve. TEE provides higher resolution than transthoracic echocardiography, and attempts have been made to measure aortic valve area by planimetry in the short-axis views. However, the anatomy of the stenotic orifice is complex in three dimensions, so that it is not always possible to obtain an accurate reliable valve orifice for planimetry (Fig. 8.5A). Because of the improved image resolution, a stenotic bicuspid aortic valve is easily identified by TEE (Fig. 8.6). The same image quality makes TEE an excellent tool for detection of subvalvular and supravalvular aortic stenoses (Fig. 8.8A).

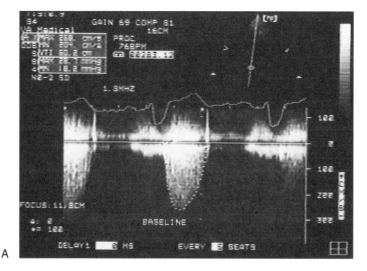

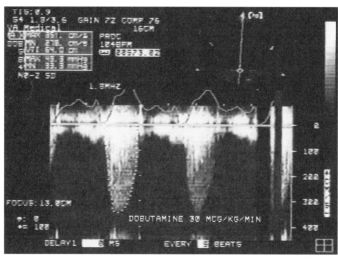

**FIG. 8.9.** Low-gradient aortic stenosis. **A:** Baseline continuous wave Doppler tracing across the aortic valve in a 74-year-old man with a degenerative, calcific aortic valve and left ventricular ejection fraction of 30%. Baseline peak velocity is 2.69 m/s and mean pressure gradient 18.2 mm Hg. **B:** Same patient after intravenous administration of dobutamine 30 μg/kg/min demonstrating an increase in peak velocity of 0.82 m/s and an increase in mean gradient to 33.3 mm Hg. Ejection fraction increased to 45%, although the stroke volume only increased by 20%. Calculated aortic valve area changed from 0.93 to 1.0 cm$^2$. All these findings are consistent with severe aortic stenosis in a patient with low cardiac output.

## SUMMARY

### Diagnostic Value of History and Physical Examination in Aortic Valve Sclerosis and Stenosis

Aortic valve sclerosis and stenosis are prevalent in the general population, particularly in patients with atherogenic risk factors.

These patients have an increased risk for cardiovascular morbidity and mortality. Patients with aortic valve sclerosis do not manifest any symptoms related to the valve, but they may show evidence of cardiovascular disease. The cardinal manifestations of severe aortic valve stenosis are angina pectoris, syncope, and heart failure. Left heart failure symptoms and

**TABLE 8.1.** *Assessment of aortic valve sclerosis and stenosis by physical examination*

| Severity | Carotid pulses | $A_2$ | $S_4$[a] | Ejection click[b] | Murmur[c] |
|---|---|---|---|---|---|
| Sclerosis | Normal | Normal | Absent | Absent | II–III/VI SEM, early peaking |
| Mild AS | Normal | Normal to mildly attenuated | Absent | Present | II–IV/VI SEM; early peaking |
| Moderate AS | Normal | Moderately attenuated | Audible | Present in <50% of patients | III–IV/VI SEM; mid peaking |
| Severe AS | ↓ and delayed/normal | Severely decreased/absent | Audible and palpable | Absent | III–VI/VI SEM; late peaking |

[a]In the absence of hypertension and younger than 40 yr.
[b]In bicuspid aortic valve stenosis.
[c]In patients with normal stroke volume.
$A_2$, second heart sound over the aortic valve; AS, aortic stenosis; $S_4$, fourth heart sound; SEM, systolic ejection murmur.

manifestations of low cardiac output are late symptoms, and sudden death usually occurs in symptomatic patients. Therapeutic decisions are based largely on the presence or absence of symptoms. Thus, the absolute valve area usually is not the primary determinant of the need for valve replacement.

Physical examination is a valuable tool in diagnosing and assessing the severity of aortic valve sclerosis or stenosis and defining which patients require closer clinical and echocardiographic evaluations (Table 8.1). Aortic sclerosis produces a systolic ejection murmur of less than grade 3/6 intensity, best heard at the base and right second intercostal space, and a normal carotid pulse. The hallmark of significant aortic stenosis is the typical slow-rising, small-volume arterial pulse, also labeled pulsus parvus et tardus (slow and late), which is best detected by palpating the carotid pulses. Hemodynamically significant aortic stenosis causes abnormal splitting of $S_2$. The characteristic alteration of $S_2$ is an increase in the $Q$–$A_2$ interval with $A_2$ occurring later (therefore coming closer to $P_2$) and a tendency for $S_2$ to become single. If LV ejection time is delayed substantially, reversed or paradoxic splitting of $S_2$ occurs. As the aortic valve becomes thickened, calcified, and rigid, the amplitude of $A_2$ decreases; in severe aortic stenosis, $A_2$ may be totally inaudible. Aortic stenosis produces the prototype of the classic systolic ejection murmur: a crescendo-decrescendo murmur that begins after $S_1$ and ends before $S_2$ and usually is heard best at the second right intercostal space. The murmur typically radiates upward and to the right and often is well heard over both carotid arteries. In general, the loudness of the murmur is proportional to the severity of the valvular obstruction in the absence of other factors that modify stroke volume or the rate of ejection. Some studies have shown that the time to peak intensity of the murmur is a better predictor of severity of aortic stenosis than its overall loudness. A murmur that peaks within the first third or half of systole suggests mild aortic stenosis. A murmur that peaks within the second half of systole indicates severe disease.

## Diagnostic Value of Echocardiography in Aortic Valve Sclerosis and Stenosis

Two-dimensional echocardiography provides excellent morphologic characterization of the sclerotic and stenotic aortic valve that, at least in the earlier stages of the disease, can help to define its etiology. Doppler echocardiography is highly accurate in defining the presence and is the best method to quantitate the severity of aortic valve stenosis.

The average rate of change in aortic valve area in patients with aortic stenosis is 0.12 $cm^2$ per year. More than half of patients will show little or no progression over a 3- to 9-year period, whereas others will have rapid progression with increases in pressure gradients of 15 to 19 mm Hg per year and decrease of aortic valve area of 0.1 to 0.3 $cm^2$ per year.

**TABLE 8.2.** *Stratification of aortic valve sclerosis and stenosis by echocardiography*

| Severity | Two-dimensional echocardiography | Peak gradient (mm Hg)[a] | Mean gradient (mm Hg)[b] | AVA (cm$^2$) | AVAi (cm$^2$/m$^2$) |
|---|---|---|---|---|---|
| Sclerosis | Thickened, hyperreflectant cusps | <16 | <10 | >2.0 | >1.1 |
| Mild AS | Thickened/Ca$^{2+}$ cusps with moderately decreased mobility | 16–25 | <20 | >1.5–2.0 | >0.9–1.1 |
| Moderate AS | Thickened/Ca$^{2+}$ cusps with moderately decreased mobility | 26–64 | 20–50 | >1.0–1.5 | >0.6–0.9 |
| Severe AS | Heavily thickened/Ca$^{2+}$ cusps with fixed cusps | >64 | >50 | ≤1.0 | ≤0.6 |

[a,b]In patients with normal stroke volumes.
AS, aortic stenosis; AVA, aortic valve area; AVAi, aortic valve area index.

For these reasons, careful echocardiographic follow-up is advised in patients with moderate to severe aortic stenosis.

Aortic stenosis is graded as mild, moderate, or severe according to valve morphology, peak and mean valve gradients, and aortic valve area and index (Table 8.2).

### Limitations of Physical Examination and Echocardiography in Patients with Aortic Valve Sclerosis or Stenosis

#### *Physical Examination*

Contrary to popular belief, systemic arterial hypertension can be associated with significant aortic valve stenosis, particularly in the older population. Even in severe aortic stenosis, only a minority of patients will have a systolic blood pressure of ≤100 mm Hg.

It is not uncommon to seriously underestimate or overestimate the severity of aortic stenosis by carotid artery palpation. In an adult >60 years of age with clinically normal LV function, completely normal carotid pulse contour and arterial pulse pressure do not exclude moderate to severe aortic stenosis. Also, in patients with LV dysfunction or other reasons for low cardiac output, a diminished and delayed carotid pulse does not necessarily signify severe aortic stenosis. Factors that can mask or underestimate the apparent severity of aortic stenosis in the carotid arterial examination are high cardiac output; elastic vessel in children and young patients; increased stiffness of the vessel in the elderly; associated aortic regurgitation; and systemic hypertension. Factors that

can exaggerate the apparent severity are low stroke volume of congestive heart failure, decreased LV function; hypovolemia; and mitral stenosis. *Practical Point: The presence of a normal or increased amplitude carotid arterial upstroke in the elderly does not rule out significant aortic stenosis.*

In patients with low cardiac output, a softer systolic murmur does not exclude moderate or worse stenosis. In addition, A$_2$ commonly is soft or absent in the absence of significant aortic stenosis in low cardiac output. A normal or increased P$_2$ (due to commonly associated pulmonary hypertension) can readily be mistaken for a normal A$_2$ and therefore underestimate its severity.

#### *Echocardiography*

Morphology and mobility of the cusps assessed by M-mode or 2-D echocardiography are not accurate for determining the severity of aortic stenosis. Also, a normal systolic excursion of the cusps in the short-axis view may lead to underestimation of the severity of a bicuspid or rheumatic stenotic aortic valve in the middle-aged or young patient.

Several important limitations must be kept in mind when using Doppler echocardiography to evaluate the severity of aortic valve stenosis. One of the major problems in obtaining the highest peak velocities is alignment of the ultrasonic beam as parallel as possible to a small, high-velocity jet. A misalignment of >20 degrees can result in significant underestimation of peak velocities and valve stenosis severity. In addition, the

**TABLE 8.3.** *Pitfalls of the physical examination and echocardiography in evaluation of aortic stenosis*

| AS severity | Physical examination | Echocardiography |
|---|---|---|
| Underestimation | 1. Normal carotid upstrokes in elderly patients<br>2. Low intensity murmur in low cardiac output<br>3. Low intensity murmur in patients with COPD/large chests<br>4. Gallavardin murmur confused for MR | 1. Depressed LV function<br>2. Moderate or severe MR<br>3. Malalignment (>20 degree) of sample volume to vena contracta<br>4. Patients with atrial fibrillation and poorly controlled ventricular response |
| Overestimation | 1. Hyperdynamic state<br>2. Anemia<br>3. Moderate or severe AR<br>4. Concomitant LV outflow gradient | 1. Pressure recovery in patients with small aortas<br>2. Hyperdynamic LV<br>3. Moderate or severe AR<br>4. Concomitant LV outflow gradient |

AR, aortic regurgitation; AS, aortic stenosis; COPD, chronic obstructive pulmonary disease; LV, left ventricular; MR, regurgitation.

pressure gradient does not always reflect the severity of aortic stenosis. In the presence of low cardiac output states, the amount of blood flowing through the stenotic valve is reduced and the peak velocities are lower; therefore, the valve gradient is underestimated. On the other hand, when coexisting aortic regurgitation or a hyperdynamic LV are present, there is a high transaortic volume flow rate and aortic jet velocity is higher; therefore, the severity of aortic stenosis is overestimated.

Another clinically relevant factor to be considered in the assessment of aortic stenosis by Doppler echocardiography is the phenomenon of pressure recovery (23–25). As the aortic jet decelerates and expands beyond the vena contracta, the associated turbulence results in an increase in aortic pressure (pressure recovery). If the aortic pressure is measured in the distal ascending aorta (as is the case in the cardiac catheterization laboratory), the LV pressure to aortic pressure difference is less than if the aortic pressure is measured in the vena contracta. Therefore, Doppler gradients and valve area severity may be overestimated by echocardiography as compared with gradients obtained during cardiac catheterization. The magnitude of pressure recovery is greater in patients with small aortic roots and moderate aortic stenosis. However, a recent series reported that the prevalence of small aortic roots (defined as <2.30 cm at the sinotubular portion and <2.85 cm at the si-

nuses) in patients with degenerative aortic valve stenosis is low (<5%) (26).

The peak-to-peak gradient measured in the catheterization laboratory is a measure of the difference between peak LV pressure and peak aortic pressure. The echo Doppler technique measures the maximum instantaneous pressure gradient across the valve, which occurs before the peak aortic pressure and is larger than the peak-to-peak gradient. Therefore, the Doppler gradient consistently overestimates the peak gradient and severity of aortic stenosis when compared with catheterization measurements. However, the mean pressure gradients (average pressure difference during the systolic ejection period) from both the Doppler technique and direct pressure recordings are true gradients and are better for comparison purposes.

Therefore, accurate interpretation of a Doppler echocardiogram and its integration into the management of a patient with suspected or known aortic valve stenosis require an understanding and awareness of its limitations or pitfalls (Table 8.3) (27,28).

## Indications for Echocardiography in Patients with Suspected Aortic Valve Sclerosis or Stenosis

If aortic sclerosis cannot be separated from stenosis by physical examination, an echocardiogram should be performed to con-

**TABLE 8.4.** *Class I indications for echocardiography in patients with aortic stenosis*

1. Diagnosis and assessment of severity of aortic stenosis
2. Assessment of left ventricular function, size, and/or hemodynamics
3. Reevaluation of patients with known aortic stenosis and changing symptoms or signs
4. Assessment of changes in hemodynamic severity and ventricular function in patients with known aortic stenosis in pregnancy
5. Reevaluation of asymptomatic patients with severe aortic stenosis

firm the diagnosis. If there is no significant gradient across the valve on initial echocardiogram, no additional follow-up echocardiograms are needed. Echocardiography is indicated in patients with aortic valve stenosis in order to assess its severity; its impact on LV function and hemodynamics; its rate of progression in symptomatic or asymptomatic patients (Table 8.4) (19).

Use of echocardiography for reevaluation of asymptomatic patients with mild to moderate aortic stenosis and evidence of LV dysfunction or hypertrophy and for routine evaluation of asymptomatic patients with mild aortic stenosis having stable physical signs and normal LV size and function lack supportive data.

In patients with severe aortic stenosis, an echocardiogram every 6–12 months may be appropriate; in patients with moderate stenosis, serial studies every 2 years may be adequate; and in patients with mild aortic stenosis, echocardiograms can be performed every 5 years. Echocardiograms should be performed more frequently if there is a change in clinical findings. Patients with a new diagnosis of severe aortic stenosis by echocardiogram are suggested to have a follow-up echocardiogram after 3 months. If they are found not to have progressed in severity on follow-up echocardiogram, then yearly follow-ups are recommended.

## REFERENCES

1. Boon A, Cheriex E, Lodder J, et al. Cardiac valve calcification: characteristics of patients with calcification of the mitral annulus or aortic valve. Heart 1997;78: 472–474.
2. Stewart BF, Siscovick D, Lind BK, et al. Clinical factors associated with calcific aortic valve disease: cardiovascular health study. J Am Coll Cardiol 1997;29: 630–634.
3. Otto CM, Lind BK, Kitzman DW, et al. Association of aortic valve sclerosis with cardiovascular mortality and morbidity in the elderly. N Engl J Med 1999;341:142–147.
4. Aronow WS, Ahn C, Shirani J, et al. Comparison of frequency of new coronary events in older subjects with and without valvular aortic sclerosis. Am J Cardiol 1999;83:599–600.
5. Lindroos M, Kupari M, Heikkilä J, et al. Prevalence of aortic valve abnormalities in the elderly: an echocardiographic study of a random population sample. J Am Coll Cardiol 1993;21:1220–1225.
6. Tolstrup K, Roldan CA, Qualls CR, et al. Aortic valve sclerosis, mitral annular calcification, and aortic root sclerosis are markers of atherosclerotic disease. J Am Coll Cardiol 2000;35:282A.
7. Otto CM, Burwash IG, Legget ME, et al. Prospective study of asymptomatic valvular aortic stenosis. Clinical, echocardiographic, and exercise predictors of outcome. Circulation 1997;95:2262–2270.
8. Faggiano P, Ghizzoni G, Sorgato A, et al. Rate of progression of valvular aortic stenosis in adults. Am J Cardiol 1992;70:229–233.
9. Mohler ER, Sheridan MJ, Nichols R, et al. Development and progression of aortic valve stenosis: atherosclerosis risk factors—a causal relationship? A clinical morphologic study. Clin Cardiol 1991;14:995–999.
10. Wierzbicki A, Shetty C. Aortic stenosis: an atherosclerotic disease? J Heart Valve Dis 1999;8:416–423.
11. Novaro GM, Tiong IY, Pearce GL, et al. Effect of HMG-CoA reductase inhibitors on the progression of valvular aortic stenosis. Circulation 2000;102:II-759(abst).
12. Shively BK, Charlton GA, Crawford MH, et al. Flow dependence of valve area in aortic stenosis: relation to valve morphology. J Am Coll Cardiol 1998;31:654–660.
13. Rosenhek R, Binder T, Porenta G, et al. Predictors of outcome in severe, asymptomatic aortic stenosis. N Engl J Med 2000;343:611–617.
14. Lester SJ, McElhinney DB, Miller JP, et al. Rate of change in aortic valve area during a cardiac cycle can predict the rate of hemodynamic progression of aortic stenosis. Circulation 2000;101:1947–1952.
15. Currie PJ, Seward JB, Reeder GS, et al. Continuous-wave Doppler echocardiographic assessment of severity of calcific aortic stenosis: a simultaneous Doppler-catheter correlative study in 100 adult patients. Circulation 1985;6:1162–1169.
16. Oh JK, Taliercio CP, Holmes DR, et al. Prediction of the severity of aortic stenosis by Doppler aortic valve area determination: prospective Doppler-catheterization correlation in 100 patients. J Am Coll Cardiol 1988;11: 1227–1234.
17. Burwash IG, Thomas DD, Sadahiro M, et al. Dependence of Gorlin formula and continuity equation valve

areas on transvalvular volume flow rate in valvular aortic stenosis. Circulation 1994;89:827–835.

18. Richards KL, Cannon SR, Miller JF, et al. Calculation of aortic valve area by Doppler echocardiography: a direct application of the continuity equation. Circulation 1986;5:964–969.

19. Carabello B, Leon AC, Edmunds LH, et al. ACC/AHA guidelines for the management of patients with valvular heart disease. J Am Coll Cardiol 1998;32:1486–1588.

20. Lin SS, Roger VL, Pascoe R, et al. Dobutamine stress Doppler hemodynamics in patients with aortic stenosis: feasibility, safety, and surgical considerations. Am Heart J 1998;136:1010–1016.

21. Connolly HM, Oh JK, Orszulak TA, et al. Aortic valve replacement for aortic stenosis with severe left ventricular dysfunction. Prognostic indicators. Circulation 1997;95:2395–2400.

22. Bermejo J, Garcia-Fernandez MA, Torrecilla EG, et al. Effects of dobutamine on Doppler echocardiographic indexes of aortic stenosis. J Am Coll Cardiol 1996; 28:1206–1213.

23. Niederberger J, Schima H, Maurer G, et al. Importance of pressure recovery for the assessment of aortic stenosis by Doppler ultrasound. Role of aortic size, aortic valve area, and direction of the stenotic jet in vitro. Circulation 1996;94:1934–1940.

24. Voelker W, Reul H, Stelzer T, et al. Pressure recovery in aortic stenosis: an in vitro study in a pulsatile flow model. J Am Coll Cardiol 1992;20:1585–1593.

25. Baumgartner H, Khan S, DeRobertis M, et al. Discrepancies between Doppler and catheter gradients in aortic prosthetic valves in vitro. A manifestation of localized gradients and pressure recovery. Circulation 1990;82: 1467–1475.

26. Crawford MH, Roldan CA. Prevalence of aortic root dilatation and small aortic roots in valvular aortic stenosis. Am J Cardiol 2001;87:1311–1313.

27. Otto CM. Valvular aortic stenosis: which measure of severity is best? Am Heart J 1998;136:940–942.

28. Bednarz JE, Krauss D, Lang RM. An echocardiographic approach to the assessment of aortic stenosis. J Am Soc Echocardiogr 1996;9:286–294.

# 9

# The Patient with Aortic Regurgitation

Carlos A. Roldan and *Jonathan Abrams

*Department of Internal Medicine, University of New Mexico School of Medicine; and
Department of Internal Medicine, Veterans Affairs Medical Center, Albuquerque, New Mexico;
*Cardiology Division, University of New Mexico School of Medicine; and
Department of Internal Medicine, University Hospital, Albuquerque, New Mexico*

## INTRODUCTION

The physical findings in severe chronic aortic regurgitation (AR) are striking and have fascinated physicians for centuries. Although the diagnosis of chronic moderate or worse AR can be made based on the presence of a diastolic murmur, displaced impulse of the left ventricle (LV), wide pulse pressure, third heart sound (S3; indicative of volume overload rather than LV dysfunction), and occasionally an Austin Flint rumble, the physical examination commonly is inaccurate in determining the severity and prognosis of AR. In addition, acute and se-

vere AR leading to rapid equilibrium between LV and aortic pressures is manifested mainly by heart failure, and physical findings of AR may not be easily identified. Therefore, echocardiography frequently is indicated to confirm the diagnosis and etiology of AR; assess aortic valve and root morphology; and provide a semiquantitative estimate of its severity and hemodynamic impact on LV size and function (1,2).

## ETIOLOGY

The prevalence of AR in young healthy subjects is ≤2% and almost always is trivial

(3). In obese but otherwise healthy middle-aged subjects (predominantly women), its prevalence increases up to 7% and is predominantly of mild degree (4). Finally, the prevalence of AR increases with age and is typically of trivial to mild degree.

The most common causes of chronic AR include degenerative aortic valve disease, bicuspid aortic valve, rheumatic heart disease, idiopathic aortic root dilation, aortic annuloectasia, healed infective endocarditis, and systemic hypertension. Uncommon causes of chronic and rarely of acute AR include noninflammatory connective tissue diseases (Marfan syndrome, Ehlers-Danlos syndrome, and osteogenesis imperfecta); inflammatory aortic root and aortic valve diseases (ankylosing spondylitis, rheumatoid arthritis, systemic lupus erythematosus, Reiter syndrome, giant cell aortitis, and syphilis); and, recently, use of anorexigens.

Infective endocarditis, aortic dissection, and aortic trauma are the most common causes of acute AR.

## PATHOPHYSIOLOGY

### Chronic Aortic Regurgitation

AR produces a classic volume overload state. The LV initially dilates and ejects more blood per beat. Stroke volume remains proportional to the regurgitant volume until LV decompensation occurs. Eccentric LV hypertrophy results, with prominent chamber enlargement and a proportionately smaller increase in wall thickness. There is an increase in LV compliance in chronic AR. LV filling pressure may remain relatively normal in the presence of considerable ventricular dilation. Cardiac output is maintained, and ejection rate and fraction actually are increased in early or mild AR. In time, however, severe AR results in a decrease in LV compliance, with subsequent elevation of filling pressure. At this point, patients typically become symptomatic, and congestive heart failure may result when LV contractility becomes sufficiently impaired.

### Acute Aortic Regurgitation

When the LV is challenged abruptly with a severe diastolic overload, normal compensatory mechanisms do not have time to develop. The LV is unable to adequately handle the large regurgitant flow, and the filling pressure becomes markedly elevated. The effective forward cardiac output falls. Peripheral vascular signs of severe AR are attenuated or may never appear due to marked systemic vasoconstriction. The heart rate usually is increased. LV failure in this clinical context carries a grave prognosis.

The hemodynamic changes of acute AR are more rapidly progressive and worse in patients with preexisting LV hypertrophy (patients with systemic hypertension and aortic dissection; infective endocarditis in patients with aortic stenosis; acute AR after balloon valvuloplasty, or surgical commissurotomy for congenital aortic stenosis). Therefore, early recognition of acute AR is imperative.

## NATURAL HISTORY AND PROGNOSIS

In asymptomatic patients with chronic severe AR, the rate of progression to symptoms or to asymptomatic LV systolic dysfunction ranges from 1.3% to 3.5% per year, but their rate of sudden death is <0.2% per year (5–8). In contrast, >25% of patients with LV systolic dysfunction develop cardiac symptoms per year (9,10). Also, patients with angina pectoris or heart failure have >10% and >20% mortality per year, respectively (11). Finally, >25% of patients who die or develop systolic dysfunction do so before the onset of warning symptoms (6,7,12). Thus, in patients with chronic moderate or worse AR, serial clinical and echocardiographic follow-up is necessary for evaluation of LV function and size. Age, LV ejection fraction, and LV end-systolic and end-diastolic dimensions or volumes are predictive of cardiovascular morbidity and mortality. Other predictors of outcome are the rate of increase in end-systolic dimension and the decrease in resting ejection fraction during serial longitudinal studies (12,13). During a mean follow-up period of 8 years, patients with an initial end-systolic dimension of >50 mm had a 19% per year rate of death, symptoms, and/or LV dysfunction compared to 6% in patients with end-systolic dimensions of 40 to 50 mm, and 0% in patients with LV dimension <40 mm (13).

Elderly patients with aortic valve disease frequently have combined aortic stenosis and regurgitation; are more likely to develop symptoms or LV dysfunction at earlier stages of LV dilation; have more persistent ventricular dysfunction and heart failure symptoms after surgery; and have worse postoperative survival rates than younger patients or those with isolated AR (14). Also, elderly patients frequently have earlier indications for surgery due to concomitant coronary artery disease that contributes to their symptoms and LV dysfunction.

## PHYSICAL EXAMINATION

### Blood Pressure

Systemic blood pressure is a valuable clue to the degree of AR. With progressive severity of AR, systolic blood pressure increases and aortic diastolic pressure declines (Fig. 9.1). *Practical Point: The presence of a completely normal blood pressure in a patient with AR and normal LV function virtually excludes the diagnosis of moderate to severe AR.* In hemodynamically significant AR, diastolic pressure typically falls below 70 mm Hg and systolic pressure may rise to 140 to 150 mm Hg.

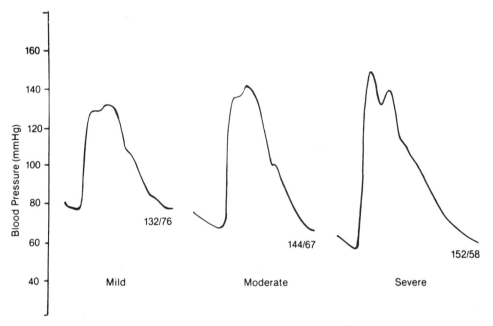

**FIG. 9.1.** Arterial pulse and blood pressure in aortic regurgitation. There is little alteration in arterial pulse and pressure in mild aortic regurgitation. With increasing reflux across the aortic valve, systolic blood pressure increases and diastolic blood pressure decreases, resulting in widening of the pulse pressure. The increased left ventricular stroke volume results in a high-amplitude, palpable arterial pulsation with rapid falloff in late systole. This produces a collapsing quality to the pulse. In severe aortic regurgitation, arterial pulsations may be very prominent and often visible in the carotid and peripheral circulation. (From Abrams J. Prim Cardiol 1983;9:16–30, with permission.)

*The degree of decrease in diastolic blood pressure is a better benchmark for assessing the severity of AR than the increase in systolic pressure.* In severe or "free" AR, diastolic blood pressure typically is 40 to 50 mm Hg, approaching or equaling the markedly elevated LV end-diastolic pressure. It is best to use the point of *muffling* of Korotkoff sounds as the indication of diastolic blood pressure in subjects with AR; audible sounds may be detected to zero.

*Practical Point: Severe isolated AR uncommonly will be present in a patient with diastolic blood pressure >60 mm Hg if there is no evidence of reduced LV function or systemic hypertension. Conversely, diastolic blood pressure ≤50 mm Hg almost always indicates a major degree of AR, irrespective of the level of systolic pressure.*

## Arterial and Carotid Pulses

The large stroke volume and enhanced rate of ejection produced by hemodynamically significant AR results in a characteristic *high-amplitude arterial pulse* (Fig. 9.1). The pulse has a *collapsing* quality caused by the low systemic vascular resistance and early diastolic reflux of blood into the LV. With a very large stroke volume, the pulse is full, literally swelling under the examining finger, then rapidly abating. Pulsations of proximal carotid arteries may be visible (Corrigan sign). Arterial pulses throughout the body are increased in force and amplitude and display a typical bounding quality.

### *Bisferiens Pulse*

One of the hallmarks of AR is the bisferiens or double systolic arterial pulse (Fig. 9.2). This bifid pulsation is best felt with light finger pressure over the carotid arteries. A transmitted systolic thrill or bruit also is felt. In severe AR, a systolic shudder of the carotid artery may be noted with or without associated aortic stenosis. The bisferiens pulse is present in moderate to severe AR or

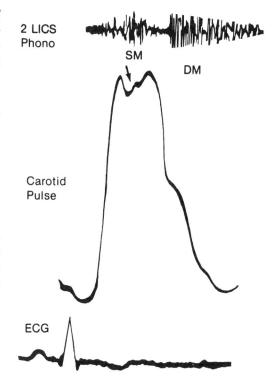

**FIG. 9.2.** Bisferiens pulse of aortic regurgitation. Note the bifid or double systolic pulse wave, which is detected best using light finger pressure over the carotid arteries. This contour is associated with an increased pulse volume. The bisferiens pulse must be differentiated from a transmitted systolic murmur or palpable thrill. Note the soft $S_1$ and $S_2$. 2 LICS, second left intercostal space; DM, diastolic murmur; SM, systolic murmur. (From Abrams J. Prim Cardiol 1983;9: 16–30 with permission.)

in patients with AR and associated mild aortic stenosis.

## Peripheral Signs

Major degrees of AR produce a variety of abnormalities on physical examination that are directly related to ejection of an increased stroke volume into a dilated and compliant arterial bed. The abrupt rise and fall of the arterial pulse wave causes a distinctive pounding or collapsing quality that is accentuated in the peripheral arteries.

**TABLE 9.1.** *Peripheral or nonauscultatory signs of severe aortic regurgitation*

| | |
|---|---|
| Bisferiens pulse | Double or bifid systolic impulse felt in the arterial pulse |
| Corrigan sign | Visible pulsations of the supraclavicular and carotid arteries |
| Pistol shot of Traube | Loud systolic sound heard with the stethoscope lightly placed over the femoral arteries |
| Palmar click | Palpable, abrupt flushing of the palms in systole |
| Quincke pulse | Exaggerated sequential reddening and blanching of the fingernail beds when light pressure is applied to the tip of the fingernail. A similar observation can be made by pressing a glass slide to the lips. |
| Duroziez sign | To-and-fro bruit heard over the femoral artery when light pressure is applied to the artery by the edge of the stethoscope head. This bruit is caused by the exaggerated reversal of flow in diastole. |
| De Musset sign | Visible oscillation or bobbing of the head with each heartbeat |
| Hill sign | Abnormal accentuation of leg systolic blood pressure, with popliteal pressure ≥40 mm Hg than brachial artery pressure. |
| Water-hammer pulse | High-amplitude, abruptly collapsing pulse of aortic regurgitation. This term refers to a popular Victorian toy comprised of a glass vessel partially filled with water, which produced a slapping impact when turned over. |
| Muller sign | Visible pulsations of the uvula |

Many well-known eponyms have been given to these *nonauscultatory signs of AR.* In general, the presence of such peripheral abnormalities correlates well with the increased systolic and pulse pressure and decreased diastolic pressure common to advanced AR. *Practical Point: These nonauscultatory signs are never seen in mild AR but are the rule in chronic severe AR in the absence of congestive heart failure.* Low cardiac output or the onset of heart failure may attenuate these signs. Table 9.1 lists most of the peripheral abnormalities that have been described in AR.

### Precordial Motion

The quality of the LV impulse parallels the severity of AR. In mild to moderate AR, the LV impulse is normal in size but often is hyperdynamic (Fig. 1.14B). Thus, the amplitude is exaggerated, but there is no leftward displacement of the apex beat; the apical impulse falls away from the palpating finger by mid systole. With greater degrees of AR, the hyperkinetic impulse becomes more prominent, and the cardiac apex is displaced inferolaterally. When LV dilation or a decrease in the ejection fraction occurs, typically with an increased end-systolic volume, the apex beat becomes *sustained* (Fig. 1.14 C). In patients with very large hearts or significant depression of LV function, a prolonged and force-ful LV lift or heave is predictable, and this finding may be impressive. In severe chronic AR, the apex impulse typically is found in the left anterior axillary line at the fifth or sixth interspace, usually occupies at least two interspaces, and is sustained into late systole. A palpable fourth heart sound ($S_4$; presystolic distension) may be noted in the left decubitus position (Fig. 1.15). A visible and palpable rapid LV filling wave ($S_3$) may be detected in severe AR.

### Heart Sounds

#### *First Heart Sound*

The first heart sound ($S_1$) has a normal intensity in mild to moderate cases but often is decreased in severe AR (Fig. 9.3). An aortic ejection sound is easily mistaken for $S_1$ in AR. Whenever "$S_1$" is particularly prominent at the base, it is likely due to an aortic ejection click instead of $S_1$.

#### *Second Heart Sound*

##### *Intensity*

The aortic component ($A_2$) of the second heart sound ($S_2$) is variable in intensity. $A_2$ may be *softer* than usual in AR because of a decreased ability of the valve leaflets to vibrate after aortic valve closure.

*Splitting of S₂*

In patients with moderate to severe AR, $S_2$ often is single.

### Third Heart Sound

A third heart sound ($S_3$) is not a feature of mild to moderate AR; however, an $S_3$ is common in severe AR (Fig. 9.3). The increase in LV diastolic blood volume is in part responsible for the prominent $S_3$. LV di-

lation and decreased contractility may be significant additive factors. The $S_3$ frequently is a visible and palpable event, coinciding with the rapid filling phase of LV diastole. An $S_3$ is more likely to be heard in younger patients.

### Fourth Heart Sound

Although an atrial sound is an uncommon finding in mild AR, it may be found occa-

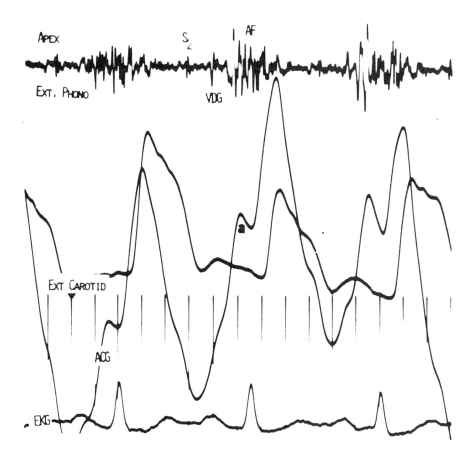

**FIG. 9.3.** Third heart sound and Austin Flint murmur (AF) in acute aortic regurgitation. The phonocardiogram demonstrates an $S_3$ or ventricular diastolic gallop (VDG) followed by a loud AF extending into late diastole. Note the accentuation of this murmur with atrial systole. The apex cardiogram (ACG) reveals a markedly augmented A wave and hyperdynamic LV impulse. $S_1$ is virtually absent. The auscultatory findings in such a patient may be extremely difficult to interpret. The presence of an $S_3$ and AF in acute or chronic aortic regurgitation indicates a major degree of aortic reflux. (From Reddy PS, et al. Syndrome of acute aortic regurgitation. In: Leon DF, Shaver JA, eds. Physiologic principles of heart sounds and murmurs. American Heart Association Monograph No. 46, 1975, with permission.)

sionally in moderate AR and is common in severe disease. The long PR interval common in many patients with AR increases audibility of an $S_4$. The $S_4$ may be manifest at the apex as palpable presystolic distention when the patient is turned onto his or her left side.

### Ejection Sound

An aortic ejection click or sound is detectable in many subjects with AR. More commonly it is heard in mild disease when there is good LV function. The ejection click may be of valve or root origin. When there is a bicuspid aortic valve, the ejection click is produced by the maximal opening excursion of the abnormal valve cusps. In subjects with an enlarged, abnormal aortic root, the ejection sound most likely is produced by sudden systolic expansion of the ascending aorta itself during early ejection (Fig. 1.19). A snappy or prominently split $S_1$ or an $S_1$ that is well heard at the base in a patient with AR should suggest to the clinician that the $S_1$ is actually an aortic ejection click.

### Cardiac Murmurs

Three different murmurs may be found in patients with AR: (i) the classic decrescendo diastolic murmur resulting from reflux of blood into the LV; (ii) a systolic ejection murmur produced by the large stroke volume, increased rate of ejection, and abnormal valve anatomy; and (iii) the Austin Flint murmur, a low-pitched diastolic murmur beginning in mid diastole and found only in major degrees of AR.

### Diastolic Murmur

The typical diastolic murmur of AR has a decrescendo shape (Figs. 9.2 and 9.4), beginning immediately with $A_2$. The volume and velocity of refluxing blood across the incompetent aortic valve tapers off in mid to late diastole. *In general, the length of the AR murmur is dependent on the severity of the leak except in very severe lesions.* The classic finding in AR is a diastolic murmur beginning with $S_2$ that tapers during diastole and may extend to $S_1$.

### Frequency

The diastolic murmur typically is high frequency or "blowing" in quality in mild to moderate AR. It is important to listen with the breath held in end-expiration so as not to confuse the AR murmur with the noise of breathing. *Practical Point: The high-frequency murmur of mild AR frequently is soft. As most physicians are unaccustomed to hearing sounds of such high pitch, this faint AR murmur is easily missed by the unsuspecting examiner.*

With more severe degrees of AR, low- to medium-frequency sound vibrations occur, and the murmur may be surprisingly low pitched.

### Duration

In mild degrees of AR, the diastolic murmur may not be audible in late diastole. In fact, the murmur of mild AR may be so short as to be little more than a blurring sound off $A_2$ (Fig. 9.4A). Such murmurs typically are low amplitude and high frequency and are hard to hear without selective focus on early diastole. With increasing degrees of aortic reflux, the murmur may become truly holodiastolic but remains decrescendo in quality (Fig. 9.4B–C). Thus, with a diastolic blood pressure ≤60 mm Hg, a pandiastolic murmur would be anticipated. Some patients with *severe* AR may actually have a *shorter* decrescendo diastolic murmur than those with milder disease (Fig. 9.4D). "Free" AR commonly is associated with a very high late LV diastolic filling pressure and a low aortic diastolic pressure. This results in a small aortic–LV gradient so that the amount of reflux may be small or nil at end-diastole (Fig. 9.4D).

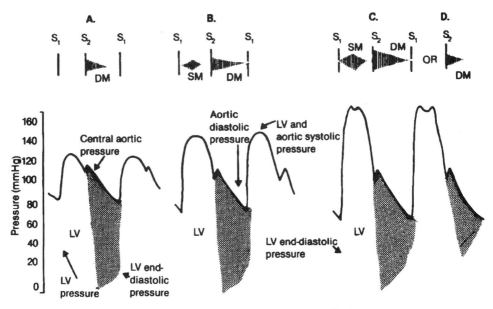

**The Murmurs of Aortic Regurgitation**

**FIG. 9.4.** Diastolic and systolic murmurs of aortic regurgitation. Diagram shows the relationship between the severity of aortic regurgitation, hemodynamic findings, and the characteristic murmurs of mild, moderate, and severe aortic regurgitation. **A:** Mild aortic regurgitation. The diastolic gradient between the aorta and left ventricle is large. Reflux of blood is high velocity and small in volume. The resultant diastolic murmur (DM) is of variable length and typically high frequency. A systolic ejection murmur (SM) may not be present. **B:** Moderate aortic regurgitation. The diastolic murmur is decrescendo and invariably long. The murmur may have medium- or high-frequency vibrations. A systolic ejection (flow) murmur is common. **C,D:** Severe aortic regurgitation. The length of the diastolic murmur is variable. With preserved left ventricular function **(C)**, the murmur usually is pandiastolic and medium frequency (high velocity, large volume reflux). The systolic murmur may be very prominent and lengthy in duration, even in the absence of aortic stenosis. If there is left ventricular failure or the late end-diastolic pressure is markedly elevated (resulting in narrow pressure gradient between the aorta and left ventricle during the last third of diastole), the diastolic murmur may be short and unimpressive **(D)**. The systolic murmur may be unremarkable in this setting. This combination can result in a serious underestimation of the severity of aortic regurgitation. (From Abrams J. Prim Cardiol 1983;9:16–30 with permission.)

*Intensity*

The AR murmur ranges in loudness between very faint to quite prominent, but is rarely of grade 4/6 to 5/6 intensity. Mild degrees of AR produce murmurs that typically are soft. It is important not to miss such a faint murmur, as the presence of audible AR supports the diagnosis of organic heart disease. *Doppler echocardiography confirms that trivial to mild AR (1 to 2+) commonly is inaudible.*

Patients in heart failure resulting from severe AR occasionally may have no more than a faint, short murmur. Severe AR can actually

be silent in acute regurgitation or with depressed LV function.

*Optimal Sites for Auscultation*

The murmur of AR usually is best heard adjacent to the sternum between the second and fourth left interspace. In mild AR, the murmur may be localized only to the second left interspace at the left sternal edge. With increasing severity of AR, the maximal intensity of the murmur may be as low as the fourth or fifth interspace. The murmur often is audible at the apex when its intensity is grade 2/6 to 3/6 or more, and in some subjects it actually may be best heard at the apex. This finding is more likely to occur in elderly patients.

### Aortic Regurgitation Heard to the Right of the Sternum

The typical AR murmur may be heard easily at the second to third right interspace where it can be quite prominent (Table 9.2). However, the murmur usually is not detectable lower down the right side of the sternum. Many years ago, Levine and Harvey observed that, on occasion, an AR murmur is very well heard at the *lower right sternal border* (third to fifth right interspace). They noted that this phenomenon occurred commonly in patients who had *disease of the aortic root* rather than at the valve level.

### Aids to Auscultation

Special techniques are not necessary to increase the audibility of a loud regurgitant murmur. However, the elusive, faint, high-pitched blowing murmur of AR can be made more audible by certain maneuvers. *Practical Point: The examination should take place in a quiet room with the patient sitting, standing, or leaning forward with the breath held in mid or full expiration. Use firm pressure with the diaphragm of the stethoscope (enough to leave an imprint on the skin).* Background noise, such as that from air conditioning or the patient's own breath sounds, can readily mask detection of a high-pitched, grade 1/6 to 2/6 aortic murmur. Sustained handgrip or squatting may "bring out" a faint murmur.

**TABLE 9.2.** *Conditions resulting in aortic regurgitation murmur heard best on the right side of the sternum*

Aortic aneurysm
  Cystic medial necrosis
  Syphilis
  Idiopathic
Sinus of Valsalva aneurysm
Aortic dissection (acute or chronic)
Selective perforation or eversion of the right coronary
  cusp

In some patients, particularly younger persons, the AR murmur may be heard more easily in the supine position. Remember that in older adults, especially those with chronic lung disease or congestive heart failure, the AR murmur occasionally may be maximal or heard only at the LV apex.

### Systolic Murmur

A systolic ejection murmur is common in moderate to severe AR. It is caused by a large stroke volume ejected with rapid force, often across an anatomically deformed aortic valve into an enlarged proximal aorta. *Practical Point: A prominent systolic murmur in a patient with severe AR does not necessarily imply coexisting aortic stenosis; typically, this systolic murmur is short and peaks before the second half of systole* (Fig. 9.4B–C). However, a very large stroke volume and/or thickened aortic valve leaflets may accentuate the intensity and duration of the systolic murmur.

### Associated Valve Lesions

Patients often have both aortic stenosis and regurgitation, particularly with rheumatic disease. In these instances, the systolic murmur also will reflect the presence of aortic valve obstruction. Typically, this results in a prominent systolic *and* diastolic murmur, the so-called bellows murmur. When both the aortic systolic and diastolic murmurs are long, this combination may mimic a continuous murmur.

When mitral stenosis coexists with AR, the obstruction to LV filling may attenuate the full expression of AR on clinical examination. The diastolic murmur of AR may be less prominent, and evidence for LV dilation will be less impressive than that usually produced by a comparable degree of AR.

### Austin Flint Murmur

The Austin Flint murmur is a low-pitched, rumbling apical diastolic murmur that sounds exactly like the murmur of mitral stenosis (Fig. 9.3). Its presence generally indicates a large diastolic leak with a regurgitant fraction >50%. The Austin Flint murmur usually is found in association with the peripheral signs of severe AR (Table 9.2).

### Pathogenesis

Many theories have been proposed to explain the Austin Flint murmur. The mechanism appears to be related to incomplete opening of the anterior leaflet of the mitral valve during diastole as a result of the impact of the regurgitant stream of blood into the LV cavity. The resultant low-pitched murmur may persist into late diastole as a result of turbulence within the LV cavity. Typically, the Austin Flint murmur is found in patients with a greatly increased LV end-diastolic volume and a very large aortic regurgitant fraction.

### Auscultatory Features

The Austin Flint bruit is a rumbling diastolic murmur that usually begins in early to mid diastole (Fig. 9.3). If a presystolic component is present, a crescendo low-frequency murmur in late diastole extends to $S_1$. The pitch of the Austin Flint murmur is identical to the rumble of mitral stenosis. Typically, the murmur begins with a prominent $S_3$ (Fig. 9.3).

### Austin Flint or Diastolic Murmur of Mitral Stenosis?

Patients with rheumatic heart disease frequently have combined AR and mitral stenosis. Therefore, it is important to accurately identify the etiology of a low-frequency, apical diastolic murmur. Evidence of associated mitral valve disease implies that the rumble is due to organic mitral stenosis and not sec-

ondary to severe AR. Table 9.3 lists a number of differentiating features.

### Differential Diagnosis

#### Pulmonic Regurgitation

In severe pulmonic hypertension, a high-pitched blowing murmur may be audible (the Graham Steell murmur). Its acoustic characteristics are identical to those of mild AR. The Graham Steell murmur invariably is associated with other signs of pulmonary hypertension, such as a right ventricular lift and increased pulmonic valve component ($P_2$).

#### Mitral Stenosis

Occasionally, the diastolic murmur of mitral stenosis is medium to high frequency and may simulate AR if it radiates well to the lower, left sternal border. Careful auscultation should identify a clear-cut interval between $A_2$ and the onset of the mitral stenosis murmur; an opening snap and an increased $S_1$ typically will be present.

#### Acute Aortic Regurgitation

The unusual syndrome of acute massive AR is well known. Often this is a dramatic, life-threatening condition resulting from the sudden influx of an excessive amount of blood into a LV unable to accommodate the large regurgitant volume. The aortic valve usually is normal or only mildly abnormal prior to the onset of the sudden regurgitation. Acute or subacute bacterial endocarditis, aortic dissection, aortic valve perforation or rupture secondary to trauma, and myxomatous degeneration are the most common causes of this syndrome.

**TABLE 9.3.** *Helpful differentiating features of an apical diastolic murmur in aortic regurgitation: Austin Flint murmur versus mitral stenosis*

|  | Austin Flint | Mitral stenosis |
|---|---|---|
| Rhythm | Normal sinus | Atrial fibrillation |
| Left ventricular heave | Common | Absent |
| Right ventricular lift | Absent | Present |
| $S_1$ | Normal to decreased | Loud |
| Opening snap | Absent | Present |
| $S_3$ | Present | Absent |

Prompt and accurate diagnosis of acute AR is of great importance, as urgent surgical intervention usually is mandatory. However, the typical physical signs of severe chronic AR often are absent in such patients, and the AR murmur itself may be unimpressive in these severely ill patients. Why is this so? (i) The voluminous regurgitant volume often precipitates acute LV failure, with secondary systemic vasoconstriction and tachycardia. The arterial tree "clamps down," preventing or attenuating the classic blood pressure alterations and peripheral signs of chronic severe AR. (ii) Sinus tachycardia is common in acute AR. The increase in heart rate results in a relative shortening of diastole, which hampers accurate auscultation by making identification of systole and diastole difficult. (iii) Because the LV usually is of normal thickness and diameter prior to the onset of the acute AR, it is unable to quickly dilate. LV filling pressure becomes markedly elevated. $S_1$ is soft and there is no $S_4$ or presystolic component to the Austin Flint murmur. LV function may be acutely depressed. The tremendously elevated LV pressure in late diastole causes shortening of the AR murmur, which also is often surprisingly soft.

### Physical Findings of Acute Aortic Regurgitation

#### General Appearance

Patients with acute AR usually appear seriously ill and may be in acute heart failure (Table 9.4). Resting tachycardia and orthopnea are common. The skin may be pale, cool, and moist, reflecting intense sympathetic vasoconstriction.

TABLE 9.4. *Features of acute versus chronic severe aortic regurgitation*

|  | Chronic | Acute |
|---|---|---|
| Resting heart rate | Normal | Sinus tachycardia common; easy to confuse systole for diastole |
| Blood pressure | Increased systolic BP (>140 mm Hg) Decreased diastolic BP (<70 mm Hg) Increased pulse pressure | Normal or slight reduction in systolic BP Diastolic BP may or may not be low |
| Peripheral pulses | Bisferiens contour Increased amplitude and volume Peripheral signs of severe AR | Pulsus alternans Can have unremarkable contour with little to no evidence for peripheral vasodilation |
| Jugular venous pulse | Normal | Mean pressure may be elevated V wave if functional tricuspid regurgitation |
| Precordial motion | LV impulse at fifth to sixth intercostal space; left anterior axillary line hyperdynamic or heaving contour Palpable $S_3$ or $S_4$ common | Normal to slight LV enlargement Bifid diastolic impulse with palpable $S_3$ and $S_4$ sustained late diastolic motion Right ventricular impulse if severe pulmonary hypertension |
| Heart sounds | $S_1$ normal to decreased $S_2$ often unremarkable; increased to decreased $A_2$ $S_3$ very common $S_4$ uncommon Ejection click possible | $S_1$ decreased to absent $S_2$ single; soft to absent $A_2$; increased P2 $S_3$ "always" $S_4$ common Ejection sound common Mid-diastolic mitral valve closure sound |
| Aortic regurgitation murmur | Medium frequency Usually holodiastolic May be short, with rapid decrescendo Grade 3 unless congestive heart failure present | Medium frequency, often harsh Musical if ruptured cusp Usually not holodiastolic; may be very short, rapidly decrescendo Can be quite soft |
| Austin-Flint murmur | Common mid-diastolic component with/without presystolic murmur murmur | "Always" mid-diastolic component with/without presystolic murmur |
| Systolic murmur | Typically present Can simulate aortic stenosis or mitral regurgitation | Typically present Mitral regurgitation murmur common |

BP, blood pressure; LV, left ventricular.

### Blood Pressure and Pulses

Low diastolic blood pressure that is common to severe chronic AR may be absent. The small forward stroke volume and decreased rate of ejection in these patients prevents the expected increase in systolic blood pressure. Thus, the pulse pressure may be normal, slightly increased, or wide. The nonausculatory signs of severe AR in the peripheral circulation may be unimpressive or totally absent.

### Jugular Venous Pulse

Right ventricular failure and pulmonary hypertension are common. Mean venous pressure often is elevated and tricuspid regurgitation may be present, resulting in large V waves in the neck veins.

### Precordial Motion

The LV impulse may be unimpressive in recent-onset AR or may be displaced laterally with a thrusting contour. The greatly enlarged LV impulse typical of chronic AR is absent.

### Heart Sounds

$S_1$ is soft or even absent due to the premature closure of the mitral valve (Fig. 9.3). $S_2$ may be normal or single. Either or both an $S_3$ and $S_4$ are commonly noted.

### Aortic Regurgitation Murmur

The murmur of acute AR may be unimpressive and thus clinically misleading, particularly if congestive heart failure or severe depression of LV function is present. Frequently, severe AR results in a murmur with medium- to low-frequency vibrations; the length of the murmur may be surprisingly short. If the acute AR is related to preexisting aortic root disease or isolated rupture of the right coronary cusp, the diastolic murmur may radiate best down the right sternal edge.

### Austin Flint Murmur

This murmur may be commonly found in acute AR (Fig. 9.3).

### Systolic Murmur

The systolic flow murmur common to chronic AR may be present in acute AR. If LV function is depressed, this murmur is likely to be soft and short.

## ECHOCARDIOGRAPHY

### Introduction

Color Doppler transthoracic echocardiography (TTE) can not only determine the presence, severity, and etiology of AR, but also help to define the natural history, prognosis, and timing of surgery for moderate or worse acute or chronic AR. Transesophageal echocardiography (TEE) is indicated when acute severe AR is suspected to be due to aortic dissection or infective endocarditis. This technique not only determines need for surgery, but also may help in the surgical approach.

In asymptomatic patients with moderate or worse AR and preserved LV systolic function, an initial color Doppler echocardiogram represents the information against which future serial studies should be compared. Measurements of LV cavity size and systolic function (fractional shortening) from M-mode tracings are reproducible and preferable to those obtained from two-dimensional (2-D) images. Indirect parameters of the severity of AR include the rate of decline in the regurgitant gradient measured by the slope of diastolic flow velocity by continuous wave Doppler. The degree of flow velocity reversal in the descending aorta by pulse wave Doppler also can help to define the severity of AR. Finally, comparison of the stroke volume at the aortic valve with that of an uninvolved valve may provide a quantitative measurement of regurgitant volume and fraction. However, these measurements are time consuming, require experience, and are more prone to significant intraobserver and interobserver variability.

Semiquantitative parameters of the severity of AR by color Doppler include assessment of AR jet width and area; determination of vena contracta width and area; and estimation of regurgitant volume and fraction and regurgitant orifice area using the proximal isoelectric velocity area (PISA).

## M-Mode and Two-Dimensional Echocardiography

M-Mode and two-dimensional echocardiography provide some characterization of the common causes of AR, such as degenerative valve disease, bicuspid aortic valve, rheumatic heart disease, and endocarditis.

By M-mode echocardiography, the thickness and mobility of the aortic valve cusps can be assessed accurately. Although the etiology of AR (degenerative, congenital, or rheumatic) cannot be determined by this technique, an eccentric valve closure in relation to the aortic root walls suggests a bicuspid aortic valve. However, M-mode echocardiography is highly accurate in defining the presence and degree of aortic root dilation causing or contributing to AR. The technique also is accurate in identifying premature closure of the mitral valve in acute severe AR.

Two-dimensional echocardiography allows morphologic characterization of the aortic valve cusps and aortic root. In *degenerative aortic valve disease,* one or more of the aortic cusps are thickened, hyperreflectant, and less mobile. Cusp thickening and sclerosis can be diffuse, localized, or nodular, and involve predominantly the cusp margins and basal portions. A *bicuspid aortic valve* has two cusps of nearly equal size, a single linear commissure, and frequently a hyperreflectant raphe. An early sign of a bicuspid aortic valve is systolic doming of the cusps (curved toward the center of the aorta) due to still pliable cusps, but with restricted mobility due to their increased area of annular attachment. The usual pattern of *rheumatic aortic valve disease* is commissural fusion, thickening of the tip portions, and retraction of the cusps. Often, all commissures are affected.

TEE 2-D imaging is highly accurate in the detection of aortic valve endocarditis and associated complications.

TTE and TEE 2-D imaging also accurately detect and characterize aortic root diseases causing AR (Figs. 9.5, 9.6, 9.7A, and 9.8A).

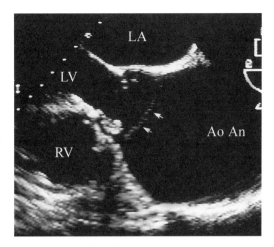

**FIG. 9.5.** Large dissecting aortic aneurysm in a 75-year-old man. Transesophageal echocardiographic longitudinal view of the aortic valve and aortic root demonstrates a large dissecting aneurysm of the ascending aorta (Ao An). The aortic root diameter exceeded 8 cm. Note the dissecting intimal flap *(arrows).* Moderate aortic regurgitation due to incomplete cusp coaptation was demonstrated by color Doppler. RV, right ventricle.

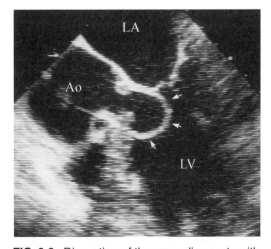

**FIG. 9.6.** Dissection of the ascending aorta with a large and prolapsing intimal flap. Transesophageal echocardiographic longitudinal view of the aortic valve and aortic root in a 57-year-old woman with syncope followed by cardiogenic shock demonstrates a large intimal flap prolapsing through the aortic valve into the outflow tract (arrows). Severe aortic regurgitation was demonstrated by color Doppler. Ao, aorta. Other abbreviations as in previous figures.

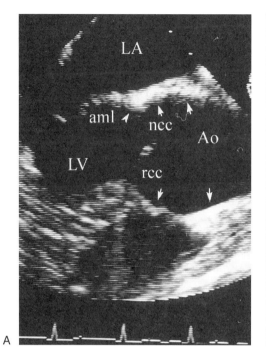 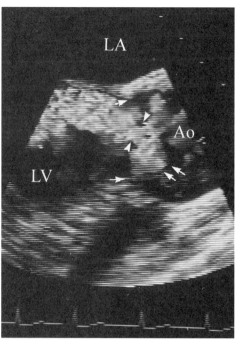

**FIG. 9.7.** Ankylosing spondylitis and symptomatic severe aortic regurgitation in a 43-year-old man. **A:** Transesophageal echocardiographic longitudinal view of the aortic valve demonstrates aortic root dilation and severe thickening and sclerosis of the aortic root predominantly of the posterior wall *(upright arrows)* extending to the base of the anterior mitral leaflet (aml) forming a characteristic subaortic bump *(arrowhead)*. Minimal thickening of the right (rcc) coronary cusp is present. **B:** Transesophageal echocardiographic longitudinal view with color Doppler imaging demonstrates moderate to severe aortic regurgitation as judged by a large (>6 mm wide) vena contracta *(arrowheads)*. Note a large flow convergence zone *(arrows)*. Using the flow convergence area method, the effective regurgitant orifice area was calculated as 1.2 cm². Ao, aorta; LA, left atrium; LV, left ventricle; ncc, noncoronary cusp. (See Color Figure 9.7B.)

Finally and most importantly, these techniques provide information on the severity and hemodynamic impact of AR, such as LV size and function. Also, by 2-D echocardiography, the total LV stroke volume using the Simpson rule can be derived as LV end-diastolic volume minus end-systolic volume.

### Pulsed Doppler

Total stroke volume is derived using pulsed Doppler as the product of the LV outflow tract (LVOT) cross-sectional area (using the LVOT diameter obtained from the TTE parasternal or TEE long-axis view) times its corresponding velocity time integral (VTI) (obtained from the TTE apical long-axis view). *Therefore, total stroke volume =* $(D^2/4)_{LVOT} \times VTI_{LVOT}$, *where D is the LVOT diameter.*

Using the same formula, but substituting the LV for the RV outflow tract or mitral annulus diameter, the forward stroke volume can be calculated from either the pulmonic or mitral valve (15,16). *Subtraction of the forward stroke volume from the total stroke volume derives the regurgitant volume. The regurgitant fraction then is calculated as the regurgitant volume divided by the total stroke volume.* In the presence of significant MR, only the pulmonic stroke volume can be used to determine the forward stroke volume.

*AR is mild if the regurgitant fraction is <20%; moderate if 20% to 35%; moderate to severe if 35% to 50%; and severe if*

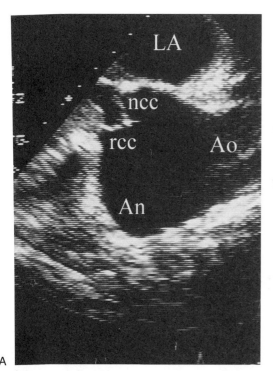
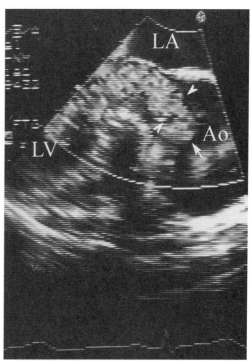

A

B

**FIG. 9.8.** Sinus of Valsalva aneurysm and symptomatic aortic regurgitation in a 58-year-old patient. **A:** Transesophageal echocardiographic longitudinal view of the aortic valve and aortic root demonstrates a large aneurysm (An) of the right coronary sinus and severe aortic root dilation (6.2 cm). **B:** Transesophageal echocardiographic longitudinal view of the aortic valve with color Doppler imaging demonstrates a large flow convergence zone *(arrow)*, vena contracta width of 7 mm *(arrowheads)*, and ratio of the color jet height to outflow tract height >75%. Because of the eccentricity of the regurgitant jet, adequate continuous wave Doppler tracings for assessing pressure half-time were not obtained by transthoracic echocardiography. Abbreviations as in previous figure. (See Color Figure 9.8B.)

>50%. *Regurgitant volume >60 mL indicates severe AR.*

The effective regurgitant orifice area also can be calculated using pulse Doppler-derived regurgitant volume, which then is divided by the regurgitant time velocity integral of the AR jet obtained by continuous wave Doppler.

Pulsed Doppler can be used to assess AR severity by determining flow characteristics in the aortic arch or descending aorta (17). Normally, systolic flow in the aorta is predominantly antegrade. With increasing severity of AR, diastolic retrograde flow is detected. Retrograde flow is proportional to the degree of AR. Although the regurgitant fraction can be calculated as the diastolic

flow divided by the antegrade systolic flow, adequate tracing are not easy to obtain, and retrograde flow can be mistaken by sampling flow in the takeoff of the branches of the arch.

**Continuous Wave Doppler**

Continuous wave Doppler allows for detection and assessment of the severity of AR. This technique provides assessment of the pressure difference between the aorta and LV during diastole. The rapidity of change of this pressure gradient is an index of the severity of AR and is assessed by the pressure half-time ($P_{1/2}$), which is defined as the time it takes for the initial transvalvular pres-

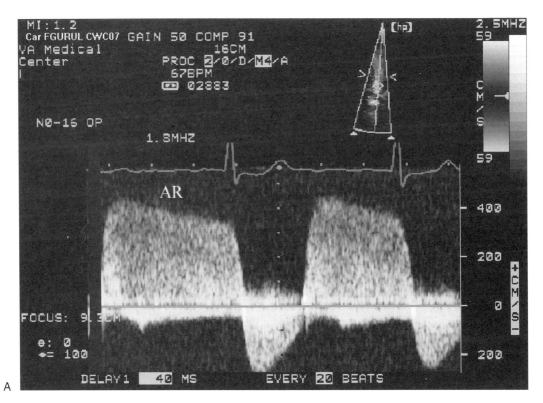

A

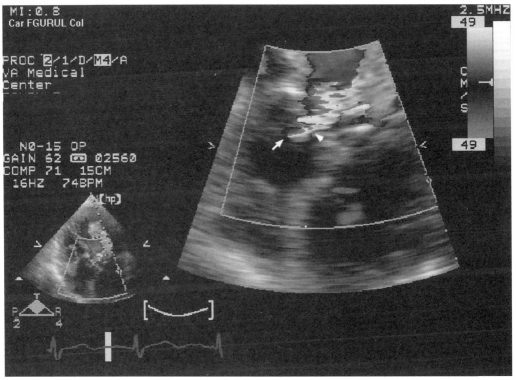

B

sure gradient to decrease by 50%. $P_{1/2}$ is best obtained from the TTE apical five- or three-chamber view. As AR severity increases, the more rapid is the decline in the aortic pressure, the more rapid is the rise in LV end-diastolic pressure, and the shorter is $P_{1/2}$ (18,19). *AR is mild if $P_{1/2}$ is >500 ms; moderate if 350 to 500 ms; moderate to severe if 200 to 350 ms; and severe if <200 ms (Fig. 9.9A).*

### Color Doppler

Probably the color Doppler method most currently used in clinical practice for assessment of AR severity is the ratio of the height of the regurgitant jet to that of the LVOT obtained from the TTE parasternal or TEE long-axis view (20). *AR is mild if the ratio is <25%; moderate if 25% to 45%; moderate to severe if 46% to 64%; and severe if >65%* (Figs. 9.8B and 9.10B).

Another commonly used method to assess AR severity is the ratio of the regurgitant jet area to the LVOT area obtained from the TTE parasternal or TEE short-axis view (20). *AR is mild if the ratio is <25%; moderate if 25% to 59%; and severe if >60%.*

The vena contracta is the smallest area of regurgitant flow through the valve. The width and area of the vena contracta of an AR jet correlate well with the effective regurgitant orifice and accurately separate severe from nonsevere AR when tested against regurgitant volume and fraction measured by intraoperative aortic flow probe (21,22). Vena contracta width and area are obtained from the TTE or TEE long- and short-axis views of the aortic valve, respectively. To maximize frame rate and line density for optimal measurements, the narrowest sector scan and lowest imaging depth possible should be used.

*By TEE, vena contracta width >6 mm or <5 mm predicts a regurgitant fraction >50% and <50%, respectively.* Also, vena contract width >6 mm or <6 mm predicts a regurgitant volume >40 mL or <40 mL with 67% and 94% accuracy, respectively. By TTE, vena contract width ≥6 mm has a sensitivity of 95% and a specificity of 90% for detecting severe AR. *By TEE, vena contracta area >7.5 $mm^2$ or <7.5 $mm^2$ predicts a regurgitant fraction >50% or <50%, respectively.* Also, vena contracta area >7.5 $mm^2$ or <7.5 $mm^2$ predicts a regurgitant volume >40 mL or <40 mL with 67% and 94% accuracy, respectively (Figs. 9.7B, 9.8B, 9.9B, and 9.10B).

Finally, the acceleration flow area or flow convergence zone proximal to the regurgitant orifice (PISA) can be used to calculate the effective regurgitant orifice area (23–25). PISA length allows for calculation of the regurgitant flow rate ($cm^3$/s) using the formula for a hemispheric or hemielliptic model as $= 2 \times \pi \times r^2 \times Vr$, where r is the radius of the flow convergence zone measured in early diastole and Vr is the corresponding color Doppler aliasing velocity (cm/s). The regurgitant orifice area ($cm^2$) is the result of the regurgitant flow rate divided by the maximal continuous wave regurgitant velocity.

*AR is mild if the regurgitant orifice area is <0.1 $cm^2$; moderate if 0.1 to 0.5 $cm^2$; moderate to severe if 0.5 to 1.0 $cm^2$; and severe if >1.0 $cm^2$.* The effective regurgitant orifice area is an accurate predictor of the severity of AR and less altered by hemodynamic variations than the regurgitant volume and fraction.

**FIG. 9.9.** Degenerative aortic valve disease with mild aortic regurgitation and stenosis. **A:** Continuous wave Doppler tracing of the aortic valve demonstrates mild aortic regurgitation (AR) based on a prolonged (>500 ms) pressure half-time. Mild aortic stenosis with a peak gradient up to 25 mm Hg is noted. **B:** Apical transthoracic echocardiographic close-up view of the aortic valve with color Doppler interrogation demonstrates a small flow convergence zone *(arrow)* and a small vena contracta width of 3 mm *(arrowhead).* (See Color Figure 9.9B.)

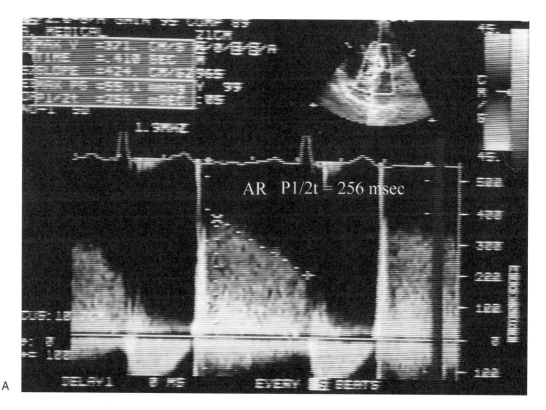

AR  P1/2t = 256 msec

A

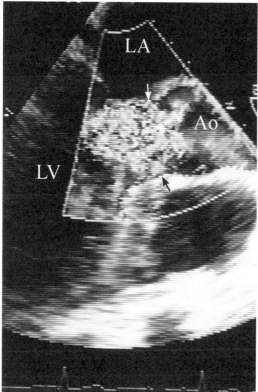

LA

Ao

LV

B

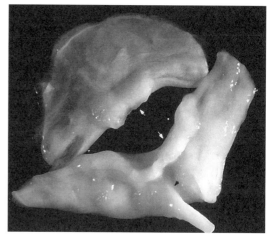

C

**TABLE 9.5.** *Echocardiographic preoperative poor prognostic predictors of surgical outcome in aortic regurgitation*

| | |
|---|---|
| LV ejection fraction | <50% |
| LV shortening fraction | <25%, in some series <30% |
| LV end-systolic diameter | >55 mm or >26 mm/m² |
| LV end-diastolic diameter | >75 mm or >38 mm/m² |
| LV end-systolic volume | >200 mL |
| LV radius to wall thickness ratio | >3.8 |

LV, left ventricular.
Data from references 26–31.

## Value of Echocardiography in Defining the Natural History and Prognosis of Aortic Regurgitation

Color Doppler echocardiography plays an important role in defining the natural history and prognosis of patients with significant AR. LV systolic function and LV end-diastolic and end-systolic sizes or volumes are the most important determinants of survival and postoperative LV function in patients undergoing valve replacement.

Echocardiographic parameters predictive of death, persistent LV dilation and dysfunction, and decreased exercise tolerance include (i) ejection fraction <50%; (ii) LV fractional shortening <25%; (iii) LV end-systolic diameter and index >55 mm and >26 mm/m², respectively; (iv) LV end-diastolic diameter and index >75 mm and >38 mm/ m², respectively; (v) LV end-systolic volume >200 mL; and (vi) LV radius to wall thickness ratio >3.8 (Table 9.5) (26–31).

The duration of preoperative LV systolic dysfunction is a poor prognostic indicator.

LV fractional shortening >26%, end-systolic diameter <55 mm, and end-diastolic diameter <80 mm predict normal LV function after aortic valve replacement and 90.5% sur-

vival at 2.5 years compared to 70% in patients with end-systolic diameter >55 mm and fractional shortening <25%.

## Clinical and Echocardiographic Follow-Up of Patients with Aortic Regurgitation

Patients with moderate or worse AR may develop LV dilation or dysfunction in the absence of symptoms. Therefore, they should have serial clinical and/or echocardiographic evaluations aimed to detect the onset of symptoms or asymptomatic LV dilation and dysfunction. The frequency of these evaluations is determined by the initial severity of AR and the degree of LV dilation and/or systolic function (Table 9.6) (1,2,26,31).

Repeat echocardiography also is recommended when a patient has new onset of symptoms, has equivocal history of changing symptoms or exercise tolerance, or has clinical findings suggesting worsening AR or progressive LV dilation.

In patients with aortic root dilation, serial echocardiograms are indicated to evaluate aortic root size as well as LV size and function. However, the degree of aortic root dilation that warrants serial and interval fre-

---

**FIG. 9.10.** Bicuspid aortic valve and severe aortic regurgitation in a symptomatic 46-year-old man. **A:** Continuous-wave Doppler recording of the aortic valve demonstrates a pressure half-time of 256 ms consistent with moderate to severe regurgitation. **B:** Transesophageal echocardiographic longitudinal view of the aortic valve with color Doppler imaging demonstrates severe aortic regurgitation as judged by a ratio of jet height and LV outflow tract height *(arrows)* >65% as well vena contracta width >6 mm. **C:** This surgically resected bicuspid aortic valve shows moderate thickening of the tip portion of the aortic cusps *(arrows)* with incomplete coaptation and an apparent large regurgitant orifice (>1 cm²). Note the raphe of the posteriorly located cusp *(black arrow).* (See Color Figures 9.10B and 9.10C.)

**TABLE 9.6.** *Clinical and echocardiographic follow-up of patients with aortic regurgitation*

| Clinical scenario | Clinical evaluation | Echocardiography |
|---|---|---|
| Asymptomatic patients with ≥ moderate AR of unknown duration | Within 3 mo | Within 3 mo |
| Asymptomatic patients with severe AR, LVEDD >70 mm, or ESD >50 mm, but normal LVEF | Every 4–6 mo | Every 4–6 mo |
| Patients with known ≥ mild AR with progressive LV dilation or declining LVEF | Every 6 mo | Every 6 mo |
| Asymptomatic patients with severe AR, normal LVEF, and LVEDD >60 mm | Every 6 mo | Every 6–12 mo |
| Asymptomatic patients with mild AR, normal or mildly dilated LV, and normal ejection fraction | Once a year | Every 2–3 yr; every year if it worsens |

AR, aortic regurgitation; LV, left ventricle; LVEDD, left ventricular end-diastolic diameter; LVEF, left ventricular ejection fraction.

quency of echocardiography has not been defined.

### Value of Echocardiography in Defining Need for Aortic Valve Replacement

Symptoms are the most important guide to whether or not aortic valve replacement should be performed (Table 9.7). However, symptoms frequently are difficult to assess, and asymptomatic patients commonly develop LV dilation and dysfunction. Therefore, echocardiographic parameters in asymptomatic patients will help to select and risk stratify patients for undergoing aortic valve replacement (Table 9.8) (27–31).

The degree of AR and LV function or size is less important in the management of patients with primary disease of the aorta. In these patients, the need and timing of aortic valve re-

placement with or without root surgery is based primarily on the degree of underlying aortic root disease (Figs. 9.5, 9.6, and 9.8A). However, when AR is severe and associated with severe LV dilation and/or systolic dysfunction, decisions regarding medical or surgical therapy should consider both conditions.

The relatively small number of asymptomatic patients with preserved systolic function but with severely increased end-systolic and end-diastolic chamber size should be considered for surgery, as these patients appear to represent a high-risk group with an increased incidence of sudden death (15,32). The results of valve replacement in such patients are excellent. In contrast, postoperative mortality is considerable once patients with severe LV dilation develop symptoms and/or LV systolic dysfunction (33). Finally, in small patients of either gender, the end-diastolic and end-sys-

**TABLE 9.7.** *Indications for aortic valve replacement in symptomatic patients*

1. Patients with normal resting systolic function (ejection fraction ≥50%) and NYHA functional class III or IV symptoms
2. New onset of mild dyspnea and severe aortic regurgitation in patients with increasing LV chamber size or declining LVEF into the low–normal range
3. Patients with NYHA functional class II–IV symptoms and LVEF 25%–49%
4. Symptomatic patients with LVEF <25% and/or end-systolic dimension >60 mm
5. Patients with NYHA functional class II–III symptoms, if (i) symptoms and LV dysfunction are of recent onset and (ii) short-term vasodilator, diuretic, and/or intravenous positive inotropic therapy result in substantial improvement in hemodynamics or systolic function
6. Patients with NYHA functional class II symptoms and ejection fraction ≥50% at rest, but with progressive LV dilation or declining ejection fraction at rest on serial studies or declining effort tolerance on exercise testing; patients with Canadian Heart Association functional class II or greater angina with/without coronary artery disease.
7. Patients with NYHA functional class IV symptoms and LVEF <25%

LV, left ventricular; LVEF, left ventricular ejection fraction; NYHA, New York Heart Association.

**TABLE 9.8.** *Indications for aortic valve replacement in asymptomatic patients*

1. Patients with LVEF below the lower limit of normal at rest or 50% on two consecutive measurements
2. Patients with LVEDD >75 mm or ESD >55 mm, even if LVEF is normal
3. Patients with LVEDD of 70–75 mm or ESD of 50–55 mm with evidence of declining exercise tolerance or abnormal hemodynamic responses to exercise
4. Patients with disease of the proximal aorta and aortic regurgitation of any degree if the aortic root dilation is ≥50 mm (valve replacement and aortic root reconstruction)
5. Asymptomatic patient with resting LVEF of 25%–49%

LVESD, left ventricular end-systolic diameter; LVEDD, left ventricular end-diastolic diameter; LVEF, left ventricular ejection fraction.

tolic dimensions recommended for valve replacement in asymptomatic patients (75 and 55 mm, respectively) may be lower.

## Echocardiography After Aortic Valve Replacement

Echocardiography should be performed soon after aortic valve replacement to assess valve function as well as LV size and function. This baseline echocardiogram serves as the comparison for subsequent echocardiograms. This initial postoperative study should be performed at the first outpatient reevaluation. Within the first week of surgery, LV ejection fraction may decrease due to reduced preload. Ejection fraction generally improves over the subsequent several weeks. Also, LV end-diastolic dimension declines significantly by the second week of operation. In fact, 80% of the reduction in LV end-diastolic dimension observed during a long-term postoperative course occurs within 10 to 14 days after valve replacement (34).

After the initial postoperative reevaluation, the patient should be clinically evaluated at 6 and 12 months and then on a yearly basis if the clinical course is uncomplicated. If the patient is asymptomatic, the early postoperative echocardiogram demonstrates significant reduction in LV end-diastolic diameter, and LV function is normal, serial postoperative echocardiograms usually are not indicated. A repeat echocardiogram is warranted if there is evidence of a new murmur, question of prosthetic valve integrity, or concerns about LV function.

Patients with persistent LV dilation on the initial postoperative echocardiogram should have a repeat echocardiogram to assess LV size and systolic function at 6 and 12 months. If LV dysfunction persists beyond this time, repeat echocardiograms should be performed as clinically indicated.

## SUMMARY

### Diagnostic Value of Physical Examination and Echocardiography

#### *Physical Examination*

The physical examination in AR is helpful in assessing the hemodynamic severity of the valve lesion in most cases (Table 9.9). However, in the presence of acute or recent-onset AR, or when LV systolic dysfunction or congestive heart failure is present, the examination may be quite misleading.

#### *Blood Pressure and Peripheral Pulses*

With progressively severe AR, the blood pressure and pulse characteristics are altered in a predictable fashion. Diastolic blood pressure falls and systolic pressure increases with increasing severity of AR. Thus, arterial pulse pressure increases as AR becomes greater. The high stroke volume of patients with moderately severe or worse AR is ejected into a compliant and dilated arterial tree, producing the classic findings of arterial peripheral manifestations (Table 9.1). However, if the AR is acute and severe, or if congestive failure is present, systemic arterial vasoconstriction may attenuate the disordered physical findings.

**TABLE 9.9.** *Summary of the physical examination in aortic regurgitation*

| Physical finding | Mild | Moderate | Severe |
|---|---|---|---|
| Blood pressure | Normal | Diastolic may be ↓ | ↑Systolic<br>↓Diastolic<br>↑Pulse pressure |
| Arterial pulse | Normal | ↑Amplitude | ↑Amplitude<br>Peripheral signs of aortic<br>  regurgitation (see text) |
| Point of maximal impulse | Normal | May be somewhat<br>  prominent | ↑Amplitude<br>May be sustained<br>May be displaced |
| Heart sounds | Normal<br>May have ejection sound | Normal<br>May have ejection sound | $S_1$ ↓<br>$A_2$ may be ↑<br>$S_3$ if severe<br>$S_4$ common |
| Murmurs<br>  Systolic<br>  Diastolic | Variable<br>Silent or soft<br>High-pitched diastolic<br>  beginning with $S_2$ | Variable<br>Decrescendo diastolic;<br>  easily heard | May be prominent<br>May be soft or loud<br>High or low frequency<br>May be surprisingly<br>  short and/or soft<br>May have apical mid-<br>  diastolic mumbling<br>  murmurs |

### Precordial Motion

The apex impulse or point of maximal impulse (PMI) is normal in mild AR. As volume overload increases, the LV impulse becomes hyperdynamic (high-amplitude, normal brief outward contour). When the degree of AR is significant (moderate or greater), the LV may dilate. Once this occurs, the PMI is displaced leftward and downward, and may become sustained. If LV systolic dysfunction ensues, the apex impulse is invariably sustained (LV heave) and displaced leftward and downward.

### Heart Sounds

Little diagnostic information is obtained from listening to normal heart sounds. $S_1$ tends to be decreased, as the PR interval often is prolonged in AR. The $A_2$ may be prominent. An ejection sound often is audible if the etiology of the AR is a bicuspid aortic valve or dilation of the aortic root (aneurysm). A fourth heart sound ($S_4$) is common in AR. An $S_3$ is found in severe AR or in the presence of associated heart failure; this is a poor prognostic sign.

### Heart Murmurs

The typical murmur of AR is a high-frequency, diastolic decrescendo murmur beginning with $A_2$. This murmur usually is relatively soft and may be hard to appreciate. Patients should be examined in held end-expiration, using firm pressure with the bell of the stethoscope, in the upright position (leaning forward helps). The diastolic murmur may be medium frequency in greater degrees of AR and may shorten in severe AR. In the setting of acute AR or in the presence of heart failure, the diastolic murmur may be quite short and unimpressive, due to the very high LV filling pressures decreasing the aortic–LV diastolic pressure gradient in mid to late diastole.

A low-frequency mid-diastolic murmur, simulating the diastolic rumble of mitral stenosis, may be present in severe AR. This is the Austin Flint murmur, which typically begins with an $S_3$. A systolic murmur, often prominent, may be audible in moderate or greater degrees if AR, due to irregularity of the aortic valve and increased stroke volume ejected across the valve. A loud systolic ejection murmur in such cases does not necessarily imply associated aortic stenosis.

**TABLE 9.10.** *Doppler echocardiographic parameters of aortic regurgitation severity*

| Method | Severity | | | |
| --- | --- | --- | --- | --- |
| | Mild | Moderate | Moderate to severe | Severe |
| Regurgitant fraction (%) | <20 | 20–35 | 35–50 | >50 |
| Pressure half-time (ms) | >500 | 350–500 | 200–350 | <200 |
| Jet/LVOT width ratio (%) | 24 | 25–45 | 46–64 | ≥65 |
| Jet/LVOT area ratio (%) | <25 | 25–59 | No criteria | >60 |
| Vena contracta width (mm) | — | <6 | ≥6 | >6 |
| Vena contracta area (cm²) | — | <7.5 | ≥7.5 | >7.5 |
| Effective regurgitant orifice (cm²) | <0.1 | 0.1–0.5 | 0.5–1.0 | >1.0 |

LVOT, left ventricular outflow tract.

## Assessment of Severity

With increasing degrees of AR, diastolic blood pressure falls; peripheral arterial pulses become bounding with increasing amplitude; the LV impulse becomes high amplitude or sustained, and often displaced if severe AR is present; and the murmur may be loud or soft, long or short. In acute AR, a diastolic rumbling murmur (Austin Flint) may be heard and the diastolic AR murmur may be unimpressive. Blood pressure changes may be little or none in the setting of recent-onset severe AR or coexisting congestive heart failure.

## Echocardiography

A complete history and physical examination should continue to be the primary screening diagnostic method in patients with cardiovascular symptoms or suspected valvular heart disease, including AR. However, color Doppler echocardiography has become essential for the final diagnosis, especially for assessment of the severity of AR (Table 9.10). Of more importance, echocardiography determines the impact of AR on LV size and function better than the physical examination (Table 9.11). This technique also defines accurately parameters that determine the natural history and prognosis of medically or surgically treated AR (Table 9.5). In addition, echocardiography helps to determine the need for aortic valve replacement, especially in asymptomatic patients (Tables 9.7 and 9.8). Finally, echocardiography defines the impact of surgery in the preservation or recovery of LV function.

## Limitations of Physical Examination and Echocardiography

### Physical Examination

1. Echocardiography has confirmed that much AR is inaudible to, or undetectable by, the examiner. The high-frequency murmur often is too soft to be audible. Thus, trivial to mild AR is not usually heard by most examiners.
2. In severe AR, recent-onset AR, or AR complicated by heart failure, the findings may be misleading. The characteristic

**TABLE 9.11.** *Class I indications for echocardiography in aortic regurgitation*

1. Confirm presence and severity of acute AR
2. Diagnosis of chronic AR in patients with equivocal physical findings
3. Assessment of etiology of AR (assess valve morphology, and aortic root size and morphology)
4. Assessment of LV hypertrophy, volumes, and systolic function
5. Semiquantitative estimate of the severity of AR
6. Reevaluation of patients with mild, moderate, or severe AR and new or changing symptoms
7. Reevaluation of LV size and function in asymptomatic patients with severe AR
8. Reevaluation of asymptomatic patients with mild, moderate, or severe AR and enlarged aortic root

AR, aortic regurgitation; LV, left ventricular.

blood pressure and pulse volume changes may not be prominent or present at all. The diastolic murmur may be attenuated or even silent. An Austin Flint murmur may simulate mitral stenosis. Obtaining an echocardiogram is critical in any patient suspected of having possible severe, recent-onset AR (e.g., possible endocarditis, dissection, and aneurysm of the aorta; overt heart failure of acute or recent-onset with any findings suggestive of AR).

### *Echocardiography*

Although color Doppler TTE or TEE echocardiography is highly accurate in the diagnosis of AR, it is important to emphasize the limitations of the technique that may lead to overestimation or underestimation of the severity of AR.

1. Errors in estimating stroke volume, regurgitant volume, and regurgitant fraction are predominantly related to overestimation or underestimation of LV or RV outflow tract diameters. Calculation of the mitral stroke volume is less accurate due to the complex morphology of the mitral annulus.
2. If the continuous wave peak velocity of the AR jet is not well defined, errors resulting in overestimation or underestimation of $P_{1/2}$ and severity of AR can occur. Also, AR severity can be overestimated by this parameter in the presence of LV diastolic dysfunction (high LV end-diastolic pressure) for reasons other than AR (i.e., hypertensive, coronary or other myocardial disease) and in patients with high systemic vascular resistance. These conditions lead to shortening of $P_{1/2}$.
3. A limitation of the ratio of the AR jet height to LVOT height is in the eccentric jets, where the severity of AR can be underestimated or overestimated. The direction of the AR jet by color Doppler assessed from multiple imaging windows can alert the interpreter to this limitation.

4. Color Doppler is dependent on gain, pulse repetition frequency, and different display approaches by the manufacturers. Unless particular attention is given to these settings, AR severity can be overestimated or underestimated (35).
5. All color Doppler echocardiographic parameters for defining the severity of AR are more accurate in determining mild or severe degrees of AR. The parameters used for defining moderate degrees of AR are less accurate and offer considerable overlap.
6. Color Doppler parameters used to assess the severity of AR are dependent on the size of the regurgitant orifice, but also of the transvalvular pressure gradient. Therefore, a high or low aortic diastolic pressure or systemic vascular resistance can result in overestimation or underestimation of regurgitant volume and jet size characteristics, respectively.

### REFERENCES

1. Cheitlin MD, Alpert JS, Armstrong WF, et al. ACC/AHA guidelines for the clinical application of echocardiography. Circulation 1997;95:1686–1744.
2. Bonow RO, Carabello B, De Leon AC, et al. ACC/AHA guidelines for the management of patients with valvular heart disease. J Am Coll Cardiol 1998;32:1486–1588.
3. Klein AL, Burstow DJ, Tajik AJ, et al. Age-related prevalence of valvular regurgitation in normal subjects: a comprehensive color flow examination of 118 volunteers. J Am Soc Echocardiogr 1990;13:1631–1636.
4. Shively BK, Roldan CA, Gill EA, et al. Prevalence and determinants of valvulopathy in patients treated with dexfenfluramine. Circulation 1999;100:2161–2167.
5. Bonow RO, Rosing DR, McIntosh CL, et al. The natural history of asymptomatic patients with aortic regurgitation and normal left ventricular function. Circulation 1983;68:509–517.
6. Tornos MP, Olona M, Permanyer-Miralda G, et al. Clinical outcome of severe asymptomatic chronic aortic regurgitation: a long-term prospective follow-up study. Am Heart J 1995;130:333–339.
7. Ishii K, Hirota Y, Suwa M, et al. Natural history and left ventricular response in chronic aortic regurgitation. Am J Cardiol 1996;78:357–361.
8. Borer JS, Hochreiter C, Herrold EM, et al. Prediction of indications for valve replacement among asymptomatic or minimally symptomatic patients with chronic aortic regurgitation and normal left ventricular performance. Circulation 1998;97:525–534.
9. Henry WL, Bonow RO, Rosing DR, et al. Observations on the optimum time for operative intervention for aortic regurgitation: II. Serial echocardiographic

evaluation of asymptomatic patients. Circulation 1980;61:484–492.

10. McDonald IG, Jelinek VM. Serial M-mode echocardiography in severe chronic aortic regurgitation. Circulation 1980;62:1291–1296.

11. Aronow WS, Ahn C, Kronzon I, et al. Prognosis of patients with heart failure and unoperated severe aortic valvular regurgitation and relation to ejection fraction. Am J Cardiol 1994;74:286–288.

12. Siemienczuk D, Greenerg B, Morris C, et al. Chronic aortic insufficiency: factors associated with progression to aortic valve replacement. Ann Intern Med 1989; 110:587–592.

13. Bonow RO, Lakatos E, Maron BJ, et al. Serial long term assessment of the natural history of asymptomatic patients with chronic aortic regurgitation and normal left ventricular function. Circulation 1991;84:1625–1635.

14. Elayda MA, Hall RJ, Reul RM, et al. Aortic valve replacement in patients 80 years and older: operative risks and long term results. Circulation 1993;88:II-11–II-16.

15. Rokey R, Sterling LI, Zoghibi WA, et al. Determination of regurgitant fraction in isolated mitral or aortic regurgitation by pulsed Doppler two-dimensional echocardiography. J Am Coll Cardiol 1986;7:1273–1278.

16. Xie GY, Berk MR, Smith MD, et al. A simplified method for determining regurgitant fraction by Doppler echocardiography in patients with aortic regurgitation. J Am Coll Cardiol 1994;24:1041–1045.

17. Touche T, Pasquier R, Nitenberg A, et al. Assessment and follow-up of patients with aortic regurgitation by an updated Doppler echocardiographic measurement of the regurgitant fraction in the aortic arch. Circulation 1985;72:819–824.

18. Teague SM, Heinsimer JA, Anderson JL, et al. Quantification of aortic regurgitation utilizing continuous wave Doppler ultrasound. J Am Coll Cardiol 1986;8: 592–599.

19. Labovitz AJ, Ferrara RP, Kern MJ, et al. Quantitative evaluation of aortic insufficiency by continuous wave Doppler echocardiography. J Am Coll Cardiol 1986;8: 1341–1347.

20. Perry GJ, Helmcke F, Nanda NC, et al. Evaluation of aortic insufficiency by Doppler color flow mapping. J Am Coll Cardiol 1987:9:952–959.

21. Willet DL, Hall SA, Jessen ME, et al. Assessment of aortic regurgitation by transesophageal color Doppler imaging of the vena contracta: validation against an intraoperative aortic flow probe. J Am Coll Cardiol 2001; 37:1450–1455.

22. Tribouilloy CM, Enriquez-Sarano M, Bailey KR, et al. Assessment of severity of aortic regurgitation using the width of the vena contracta: a clinical color Doppler imaging study. Circulation 2000;102:558–564.

23. Shiota T, Jones M, Yamada I, et al. Evaluation of aortic regurgitation with digitally determined color Doppler-imaged flow convergence acceleration: a quantitative study in sheep. J Am Coll Cardiol 1996;27:203–210.

24. Schwammenthal E, Chen C, Giesler M, et al. New method for accurate calculation of regurgitant flow rate based on analysis of Doppler color flow maps of the proximal flow field. J Am Coll Cardiol 1996;27: 161–172.

25. Tribouilloy CM, Enriquez-Sarano M, Fett SL, et al. Application of the proximal flow convergence method to calculate the effective regurgitant orifice area in aortic regurgitation. J Am Coll Cardiol 1998;32:1032–1039.

26. Daniel WG, Hood WP Jr, Siart A, et al. Chronic aortic regurgitation: reassessment of the prognostic value of preoperative left ventricular end-systolic dimension and fractional shortening. Circulation 1985;71:669–680.

27. Bonow RO, Picone AL, McIntosh CL, et al. Survival and functional results after valve replacement for aortic regurgitation from 1976 to 1983: impact of preoperative left ventricular function. Circulation 1985;72:1244–1256.

28. Michel PL, Lung B, Jaoude SA, et al. The effect of left ventricular systolic function on long term survival in mitral and aortic regurgitation. J Heart Valve Dis 1995; 4:S160–S168.

29. Sheiban I, Trevi GP, Casarotto D, et al. Aortic valve replacement in patients with aortic incompetence: preoperative parameters influencing long-term results. Z Kardiol 1986;75[Suppl 2]:146–154.

30. Carabello BA, Usher BW, Hendrix GH, et al. Predictors of outcome for aortic valve replacement in patients with aortic regurgitation and left ventricular dysfunction: a change in the measuring stick. J Am Coll Cardiol 1987; 10:991–997.

31. Bonow RO, Dodd JT, Maron BJ, et al. Long-term serial changes in left ventricular function and reversal of ventricular dilatation after valve replacement for chronic aortic regurgitation. Circulation 1988;78:1108–1120.

32. Turina J, Turina M, Rothlin M, et al. Improved late survival in patients with chronic aortic regurgitation by earlier operation. Circulation 1984;70:I-147–I-152.

33. Klodas E, Enriquez-Sarano M, Tajik AJ, et al. Aortic regurgitation complicated by extreme left ventricular dilation: long-term outcome after surgical correction. J Am Coll Cardiol 1996;27:670–677.

34. Gaasch WH, Carroll JD, Levine HJ, et al. Chronic aortic regurgitation: prognostic value of left ventricular end-systolic dimension and end-diastolic radius/thickness ratio. J Am Coll Cardiol 1983;1:775–782.

35. Sahn DJ. Instrumentation and physical factors related to visualization of stenotic and regurgitant jets by color Doppler flow mapping. J Am Coll Cardiol 1998;12: 1354–1365.

# 10

# The Patient with Prosthetic Heart Valves

Michael H. Crawford

*Department of Internal Medicine, Mayo Medical School, Rochester, Minnesota; and
Department of Cardiovascular Diseases, Mayo Clinic Scottsdale, Scottsdale, Arizona*

## INTRODUCTION

There are two basic types of prosthetic heart valves: (i) biologic valves, such as autografts, homografts and heterografts; and (ii) mechanical valves (1). Autografts and homografts usually are freestanding valves harvested from the patient or a human cadaver. Heterograft valves usually have a mechanical structure to suspend the animal valve leaflets and a sewing ring with which to attach the valve to the annulus (Fig. 10.1). Mechanical valves are made of various metals, plastics, and pyrolytic carbon (Fig. 10.2). Biologic valves rarely alter the normal cardiac physical examination, and disease of biologic valves presents with the same clinical findings as native valve disease. On the other hand, mechanical valves markedly alter the cardiac physical examination, and valve malfunction presents with unique findings not observed with native valves. Thus, this chapter will emphasize mechanical heart valves.

Mechanical valves frequently are placed in the aortic and mitral positions, as the left-sided valves are the most frequently diseased in adults. Occasionally, a mechanical valve is placed in the tricuspid position, but rarely in the pulmonic position. The major advantage of mechanical valves is their high durability in comparison to biologic valves. Their major drawback is the risk for thrombosis and thromboembolism, which is greater than that observed with biologic valves. Thus, patients with mechanical valves almost always are placed on oral anticoagulant therapy indefinitely. The next most common complication of mechanical valves is infectious endocarditis, which may occur early, within the first 60 days following surgery, due to infections that start during surgery, or may occur late following surgery (>60 days) due to factors that produce infectious endocarditis in diseased native valves, such as extensive dental work. A more detailed discussion on prosthetic valve endocarditis is given in Chapter 11. Another com-

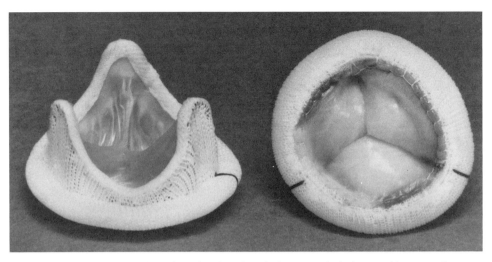

**FIG. 10.1.** Porcine bioprosthetic valve showing the cloth-covered skeleton with struts that support the porcine leaflets and the prominent sewing ring.

plication of mechanical valve placement is growth of panus from the sewing ring into the lumen of the valve, which may either obstruct the valve or interfere with the movement of the valve closure mechanism and result in severe regurgitation. A more common cause of regurgitation is a perivalvular leak, usually due to in-

complete attachment of the sewing ring to the valve annulus. Perivalvular leaks also are seen with bioprosthetic heterograft valves; some may be trivial and others may be quite significant. Perivalvular leaks and other mechanical valve abnormalities may lead to significant red cell trauma and result in hemolytic anemia. Finally, valve dehiscence is a rare but catastrophic complication of mechanical and bioprosthetic heterograft valves. It usually is due to unrecognized annular abscess formation that undermines the attachment of the valve to the annulus, resulting in partial or complete detachment. Thus, prosthetic valves have the same complications as native valves: stenosis, regurgitation, infection, and rupture (dehiscence) (Table 10.1).

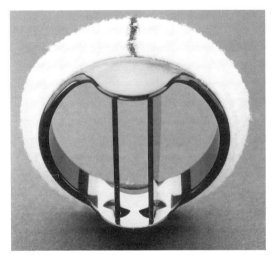

**FIG. 10.2.** St. Jude bileaflet mechanical prosthetic valve showing three flow channels in the open position: two major channels and one minor channel.

**TABLE 10.1.** *Relative incidence of prosthetic valve complications by valve type*

|  | Mechanical | Biologic |
|---|---|---|
| Thrombus | +++ | + |
| Infection | ++ | + |
| Dehiscence | ++ | + |
| Stenosis | + | ++ |
| Pannus | + | + |
| Degeneration | + | +++ |

## HISTORY

The most important history in patients with prosthetic heart valves is when the surgery was performed; the type and size of valve placed; and the cardiac position in which the valve was placed. Also important is whether the patients are taking medications, including oral anticoagulants; whether they are taking the drugs as directed; and whether they have documentation of international normalized ratios (INRs) in the therapeutic range. The major symptoms of prosthetic valve malfunction are similar to those of native valvular disease, namely, dyspnea, fatigue, chest pain, syncope, fever, and thromboembolic events. If a patient with a mechanical heart valve has not been taking oral anticoagulants properly and has symptoms suggesting valvular heart disease, valve thrombus should be suspected. Fever, sweats, and embolic phenomenon suggest infectious endocarditis. If >60 days have passed since surgery in patients with these symptoms, a source of infection should be sought, such as recent dental work or intravenous drug use. If a patient has a thoracotomy scar and does not know the type of surgery that was done, the presence of a mechanical valve and its position in the heart can be readily discerned by physical examination.

## PHYSICAL EXAMINATION

### Blood Pressure

Systemic arterial blood pressure usually is within the normal range in patients with normal or malfunctioning prosthetic valves. Moderate to severe aortic regurgitation can result in a wide pulse pressure. This sign is particularly useful when it is a change from previous measurements, which suggests the recent development of significant regurgitation. The wide pulse pressure reflects the increase in stroke volume caused by the increased regurgitant volume and is present only if the left ventricle remains able to increase stroke volume in the face of increased preload.

### Arterial Pulse

Peripheral arterial pulses usually are normal in patients with normal or malfunctioning prosthetic valves. Occasionally, severe abnormalities of mechanical aortic valve function will produce peripheral pulse findings that are similar to those encountered in native aortic valve stenosis or regurgitation. Of more importance is the finding of absent pulses and limb ischemia suggesting thromboembolic events. One unique finding is a bifid carotid impulse during systole in patients with significant encroachment of the prosthetic mitral valve on the left ventricular outflow track, similar to that observed with hypertrophic cardiomyopathy.

### Jugular Venous Pulse

The venous pulse in patients with normal or malfunctioning prosthetic valves is abnormal only if right atrial hemodynamics are affected by the malfunction. The findings in the jugular venous pulse will be predictable based on the abnormality.

### Palpation

Precordial palpation can reveal abnormalities of right and left ventricular size that may reflect changes in prosthetic valve function. Also, thrills and abnormal impulses may be felt in patients with a variety of prosthetic valve malfunctions. There may be a bifid apical impulse in the patient with outflow track obstruction. Perivalvular leaks, especially if they are associated with hemolytic anemia, often result in precordial thrills. Finally, in thin individuals, the closure of the mechanical prosthetic valve may be palpated and heard without a stethoscope.

## AUSCULTATION

### Heart Sounds

Either the first or second heart sound is accentuated with a mechanical prosthetic valve, depending on its cardiac position. The closure of the mechanical valve accentuates the normal heart sound, and the intensity of the sound is proportional to the mass of the closure device in the prosthetic valve. Ball valves produce a greater intensity closure sound than does a disk valve, which in turn is louder than a bileaflet mechanical valve. *Practical Point: Lack of accentuation of the opening or closure sound of the valve suggests an abnormality, such as the presence of thrombus, vegetation, or pannus, and should be investigated further.* The opening of a mechanical valve can produce a sound. If so, it is always less intense than the closing sound and is proportional to the mass of the valve device. *Practical Point: Carefully analyze the relative loudness or intensity of both the opening and closure sounds of any mechanical prosthesis. One (the closure sound) should be much louder than the other (opening sound). If there are two prosthetic valves in place, all the mechanical heart sounds will be loud.* Again, ball valves frequently can be heard to open when they strike the cage, whereas disk valves and bileaflet valves are less likely to produce an opening sound. Complete absence of an opening sound in a patient with a disk or bileaflet valve is not unusual, especially if the person is heavy or has a large chest. However, the absence of an opening sound of a ball valve is unusual and should be investigated further. Opening and closing sounds of mechanical valves are high-frequency events. A third heart sound can be distinguished from the opening sound of the mechanical mitral valve because it occurs later in the cardiac cycle and is a low-frequency sound. A third sound may be present if significant left ventricular dilation or dysfunction is present. Similarly, a fourth heart sound can be separated from the opening sound of a mechanical aortic valve because of its lower frequency and because it occurs before the first heart sound. The presence of a fourth heart sound suggests left ventricular hypertrophy or diastolic dysfunction, either of which may have been present since before valvular surgery and may not always disappear after successful valve surgery.

## Murmurs

Almost all prosthetic valves in the aortic position are accompanied by a systolic ejection murmur, which may be soft or prominent. This is because the prosthetic valve effective orifice area is less than that of a native valve; thus, there is a mild aortic stenosis inherent in every prosthetic valve. The absence of a systolic murmur is unusual and suggests low cardiac output, obesity, hyperinflated lungs, or the possibility of an abnormality with the prosthetic valve. The reason for lack of a systolic murmur with a prosthetic aortic valve should be determined and documented. A diastolic murmur associated with an aortic mechanical prosthesis suggests perivalvular leak, or thrombus or panus ingrowth preventing complete closure of the mechanical device. A diastolic murmur with a bioprosthetic aortic valve can be due to perivalvular or valvular regurgitation. The cause of the diastolic murmur with an aortic prosthetic valve must always be determined. The normal regurgitation through the hinges on a St. Jude bileaflet valve is trivial and usually cannot be heard by auscultation.

Mechanical mitral valves normally do not produce any murmurs. Occasionally one can hear a brief low-frequency rumble in early to mid diastole in thin individuals with prosthetic mitral valves because of the smaller size of the effective prosthetic valve orifice compared to the normal mitral valve. This is especially true in high-flow states with bioprostheses. This should not be interpreted as an abnormality if the patient is otherwise doing well. A louder, longer murmur or other abnormalities suggests prosthetic valve obstruction. A holosystolic murmur associated with mitral valve replacement suggests either malfunction of the valve or a perivalvular leak. Again, the normal trivial regurgitation through a bileaflet mitral valve usually is not audible. There are normally no murmurs associated with the mechanical tricuspid valve. Thus, any murmurs with a mechanical tricuspid valve should prompt an investigation of the etiology.

Murmurs due to perivalvular leak or malfunctioning of prosthetic valves rarely are musical. The musical quality of murmurs is due to the vibration of valve leaflet tissue at a frequency that produces a musical note. Mechanical valve prosthetic materials rarely are able to vibrate at such frequencies; thus, a musical murmur suggests native valve disease or the presence of a biologic valve that is malfunctioning. In the case of poppet escape or valve dehiscence, the patient usually is in shock, with thready pulses. There may be one area of the body with no pulses if the valve or poppet is occluding that arterial territory. Most frequently, this would be one of the two femoral artery territories, because the valve or poppet usually is lodged in the iliac arteries. Despite the profound hemodynamic abnormality, murmurs usually are absent due to a lack of a pressure gradient between the chambers that are in wide communication throughout the cardiac cycle. Of course, normal mechanical valve closure sounds are absent in this situation.

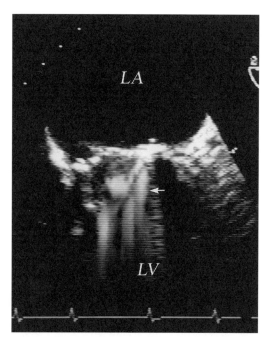

**FIG. 10.3.** St. Jude mechanical mitral valve in the closed position. Note the strong reverberations behind the valve *(arrow)* in this transesophageal echocardiographic image. LA, left atrium; LV, left ventricle.

## ECHOCARDIOGRAPHY

### M-Mode and Two-Dimensional Echocardiography

The distinction between normally and abnormally functioning prosthetic valves is difficult because ultrasound attenuation and acoustic artifacts obscure prosthetic valve imaging. Also, there are a wide variety of valve types and variations that must be recognized. The density of mechanical valve components creates intense echo reflections from the surfaces of the valve structures that may reverberate with the transducer or other valve components creating artifacts that obscure other structures near the valve (Fig. 10.3). Also, the dense valve structures create shadowing behind them, such that structures and color flow behind the valve are poorly visualized. In addition, strong reflecting surfaces overwhelm the poor lateral resolution of two-dimensional echocardiography, which results

in lateral artifacts (side lobes) emanating from the valve structures (Fig. 10.4). These problems not only obscure or hide adjacent structures, they also make it difficult to appreciate the internal working of the valve itself. This is especially true of bioprosthetic valves, where strong echoes from the struts obscure the leaflets (Fig. 10.5).Although infrequently encountered today, ball valves create the most difficult patterns on echocardiography to interpret (2). Most of the materials used in the manufacture of the ball are denser than blood or myocardial tissue. Thus, ultrasound transit time through the ball is much slower than through the surrounding tissue and blood. By the time the echoes return to the transducer from the proximal and distal surfaces of the ball, the machine interprets the ball to be much larger that it actually is. The resulting ball echoes overwhelm adjacent structures and deeper structures, obscuring everything near the ball. Also, the cage ap-

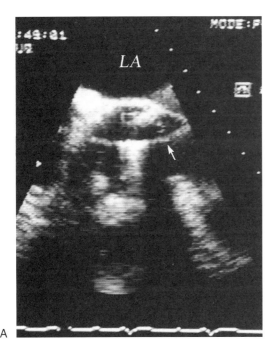
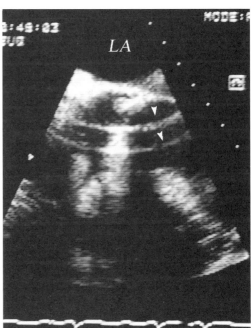

A

B

FIG. 10.4. A: St. Jude bileaflet aortic valve in the closed position. Note the side lobes from exaggerated poor lateral resolution in the transesophageal image *(arrow)*. B: Open position with the side lobes corresponding to each leaflet *(arrowheads)*.

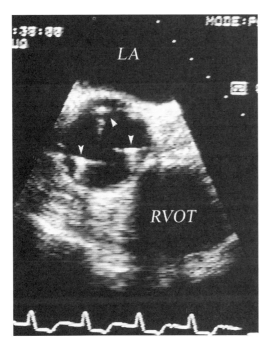

FIG. 10.5. Transesophageal echocardiographic image of a porcine aortic valve showing strong echoes from the three struts *(arrowheads)* without visible leaflet tissue. RVOT, right ventricular outflow tract.

pears to be closer to the transducer than the distal parts of the ball, resulting in truly bizarre echocardiographic patterns.

Disk valves, especially the nontilting variety, probably are the easiest mechanical valves to interpret by echocardiography. The disk makes a distinct echo produced by rapid disk motion that is readily seen. Disk opening or closing occurs in one video frame on two-dimensional echocardiography and appears instantaneous on M-mode echocardiography. M-mode echocardiography is especially useful in such valves because the movements of the disk are easily appreciated and any retardation of disk movement or unevenness of disk excursion is readily detected. Tilting disk valves involve more of a challenge because when the disk tilts open, considerable reverberations are radiated proximately and distally. However, at some point in the cardiac cycle, the disk can be made perpendicular to the transducer such that clear interrogation of its excursion can be appreciated through multiple views.

Bileaflet valves are difficult to interrogate because the supporting structures often obscure the thin bileaflets. These valves are best interrogated by transesophageal echocardiography, where echo views can be obtained that minimize interference from surrounding structures to permit visualization of the bileaflets (Fig. 10.6). Also, the omniplane capabilities of transesophageal echocardiography make it much easier to

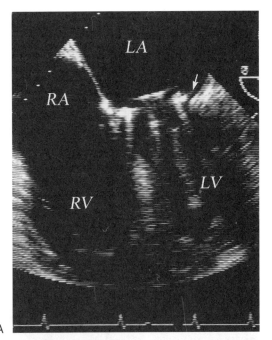

A

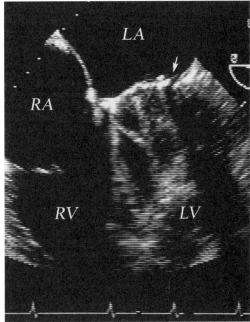

B

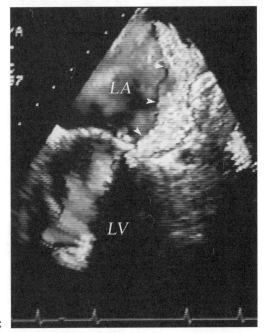

C

**FIG. 10.6.** Transesophageal four-chamber view showing a St. Jude mitral valve in the open position **(A)** and the closed position **(B)**. Note the reverberations *(bright lines)* and shadowing *(dark spaces)* on the ventricular side of the valve. Note also the perivalvular defect *(arrow)*. **C:** Color Doppler flow image showing perivalvular leak *(arrowheads)* in systole. (See Color Figure 10.6C.)

orient the valve in a plane where the functional components can best be interrogated.

In general, transesophageal echocardiography improves the imaging of all mechanical valves, but especially of the bileaflets valves (3). This is especially important in suspected valve-related thromboembolism or infectious endocarditis, because small thrombi or vegetations may be obscured by the artifacts produced by the strong reflectors on a mechanical valve. Omniplane imaging with transesophageal echocardiography can orient the structures such that the offending thrombi or vegetation can be visualized (Figs. 10.7 and 10.8). Valve thrombi occur more commonly with mitral prostheses, frequently are associated with subtherapeutic anticoagulation, usually appear as soft masses, and almost always interfere with mechanical valve leaflet motion, resulting in obstruction or regurgitation. Pannus formation is more common at the aortic position and occurs predominantly on the ventricular side of the sewing ring, leading to encroaching of the outflow tract and obstruction.

It also can interfere with valve leaflet motion, also resulting in regurgitation. Pannus, in contrast to thrombi, usually appear as dense masses. Transesophageal echocardiography is superior to transthoracic echocardiography in detecting and differentiating valve thrombi and pannus (4). Vegetations are intermediate in density, but characteristically protrude from the valve and move independently of valve. One must take care not to mistake thin, mobile, filamentous echos for vegetations or thrombi. These are a normal variant, the source of which is controversial (5–7). Also, bright fleeting echos can be seen after disk closure, especially on the atrial side of mitral valves. These are microcavitations due to valve closure and are of no consequence. Partial valve dehiscence often can be recognized by excessive rocking of the entire prosthetic valve beyond what is normally observed due to the mechanical action of the heart.

The most important consideration with bioprosthetic valves is leaflet degeneration. Early degeneration may result in marked leaflet

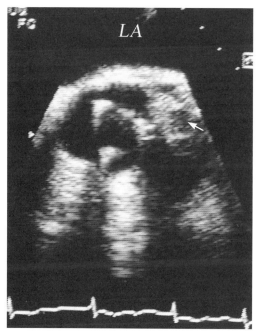
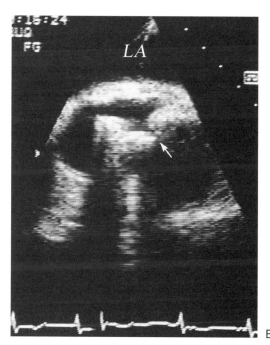

**FIG. 10.7.** Transesophageal echocardiographic image of a porcine aortic valve with a visibly thickened left coronary cusp and vegetation *(arrows).* **Left:** closed; **right:** open.

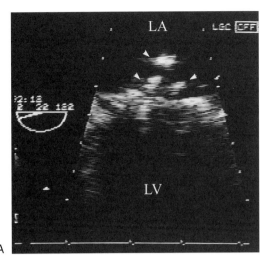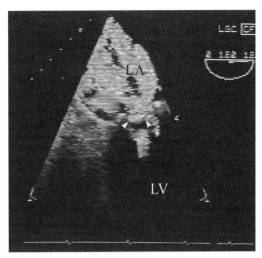

A

B

**FIG. 10.8. A:** Transesophageal echocardiogram of a porcine mitral valve with a vegetation and torn leaflet. The *lower two arrowheads* point to the torn portions of the leaflets protruding into the left atrium. The *upper arrowhead* shows a mobile vegetation. **B:** Color flow Doppler image showing severe mitral regurgitation centrally through the leaflets. Note the large jet width and acceleration zone *(arrowheads)* consistent with severe regurgitation. (See Color Figure 10.8B.)

thickening and valve stenosis, which is more common in younger individuals. Late degeneration is associated with mild leaflet thickening, especially along the commissural lines, which retracts the valve leaflet and results in regurgitation. In about 30% of cases, leaflet failure is acute and profound, often with leaflet prolapse and severe regurgitation.

### Pulsed and Continuous Wave Doppler Echocardiography

Early recognition of prosthetic valve stenosis is difficult because almost all prosthetic valves are intrinsically stenotic compared to native valves. Thus, transvalvular Doppler flow velocities are increased relative to native valves in the same position (Table 10.2) (8). In theory, using the same echo Doppler techniques as used with native valves, a valve area can be calculated and related to manufacturers' tables regarding the expected orifice area of various prosthetic valves of a certain size. This usually works reasonably well, but there are some unique problems with using echo Doppler methods to calculate the valve area of prosthetic valves. Mechanical valves may have more than one flow channel: ball valves and disk valves that do not tilt have circumferential flow; tilting disk valves have two channels: a

**TABLE 10.2.** *Peak velocity and mean gradients with common prosthetic valves*

| Prosthesis | Mean Velocity ±SD (m/s) | Mean gradient ±SD (mm Hg) |
|---|---|---|
| Aortic | | |
| St. Jude | 3.0 ± 0.8 | 11 ± 6 |
| Hancock porcine | 2.4 ± 0.4 | 11 ± 2 |
| Homograft | 0.8 ± 0.4 | 7 ± 3 |
| Mitral | | |
| St. Jude | 1.6 ± 0.3 | 5 ± 2 |
| Hancock | 1.5 ± 0.3 | 4 ± 2 |

major and a minor orifice; and bileaflet valves have three channels (Fig. 10.2). Continuous wave Doppler will favor the smallest channel with the highest velocity, resulting in underestimation of the valve orifice area. In general, valve area is greater for a comparably sized valve for mechanical versus bioprosthetic valves. Valve areas range from 1.2 cm² for small aortic bioprosthetic valves to 4.4 cm² for large mitral mechanical valves. If the same technique is used for each echocardiogram, changes in velocity or valve area over time may be more important than initial echo Doppler measures in a particular valve. Thus, an early postoperative echocardiogram as a baseline is useful at about 3 to 6 months after the operation. Earlier studies will be influenced by perioperative increases in sympathetic nervous system activity. Finally, if prosthetic valve stenosis is suspected, echocardiographic imaging is very useful because thickened bioprosthetic leaflets or masses obstructing mechanical valves may be observed.

### Color Doppler Echocardiography

Prosthetic valve regurgitation is much easier to detect with color flow Doppler echocardiography than is stenosis. However, there are a few pitfalls. Care must be taken to avoid acoustic shadowing, which can obscure a color flow regurgitant jet when the prosthetic valve is between the transducer and the regurgitant flow stream. The best example of this difficulty is prosthetic mitral valve regurgitation from an apical transducer position. If the regurgitant jet is obscured by the valve transthoracically, a proximal flow acceleration zone in systole can alert one to the possibility of significant prosthetic leak. This problem is readily solved by transesophageal echocardiography, which puts the mitral regurgitant flow between the transducer and the prosthetic valve. Prosthetic aortic regurgitation usually is readily detected by transthoracic echocardiography.

There are two types of prosthetic valve regurgitation: (i) periprosthetic leaks due to inadequate fixation of the sewing ring to the annulus, and (ii) valve leaks due to failure of the

valve leaflets or masses that prevent their closure. Some prosthetic valves, such as the St. Jude bileaflet valve, normally have a mild degree of regurgitation that must be distinguished from abnormal regurgitation (9,10). Perivalvular regurgitation is readily diagnosed by the origin of the color jet (Fig. 10.6). Also, infection or surgical difficulties can result in fistulous connection between the perivalvular area and other chambers, such as the right heart or coronary arteries. These can be readily detected by color flow imaging. Tissue valves normally do not leak, but about 10% may show mild central regurgitation, which is of no consequence (11).

### SUMMARY

Mechanical valve malfunction seems to be an all or nothing phenomenon. By the time abnormal findings or valve dysfunction are detected by echocardiography, the patient usually is symptomatic. Thus, the diagnosis of mechanical valve malfunction should not be challenging. Despite the potential of a careful physical examination and serial echocardiography to detect problems early before the patient becomes symptomatic or catastrophes occur, this rarely happens in practice. A possible reason is that the physical examination and echocardiography have such wide variances in normally functioning prosthetic valves that subtle changes in function are not easily appreciated until the problems become severe. The jaded may say that it is not worth paying much attention to the physical examination and serial echocardiography in a patient with prosthetic valves, because these examinations rarely show anything before the patient is symptomatic. On the other hand, carefully performed periodic physical examinations in a patient can detect problems early, even though this is less often the case.

Certain physical findings should prompt the physician to consider performing echocardiography (Table 10.3), as should changes in the physical examination, especially of the heart sounds and murmurs. Of note, most significant prosthetic valve complications de-

**TABLE 10.3.** *Physical examination findings that prompt consideration of echocardiography*

Blood pressure
  Wide pulse pressure (≥half systolic pressure)
  Hypotension
Pulses
  Absent limb pulses
  Bifid carotid pulse
  Slow rising, low-amplitude carotid pulse
  Elevated jugular venous pulse
Palpation
  Thrill
  Bifid apical impulse
  New right or left ventricular heaves
Auscultation
  Decreased intensity of valve closure sound
  Loss of previous heard opening sound
  New gallops
  Systolic murmur with mitral prosthesis
  Any diastolic murmur
General
  Prolonged fever without obvious source
  Embolic phenomena

tectable on physical examination also produce symptoms. Finally, symptoms or signs of possible infectious endocarditis, such as prolonged fever without an obvious source, and embolic phenomena or other peripheral manifestations (Osler nodes, Janeway lesions, Roth spots) should prompt echocardiography.

Cost constraints prevent physicians from ordering frequent serial echocardiograms, so a careful physical examination is a reasonable alternative. Inadequate anticoagulation is the main cause of mechanical valve dysfunction due to thrombus formation. As long as the patient's anticoagulation is monitored properly, valve assessments in the absence of symp-

toms can be less frequent than in patients with older bioprosthetic valves. Patients with bioprosthetic valves, which often degenerate and fail after 8 years, should be followed more closely than patients with mechanical valves, with which primary valve failure is unusual.

An echocardiogram should be obtained about 2 to 3 months after surgery to serve as a baseline, because of patient-to-patient variability in imaging and Doppler findings of normally functioning prosthetic valves. Once prosthetic valve dysfunction is suspected due to the patient's history, the physical examination is good at indicating the problem, i.e., thrombus, infection, stenosis, or regurgitation. Echocardiography is excellent at defining the pathologic anatomy and cardiac functional consequences of the problem. Thus, echocardiography should always be performed if prosthetic valve dysfunction is suspected based upon the history and physical examination (Table 10.4) (12,13). The physical examination cannot detect mild regurgitation or hemodynamically insignificant changes in valve morphology, yet such findings are common if routine follow-up echocardiography is done. When such abnormalities are found on routine follow-up echocardiograms, the frequency of follow-up with physical examination and echocardiography should be increased, because such changes suggest the beginning of valve degeneration or other complications. The ultimate goal of careful and timely follow-up is to detect and correct problems before they become catastrophic.

**TABLE 10.4.** *Indications for echocardiography in patients with prosthetic heart valves*

1. First outpatient postoperative visit 3–4 wk after hospital discharge for baseline assessment of valve function and left ventricular remodeling
2. New regurgitant murmur
3. Development of new or changing cardiovascular symptoms
4. Lack of improvement or deterioration of functional capacity or cardiovascular symptoms after valve replacement
5. Every 6 mo in asymptomatic patients with bioprosthetic valve degeneration and ≥mild regurgitation
6. Patients with suspected valve obstruction caused by thrombus or pannus ingrowth[a]
7. Patients with suspected prosthetic valve endocarditis[a]

[a]Transesophageal echocardiography is superior to transthoracic echocardiography in these conditions.
Data from references 12 and 13.

# REFERENCES

1. Wernly JA, Crawford MH. Choosing a prosthetic heart valve. Cardiol Clin 1998;16:491–504.

2. Alton ME, Pasierski TJ, Orsinelli DA, et al. Comparison of transthoracic and transesophageal echocardiography in evaluation of 47 Starr-Edwards prosthetic valves. J Am Coll Cardiol 1992;20:1503–1511.

3. Daniel WG, Mügge A, Grote J, et al. Comparison of transthoracic and transesophageal echocardiography for detection of abnormalities of prosthetic and bio-prosthetic valves in the mitral and aortic positions. Am J Cardiol 1993;71:210–215.

4. Barbetseas J, Nagueh SF, Pitsavos C, et al. Differentiating thrombus from pannus formation in obstructed mechanical prosthetic valves: an evaluation of clinical, transthoracic and transesophageal echocardiographic parameters. J Am Coll Cardiol 1998;32:1410–1417.

5. Ionescu AA, Moreno de la Santa P, Dunstan FD, et al. Mobile echos on prosthetic valves are not reproducible. Results and clinical implications of a multicentre study. Eur Heart J 1999;20:140–147.

6. Isada LR, Torelli JN, Stewart WJ, et al. Detection of fibrous strands on prosthetic mitral valves with transesophageal echocardiography: another potential embolic source. J Am Soc Echocardiogr 1994;7:641–645.

7. Orsinelli DA, Pasierski TJ, Pearson AC. Spontaneously appearing microbubbles associated with prosthetic cardiac valves detected by transesophageal echocardiography. Am Heart J 1994;128:990–996.

8. Burstow DJ, Nishimura RA, Bailey KR, et al. Continuous wave Doppler echocardiographic measurement of prosthetic valve gradients. Circulation 1989;80:504–514.

9. Flachskampf FA, O'Shea JP, Griffin BP, et al. Patterns of normal transvalvular regurgitation in mechanical valve prostheses. J Am Coll Cardiol 1991;18:1493–1498.

10. Alam M, Serwin JB, Rosman HS, et al. Transesophageal color flow Doppler and echocardiographic features of normal and regurgitant St. Jude Medical prostheses in the aortic valve position. Am J Cardiol 1990;66:873–875.

11. Alam M, Rosman HS, Lakier JB, et al. Doppler and echocardiographic features of normal and dysfunction bioprosthetic valves. J Am Coll Cardiol 1987;10:851–858.

12. Cheitlin MD, Alpert JS, Armstrong WF, et al. ACC/AHA guidelines for the clinical application of echocardiography. Circulation 1997;95:1686–1744.

13. Bonow RO, Carabello B, De Leon, AC, et al. ACC/AHA guidelines for the management of patients with valvular heart disease. J Am Coll Cardiol 1998;32:1486–1588.

# 11

# The Patient with Infective Endocarditis

Carlos A. Roldan

*Department of Internal Medicine, University of New Mexico School of Medicine; and Department of*
*Internal Medicine, Veterans Affairs Medical Center, Albuquerque, New Mexico*

## INTRODUCTION

Infective endocarditis (IE) is a clinical syndrome associated with significant morbidity and mortality. Therefore, its early recognition and treatment should impact favorably on patient outcome. Integration of clinical and echocardiographic data is critical in the diagnosis, risk stratification, and management of IE.

## DEFINITION

Infective endocarditis results from infection of the endothelial lining of the endocardium. Most commonly it involves the heart valves, mitral or aortic annulus, aortic root, and mitral chorda tendineae. Uncommonly it affects the ventricular or atrial endocardium. Endocarditis typically is characterized by fever and a heart murmur. It is confirmed by positive blood cultures or echocardiographic or pathologic evidence of valvular or paravalvular infection.

## PATHOGENESIS AND PATHOPHYSIOLOGY

Valvular and congenital abnormalities, especially those associated with abnormal high-velocity jet streams, lead to endothelial denudation, platelet aggregation, and fibrin deposition and ultimately to the formation of small nonbacterial thrombotic vegetations (NBTVs). The NBTVs are located on the atrial side of the mitral and tricuspid valves and on the ventricular side of the aortic and pulmonic valves. In the presence of bacteremia, microorganisms adhere to the NBTVs, multiply within the platelet–fibrin complex, and form an infective vegetation (1). A formed infective vegetation can lead to four major pathophysiologic phenomena. (i) Bacteremia. (ii) Growth and extension of the vegetative lesion within and into other leaflets, valve annulus, aortic–mitral junction, aortic root, and interventricular septum. This destructive process leads to severe valve distortion and malfunction (usually regurgitation) and leaflet perforation; annulus, sewing ring, root, or myocardial abscesses; and pseudoaneurysms or fistulas. (iii) Embolism with resultant septic infarcts or formation of mycotic aneurysms. (iv) Stimulation of cellular and humoral autoimmunity leading to formation and deposition of circulating immune complexes.

## PREEXISTING HEART DISEASE AND OTHER CONDITIONS

Preexisting heart disease is found in at least two thirds of cases of left-sided IE, but is uncommon in right-sided IE (Table 11.1). The prevalence of underlying heart disease varies according to patient age. In patients <30 years old, rheumatic heart disease (in underdeveloped countries) and mitral valve prolapse or intravenous drug abuse (IVDA; in developed countries) are the most common underlying heart diseases. Also, in this age group, bicuspid aortic valve, ventricular septal defect, patent ductus arteriosus, and hypertrophic obstructive cardiomyopathy are the most common congenital heart conditions associated with IE (2,3). In patients >60 years old, aortic valve sclerosis or stenosis and mitral annular sclerosis with corresponding ≥ mild degrees of regurgitation are common underlying cardiac pathologies. However, in either age group, it has been reported that at least one third of patients may have normal valves or clinically unrecognizable valve disease preceding the development of IE, most commonly in the acute type and right-sided IE. In the current era of echocardiography, most patients probably have some degree of underlying valve disease.

Decreased humoral and cellular immunity associated with acquired immunodeficiency syndrome (AIDS), renal failure, alcoholism, IVDA, and inflammatory connective tissue diseases predisposes to IE. End-stage renal disease patients on hemodialysis using dual-lumen cuffed venous catheters or polytetrafluoroethylene grafts are at higher risk of IE than patients with arteriovenous fistulas (4).

## DIAGNOSIS

The definitive histopathologic diagnosis of IE is established when microorganisms are demonstrated by culture or histology in a vegetation or there is histologic evidence of active vegetation or intracardiac abscess. A *definite* clinical diagnosis of IE according to Duke criteria requires integration of clinical, microbiologic, and echocardiographic data (Table 11.2). The diagnosis of IE is made by

**TABLE 11.1.** *Cardiovascular conditions predisposing to infective endocarditis*

| Condition | Percentage 15–60 yr old | Percentage >60 yr old |
| --- | --- | --- |
| Rheumatic heart disease | 25–30 | 8 |
| Mitral valve prolapse | 10–30 | 10 |
| Intravenous drug abuse | 15–35 | 10 |
| Congenital heart disease | 10–20 | 2 |
| Degenerative heart disease | Rare | 30 |
| Other | 10–15 | 10 |
| None | 25–45 | 25–40 |

**TABLE 11.2.** *Duke diagnostic criteria for infective endocarditis*

| Major criteria | Minor criteria |
|---|---|
| 1. Persistently positive blood cultures for typical microorganisms<br>  A. *Streptococcus viridans* and *Streptococcus bovis*<br>  B. *Staphylococcus aureus*<br>  C. Enterococci<br>  D. "HACEK" group | 1. Predisposing heart disease<br>  A. Mitral valve prolapse<br>  B. Bicuspid aortic valve<br>  C. Rheumatic heart disease<br>  D. Congenital heart disease<br>  E. Intravenous drug abuse |
| 2. Persistent bacteremia<br>  A. ≥2 positive blood cultures ≥12 hr apart<br>    or<br>  B. ≥3 positive cultures ≥1 hr apart<br>  C. 70% positive cultures if ≥4 drawn | 2. Fever |
| 3. Evidence of endocardial involvement<br>  A. Positive echocardiogram<br>    Oscillating vegetation<br>    Abscesses<br>    New partial dehiscence of prosthetic valve<br>  B. New valvular regurgitation | 3. Vascular phenomena<br>  A. Major arterial emboli<br>  B. Septic pulmonary emboli<br>  C. Mycotic aneurysm<br>  D. Intracranial hemorrhage<br>  E. Janeway lesions<br>4. Immunologic phenomena<br>  A. Glomerulonephritis<br>  B. Osler nodes<br>  C. Roth spots<br>  D. Rheumatoid factor<br>5. Other<br>  A. Positive blood cultures not meeting major criteria<br>  B. Positive echocardiogram not meeting major criteria |

Diagnosis: (i) two major criteria; (ii) one major and three minor criteria; or (iii) five minor criteria.
"HACEK" group, *Haemophilus, Actinobacillus, Cardiobacterium, Eikenella,* and *Kingella* species. These pathogens uncommonly cause infective endocarditis (<5% of all cases).

two major criteria; one major and three minor criteria; or five minor criteria. According to these criteria, IE is *possible* when findings consistent with this diagnosis fall short of "definite" but not "rejected." IE is *"rejected"* when a firm alternate diagnosis explains manifestations suggestive of endocarditis or when clinical manifestations or pathologic evidence of endocarditis are not found after ≤4 days of antibiotic therapy. The Duke criteria have high sensitivity and specificity for diagnosis of IE (5,6). The addition of other minor criteria (clubbing, splenomegaly, splinter hemorrhages, petechiae, central nonfeeding venous lines, peripheral venous lines, microscopic hematuria, high erythrocyte sedimentation rate >30 or >50 mm/h for patients <60 or >60 years old, respectively) and C-reactive protein (>100 mg/L) increases the sensitivity of the Duke criteria for the diagnosis of native and especially prosthetic valve IE from 83% and 50% to 94% and 89%, respectively (7).

## CLASSIFICATION

Endocarditis is classified into two main categories: acute and subacute.

### Acute Infective Endocarditis

Acute IE involves a normal heart valve (right heart valves frequently are affected), manifests within days to <2 weeks of onset of infection, is rapidly progressive, and often results in death within 6 weeks if unrecognized.

### Subacute Infective Endocarditis

Subacute IE usually involves a preexisting abnormal valve, manifests >2 weeks after infection, and has a more indolent clinical course. However, in an individual patient, this distinction is difficult and probably of no clinical relevance. *Chronic IE* rarely occurs and has been associated with *Legionella* and *Brucella* infection and with infection of right heart wires. Endocarditis can be subcategorized as *native* (left- or right-sided valve involvement) or *prosthetic valve IE* (*early* or *late* if it occurs <60 or >60 days after surgery, respectively).

## INCIDENCE

The incidence of native valve IE in developed countries is 1.7 to 4 per 100,000 persons per year. Endocarditis occurs more frequently in men than in women (ratio of 1.6 to 2.5:1) and in subjects 40 to 60 years old. The incidence of right-sided IE associated with IVDA ranges from 2% to 5% per year. It is more common in men than women (5.4:1 ratio) and in young subjects (<40 years old) [8]. An uncommon type of right-sided IE, with an incidence of 0.13% to 7%, occurs among patients with right heart wires or catheters [9]. The incidence of early and late prosthetic valve IE ranges from 0.4% to 1.2% and up to 4% per year, respectively. The incidence of late prosthetic valve IE probably is higher for bioprosthetic than for mechanical valves. The increased incidence of IE in industrialized countries is related to a high prevalence of degenerative valve disease, nosocomial infections, and IVDA, and to an improved diagnosis by echocardiography, especially transesophageal echocardiography (TEE).

## DISTRIBUTION OF TYPES OF INFECTIVE ENDOCARDITIS

*Subacute and acute IE of the native left heart valves* constitutes 60% to 75% and 5% to 10% of all cases, respectively. *Prosthetic valve IE* constitutes 10% to 25% of all cases of IE. The incidence of prosthetic valve IE is higher with prosthetic aortic valves and multiple valves, and in patients who have undergone replacement of an infected native valve. Infection of a prosthetic valve results from direct or extracorporeal contamination of the wound intraoperatively or from contamination of arterial, venous, or urethral catheters, or endotracheal tubes during the postoperative period. *Right-sided IE* constitutes 5% to 10% of all cases of IE, most commonly associated with IVDA.

## ANATOMY AND PATHOLOGY

The left heart valves are involved in >85% cases of IE. Isolated aortic IE is observed in 55% to 60% of cases, mitral in 25% to 30%, and both valves in 15%. In right-sided IE, the tricuspid valve is predominantly involved (80% of cases).

The *sine qua non* pathology of IE is valve vegetations. They start along the valve closure line as pinkish, red, or grayish sessile or pedunculated masses that range from 0.2 to 4 cm in diameter. They are composed of fibrin, platelets, inflammatory cells, and clumps of microorganisms. Vegetations are rarely located or extend to the ventricular or auricular endocardium. Tricuspid valve vegetations generally are larger than those of the mitral and aortic valves, but the correlation of vegetation size with outcome in right heart IE is poor.

Ulceration, tears, or perforation of a valve leaflet and rupture of a mitral or tricuspid chordae tendineae can occur and cause severe regurgitant lesions. Ruptures of mitral chordae tendineae in IE often are multiple and involve both leaflets. Leaflet perforation occurs more commonly with aortic valve IE. Perforation of the aortic–mitral intervalvular fibrosa or anterior mitral leaflet also can result from ulceration with or without a preceding pseudoaneurysm formation by metastatic infection from a regurgitant aortic valve (jet lesion).

Cardiac abscesses associated with native or prosthetic valves occur in 20% to 40% of IE cases and predominantly are seen in the aortic valve annulus, sewing ring, periannular area, aortic–mitral intervalvular fibrosa, aortic root, and interventricular septum [10,11]. They are twice as common with prosthetic than with native valve IE. The eroding effect of an abscess in the intervalvular fibrosa or aortic root leads to formation of a pseudoaneurysm or fistula communicating the aorta with the right atrium (RA) or left atrium (LA) or the left ventricle (LV) with either atrium or with the right ventricle (RV). Rarely, isolated myocardial abscess or infarction can occur because of coronary embolism. Prosthetic valve abscesses can lead to ring dehiscence.

Extracardiac lesions result from arterial emboli to the kidneys, spleen, liver, and central nervous system. Mycotic aneurysms, which occur in up to 15% of cases of IE, can involve the sinuses of Valsalva, cerebral arteries, and branches of the abdominal aorta.

## COMMON PATHOGENS

The microorganisms associated with IE vary according to patient age, acuteness of the disease, involvement of a native (left- or right-sided) or prosthetic valves (early or late type), and IVDA (Table 11.3).

*Acute IE* is caused most commonly by *Staphylococcus aureus, Streptococcus pneumoniae, Streptococcus pyogenes, Haemophilus influenza, Pseudomonas aeruginosa,* and β-hemolytic streptococcus.

*Subacute IE* of native or late prosthetic valves is predominantly (80%) caused by *Streptococcus viridans* and *S. aureus.*

*Early prosthetic valve IE* and that of patients with renal failure on hemodialysis with prosthetic vascular access lines are caused most commonly by *S. aureus* and *Staphylococcus epidermidis.*

*Right-sided IE* is caused most commonly by *S. aureus* (60% to 75%) and occurs most often in patients with IVDA. Streptococci (10%), enterococci (10%), gram-negative bacteria (5% to 10%), and fungi (5%) uncom-monly cause *right-sided IE.* Acute right-sided IE related to pacemaker or automatic implantable cardioverter-defibrillator (AICD) wires also is caused most commonly by *S. aureus* in 50% and *S. epidermidis* in 30% to 40%. The most common pathogens of chronic right-sided IE related to pacemaker or AICD wires are *S. epidermidis* (75%), *S. aureus* (15%), and Gram-negative bacteria (10%).

*Culture negative IE* is uncommon (5% to 10%) and related to antibiotic therapy before blood cultures are obtained in the majority of cases. Other causes include *Candida, Aspergillus, Coxiella burnetii,* and other fastidious slow-growing microorganisms.

*Other pathogens.* In patients with gastrointestinal or genitourinary malignancies or manipulation, *Enterococcus faecalis* and *Enterococcus faecium* are the most common pathogens. In immunocompromised patients, fungi, especially *Candida,* are common.

## HISTORY

Early clinical and echocardiographic diagnosis and treatment of IE often prevents patients from developing significant cardiac involvement. Therefore, patients with uncomplicated IE commonly lack or have nonspecific cardiovascular symptoms and physical findings. A variety of noncardiovascular symptoms, predominantly *fever, chills, anorexia, and general malaise,* occur within a few days or weeks of bacteremia in most patients with acute and subacute IE (Table 11.4) (1–3,12,13). Fever and chills often are remitting. However, fever can be absent (5%) in pa-

**TABLE 11.3.** *Microbiology of infective endocarditis of native heart valves*

| Pathogen | Percentage 15–60 yr old | Percentage >60 yr old |
|---|---|---|
| Streptococci | 45–65 | 30–45 |
| *Staphyloccocus aureus* | 30–40 | 25–30 |
| Enterococci | 5–8 | 15 |
| *Staphyloccocus epidermidis* | 3–5 | 5–8 |
| Gram-negative bacteria | 4–8 | 5 |
| Culture negative[a] | 3–10 | 5 |

[a]Includes infective endocarditis caused by fungi, fastidious slow-growing microorganisms, and *Coxiella burnetii.*

**TABLE 11.4.** *Common symptoms in patients with infective endocarditis*

| Symptom | Percentage |
|---|---|
| Fever | 80–85 |
| Chills | 42–75 |
| Anorexia | 25–55 |
| General malaise | 20–40 |
| Dyspnea | 20–30 |
| Sweats, cough, nausea, vomiting | 15–25 |
| Myalgias, arthralgias | 15–30 |
| Stroke, confusion | 10–20 |
| Fatigue, weight loss | 10–15 |

tients who had antibiotic therapy preceding blood cultures, in elderly or debilitated patients, in patients with chronic renal failure, and in individuals with other immunocompromising conditions (14). *Anorexia, general malaise, anemia,* and *weight loss* are common symptoms in patients with subacute IE. Dyspnea, cough, pleuritic chest pain, and hemoptysis are common symptoms in patients with acute right-sided IE. However, *dyspnea* also can be related to anemia, preexisting pulmonary disease, pulmonary infection, or preexisting rather than new or worsened heart disease. A new neurologic deficit or encephalopathy can be an initial manifestation of IE. The symptomatology of patients with

significant valve dysfunction will be that of acute mitral regurgitation (MR) or aortic regurgitation (AR) leading to heart failure or pulmonary edema, systemic embolism, infarction of visceral organs, or neurologic dysfunction. In conclusion, no symptom is specific for any type of IE.

## PHYSICAL EXAMINATION

The physical findings in uncomplicated IE are predominantly nonspecific. Fever and heart murmurs are the most common and often the only clinical manifestations of IE (Table 11.5). Because of the high prevalence of flow murmurs in young patients, degenerative valve disease (especially aortic valve sclerosis) in the elderly, and the common presence of fever and anemia, heart murmurs in patients with IE often are nonspecific systolic ejection murmurs and, therefore, not suggestive of valve dysfunction. Thus, the presence of a systolic heart murmur in patients with suspected IE has high sensitivity but low positive predictive value for detection of IE. In contrast, auscultation of a new diastolic murmur, changing characteristics of a preexisting systolic murmur, or a murmur

**TABLE 11.5.** *Common physical findings in infective endocarditis*

| Finding | Percentage |
|---|---|
| Nonspecific | |
|   Fever | 80–90 |
|   Anemia | 25 |
|   Clubbing | 10–20 |
|   Confusion | 10–20 |
|   Weight loss | 10–15 |
|   Polyarthritis | Rare |
| Cardiac | |
|   Heart murmur | 80–85 |
|   Changing, new, or diastolic murmur | 30–50 |
|   Aortic and/or mitral regurgitation | Most common |
|   Tricuspid regurgitation | <50 |
| Peripheral manifestations | |
|   Central nervous system abnormalities | 30–40 |
|   Embolism | 20–40 |
|   Petechia | 10–40 |
|   Splenomegaly | 5–30 |
|   Osler nodes | 10–20 |
|   Splinter hemorrhage | 5–15 |
|   Janeway lesion | 5–10 |
|   Roth spot | 5–10 |

with systolic and diastolic components is of the most diagnostic value. Patients with significant valve dysfunction will have regurgitant murmurs with characteristics similar to those of other etiologies of valvular heart disease discussed in chapters 5, 6, and 9 of this book. However, in patients with acute regurgitant lesions (MR or AR), the predominant clinical manifestations will be those of acute heart failure, pulmonary edema, or rarely cardiogenic shock. Heart murmurs in these patients frequently are not audible (up to 50%) or are of low intensity (disproportional to the severity of valve dysfunction).

*Acute IE of native left heart valves* manifests with severe sepsis, high fever (102° to 104°F), shivering, splenomegaly, and uncommonly necrotic purpura. Because these patients frequently do not have preexisting heart disease, murmurs are absent initially but develop soon after due to rapid valve destruction. Consequently, acute and severe MR or AR, left heart failure, uncontrolled sepsis, and metastatic infection can occur.

*Acute right-sided valves IE* commonly is manifested with fever, chills, dyspnea, cough, hemoptysis due to septic pulmonary emboli leading to pneumonia, lung abscesses, empyema, and pulmonary hypertension. A murmur of tricuspid regurgitation is heard in <50% of patients.

The *acute syndrome of right-sided IE related to right heart catheters or wires* manifests within 6 weeks (generally <30 days) after first lead implantation with fever (>90% of cases), local pain, inflammation or infection (>40% of cases), and commonly (35% to 40%) clinical or radiologic evidence of pneumonia, pneumonitis, pulmonary embolism, or lung abscesses. *The chronic syndrome* occurs ≥6 weeks after implantation (usually several months) and more commonly (>60% of cases) after pacemaker lead reimplantation, revision, pacemaker exteriorization, or local infection. The syndrome manifests as fever and chills (>80%), local symptoms (>50%), pulmonary manifestations of pleural effusions, pneumonia, pulmonary abscess or embolism (>40%), and immunologic mani-

festations (>15%) (9,15). Rare cases of right-sided IE related to infection of *in situ* thrombi (attached to the RA wall) induced by a central venous catheter have been reported and have clinical manifestations and microbiology similar to that related with right heart wires (16).

*Prosthetic valve IE* manifests clinically as an acute or subacute syndrome with clinical manifestations similar to those of native valve IE.

## Peripheral Manifestations

Clinical manifestations are seen predominantly in patients with subacute IE.

*Petechiae* are found on the upper and lower extremities; buccal and palatal mucosa; and palpebral conjunctiva. *Splinter or subungual hemorrhages* are dark, red, linear, or sometimes flame-shaped streaks seen in the finger or toenails. *Osler nodes*, believed to be immune-mediated vasculitic lesions, are bluish red and pinhead to pea-sized tumefactions that are characteristically painful to pressure and usually are seen on the pulps of the fingers or toes. They usually disappear after a few days of antibiotic therapy. *Janeway lesions* result from septic microembolism. They are erythematous, have irregular borders, and are small (1 to 5 mm) nontender macules located predominantly on the palms and soles. These lesions are common in patients with acute IE. *Roth spots* are oval retinal hemorrhages with a pale center. *Asymmetric polyarthritis and clubbing* are uncommon manifestations in patients with subacute IE (17).

## Clinical Manifestations of Infective Endocarditis Complications

### Cardiac

Heart failure is caused by severe valve destruction (including leaflet perforation) and extension of valve infection to contiguous structures, including the myocardium (10,18). Acute and severe AR, MR, or both are the most common causes. Cardiac abscesses most commonly associated with prosthetic or native aortic valve IE can lead to heart failure as a result of fistulas formation (more commonly, aorta to RA, LA, or RV) (11,19). Myocardial infarction or abscesses resulting from extension of perivalvular infection or from septic emboli to the coronary arteries can lead to heart failure, high-degree atrioventricular block, and ventricular arrhythmias. Heart failure and frequently related sepsis are associated with 50% to 75% mortality unless cardiac surgery is performed.

### Extracardiac

#### Systemic Arterial Embolism

Systemic arterial embolism is the most common extracardiac complication of IE, occurring in 20% to 40% of cases. It involves the brain and less often the lower limbs, kidneys, spleen, liver, coronary arteries and bone. It can be multiple and frequently (>50%) recurs within 30 days. Embolism more commonly occurs within 2 weeks of the diagnosis of IE. High-risk predictors include large (>10 mm), elongated, and mobile vegetations; *S. aureus* infection; mitral valve IE (two times higher incidence than the aortic or other valves); and double valve IE (20).

*Cerebral emboli* (stroke or transient ischemic attack) present with a focal neurologic deficit having clinical features particular to the cerebral artery territory involved (21). Occlusion of an ophthalmic artery leads to total or partial monocular blindness. Embolism to the anterior cerebral artery causes contralateral weakness, predominantly of the leg. Occlusion of the anterior branch of the middle cerebral artery leads to contralateral motor and sensory loss of the face, hand and arm, and nonfluent (Broca) aphasia. Occlusion of the posterior branch of the anterior cerebral artery leads to contralateral hemisensory loss, homonymous hemianopsia, and fluent (Wernicke) aphasia. Occlusion of the vertebral artery manifests with binocular visual loss, quadriparesis, altered consciousness, ipsilateral cranial nerve or contralateral limb abnormalities, dysarthria, diplopia, vertigo, and ataxia.

*Peripheral arterial embolism* occurs predominantly to the legs (60%), then to the arms (20%) and visceral arteries (20%) (20,21). Acute limb ischemia manifests as pain, paresthesias, motor dysfunction, and loss of distal pulses. Mesenteric artery ischemia manifests with symptoms of severe abdominal pain with or without peritoneal signs. Splenic infarction may present with left upper quadrant or left shoulder pain and a left pleural effusion. Infarction of a renal artery causes flank pain and gross or microscopic hematuria.

#### Circulating Immune Complexes

Circulating immune complexes are most common in patients with positive blood cultures, but also are seen in half of patients with culture-negative IE. Deposition of these complexes along the glomerular basement membrane leads to a focal or diffuse glomerulonephritis.

#### Abscesses

Abscesses resulting from septic embolism and infarction more frequently involve the spleen and kidney and rarely the brain. In right-sided IE, pulmonary abscesses resulting from septic embolism are common.

#### Mycotic Aneurysms

Mycotic aneurysms are a late complication of IE and have an incidence of 2% to 15%. Cerebral mycotic aneurysms (25% of all cases) account for 2.5% to 6.2% of all intracranial aneurysms (22). They commonly are asymptomatic, but they can manifest as severe localized headaches or sudden subarachnoid hemorrhage. Aneurysmal rupture may happen during active disease or several months or years later.

#### Other Neurologic Complications

Other neurologic complications resulting from diffuse vasculitis and metastatic infection can occur (21). Intracranial hemorrhage, brain abscess, meningitis, and meningoencephalitis are uncommon. Patients with neurologic complications have a mortality rate of about 40%.

## Clinical Differential Diagnosis

### *Rheumatic Valvulitis*

In the appropriate geographic areas, the clinical syndrome of acute rheumatic endocarditis may mimic that of endocarditis. Both diseases have similar clinical and serologic markers, except for elevation of antistreptolysin antibodies in rheumatic carditis (23).

### *Libman-Sacks Endocarditis*

Pseudo-IE is a clinical syndrome of active systemic lupus erythematosus (SLE) that mimics IE. It consists of fever, cardiac murmurs, splinter hemorrhages, valvular masses on echocardiography, high titers of antibodies to DNA, low complement, and moderate to highly positive antiphospholipid antibodies, but negative blood cultures. Low white count, moderate or high elevations of antiphospholipid antibodies, and negative or low positive C-reactive protein indicates active SLE (24,25). In these patients, noninfective and infective endocarditic may coexist (25). Rarely, IE may initially manifest with polyarthritis and mimic a connective tissue disease (i.e., SLE) (17).

## ECHOCARDIOGRAPHY

### Introduction

Infective endocarditis is associated with high morbidity and mortality if not recognized promptly and treated appropriately. Therefore, a technique used for its diagnosis must be highly accurate with low false-negative (high sensitivity and positive predictive value) and false-positive rates (high specificity and negative predictive value). Color Doppler transthoracic echocardiography (TTE) and especially TEE are highly accurate and cost effective for the diagnosis, risk stratification, and determination of the need for surgery in patients with IE (12,13,26). In a patient with a suggestive clinical syndrome, echocardiography can confirm the diagnosis of IE by detecting vegetations (the *sine qua non* of this condition). In this type of patient, the absence of vegetations does not exclude IE. The Bayesian theorem may be applic-

able to echocardiography in the diagnosis of IE. In patients with a high pretest likelihood of IE, echocardiography may have limited additive diagnostic value, but it adds information of prognostic importance, especially TEE. The detection (or exclusion) of valve vegetations and their characterization, as well as the detection (or exclusion) of valve complications, such as abscesses, leaflet perforation, or fistulas, helps stratify patients into those with low or high morbidity and mortality. In patients with a low likelihood of IE, echocardiography may have limited additive diagnostic and prognostic value. In patients with intermediate likelihood of IE, echocardiography, and especially TEE, may play the most important diagnostic and prognostic role (13,26). However, in clinical practice, stratification of patients into these categories is difficult and probably arbitrary.

Echocardiography can define the mechanism and severity of valve dysfunction (generally valve regurgitation) as well as the hemodynamic impact of regurgitant lesions (assesses LV size and function, and LA size, and provides an estimate of LA and pulmonary artery pressures).

Thus, echocardiography is essential for risk stratification and decision-making regarding medical or surgical management of patients with IE. The absence of valve disease or detection of small vegetations with no or mild valve dysfunction indicates a good prognosis with medical therapy. In contrast, detection of large or multiple vegetations (>10 mm) or severe valve dysfunction (moderate to severe regurgitation, abscess, leaflet perforation, fistula, ring dehiscence, etc.) indicates high morbidity and mortality with medical therapy and, therefore, points to the need for surgical intervention.

However, echocardiography may not detect valve vegetations in a patient with other clinical data diagnostic of IE. Also, in patients with suspected IE, echocardiography might detect valve lesions that mimic vegetations (see Differential Diagnosis section). Therefore, echocardiography by itself does not supplant (confirm or exclude) but rather complements the clinical and microbiologic diagnosis of IE.

## Echocardiographic Criteria for Diagnosis

### *General Considerations*

A systematic approach to the performance and interpretation of TTE and TEE in a patient with suspected IE is essential to the diagnostic accuracy of echocardiography. Careful scanning of one heart valve at a time should be performed in multiple planes at short depth settings (12 cm for TTE and 4 to 8 cm for TEE) and with narrow sector scans to improve image resolution. For TEE, for each valve and especially from the basilar views, two-dimensional followed by color Doppler imaging should be done at different valve or subvalvular levels by slowly advancing or withdrawing the probe.

In our laboratory, TEE interrogation of all heart valves is performed with the following views sequence: transgastric four chamber; transgastric short and long axis of the mitral and tricuspid valves (this is the only view that allows assessment of the tricuspid posterior leaflet); short axis of the mitral valve as the TEE probe is withdrawn form the transgastric to the basilar level; basilar four chamber with a sector scan limited to the mitral valve and scanning of the valve at multiple planes and levels; basilar short axis and multiplane interrogation of the aortic and then of the pulmonic valve; and finally assessment of the anterior and septal tricuspid leaflets from the basilar four-chamber view at multiple planes and levels.

In addition to characterizing valve masses and associated complications, valve leaflets and subvalvular apparatus are assessed for the presence of thickening, hyper-reflectance, retraction, presence of calcification, and abnormal mobility. These characteristics help to categorize an underlying valve morphology/etiology as myxomatous, degenerative, rheumatic, or congenital. Then, the presence and severity of valve regurgitation are defined according to criteria also described in chapters 5, 6, and 9 of this book.

## Detection of Valve Vegetations and Associated Complications

### *Valve Vegetations*

Valve vegetations are the *sine qua non* of IE and the most common echocardiographic abnormality of IE. They are well-defined or discrete masses attached to the valve leaflets. Valve vegetations are characterized by their location, size, shape, echo-reflectance, mobility, and extent (Fig. 11.1) (27).

*Location:* Valve vegetations characteristically are located at the leaflet coaptation point and on the upstream side of the valve (on the atrial side of atrioventricular valves and ventricular side of semilunar valves). Uncommon locations of valve vegetations

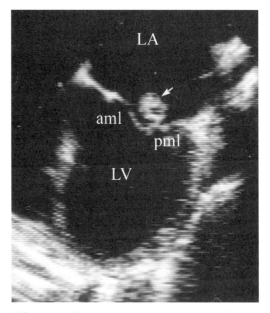

**FIG. 11.1.** Mitral valve infective endocarditis due to *Streptococcus viridans* in a 20-year-old woman. Transesophageal echocardiographic four-chamber view demonstrates a large (1 × 1 cm) oval vegetation located on the atrial side and distal portion of the posterior mitral leaflet (pml) *(arrow)*. Note the echo-lucency within this mass suggestive of an *in situ* abscess. The appearance of the underlying leaflet is unremarkable. Associated severe mitral regurgitation (MR) was demonstrated by color Doppler. aml, anterior mitral leaflet; LA, left atrium; LV, left ventricle.

include the ventricular side of the mid to distal portion of the anterior mitral leaflet or chordae tendineae as a result of an AR jet lesion or from a contact lesion with the basal septum in patients with obstructive hypertrophic cardiomyopathy. Also, in patients with hypertrophic cardiomyopathy, vegetations can be seen on the basal septum as a result of a contact lesion with the mitral valve (McCallum plaques) (28).

*Size:* Vegetations are of variable size, but generally >3 mm. A vegetation is small if it measures <5 mm; moderate if 5 to 10 mm; and large if >10 mm. The size of a vegetation has important prognostic implications (20,28).

*Shape:* Vegetations are of variable shape. Although commonly of globular shape, they can be polypoid, tubular, frondlike, elongated, pedunculated, unilobulated, or multilobulated.

*Echo-reflectance:* The echo-reflectance of recently formed vegetations is that of the myocardium (soft tissue echo-reflectance) and less frequently of heterogeneous appearance. Vegetations denser than the myocardium or partially or completely calcified denote chronicity and likely healed lesions. Infrequently, recent and large vegetations can have discrete areas of echo-lucency that suggest *in situ* abscess formation.

*Mobility.* The mobility of a sessile lesion is that of the underlying leaflet, an elongated mass has partial independent mobility, and a pedunculated or prolapsing mass has a characteristic independent rotatory mobility.

### Valve Perforation

Perforation of a leaflet appears as a leaflet tissue discontinuity of variable size (Figs. 11.2 and 11.3). Demonstration of a color Doppler jet through the leaflet discontinuity make this diagnosis almost certain. Perforation can occur on any leaflet portion, but commonly adjacent to vegetations or leaflet thickening. The aortic noncoronary cusp, aortic–mitral junction or intervalvular fi-

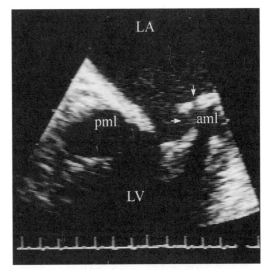

A

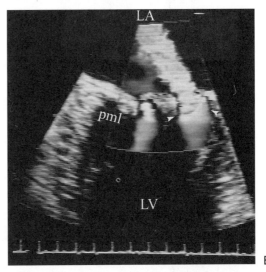

B

**FIG. 11.2.** Mitral valve infective endocarditis due to *Staphylococcus aureus* in a 43-year-old woman with underlying mitral stenosis. **A:** Transesophageal echocardiographic two-chamber view demonstrates severe and diffuse thickening of the posterior mitral leaflet (pml) and severe thickening of the anterior mitral leaflet tip. Note on the base and mid portion of the anterior mitral leaflet two discrete areas of tissue discontinuity consistent with leaflet perforations *(arrows).* **B:** Color Doppler demonstrates a wide regurgitant jet through a perforation *(arrowheads).* (See Color Figure 11.2B.)

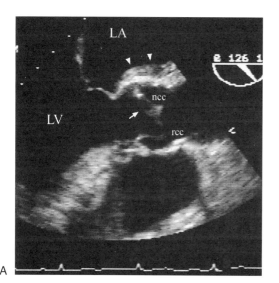

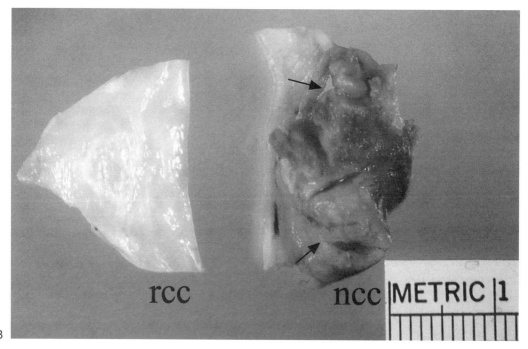

**FIG. 11.3.** Aortic valve infective endocarditis due to β-hemolytic streptococcus in a 63-year-old man. **A:** Transesophageal echocardiographic long-axis view of the aortic valve demonstrates moderate soft tissue thickening of the aortic noncoronary cusp (ncc) with a small area of echo-lucency on its mid portion *(arrow)* suggestive of a perforation. Note the contrasting unremarkable appearance of the right coronary cusp (rcc). Also note the severe soft tissue thickening of the posterior aortic annulus and root *(arrowheads)* suggestive of an early abscess. Color Doppler demonstrated two regurgitant jets, one at the leaflet coaptation point and the second one through the echo-lucent portion. **B:** Note the thickening and distortion of the ncc with two discrete perforations *(arrows)*. Also note the contrasting minimal sclerosis of the rcc. Other abbreviations as in previous figures. (See Color Figure 11.3B.)

brosa, and basilar to mid portions of the anterior mitral leaflet are involved more commonly. Up to 50% of leaflet perforations, especially those of the mitral valve, are associated with or preceded by a pseudoaneurysm (11,18). Scanning of the valve leaflets without and with color Doppler in multiple planes is essential for accurate diagnosis.

### Valvular, Annular, Aortic Root, or Myocardial Abscesses

An abscess appears as an amorphous soft tissue echo-reflectant mass (if solid) or with areas of echo-lucency (if cystic), of variable size, located more commonly on the posterior aortic valve annulus and periannular area (intervalvular fibrosa), then on the aortic root, and uncommonly on the myocardium (predominantly the proximal septum) (Figs. 11.3 and 11.4) (11,19,29,30). Cystic abscesses, unlike pseudoaneurysms, do not expand and collapse during the cardiac cycle and do not show flow by color Doppler. In prosthetic valves, abscesses are characteristically seen around the sewing ring (31).

### Valve Pseudoaneurysm

Pseudoaneurysms are seen predominantly (50% to 75%) in the aortic–mitral intervalvular fibrosa, then on the aortic annulus (most commonly posterior), and rarely on the base or mid portions of the aortic or mitral leaflets (Fig. 11.5). They appear as a narrow discontinuity (neck) communicating with a sac or pouchlike structure. The neck of the lesion opens to the LV outflow tract and the saccular portion bulges or expands during systole and collapses during diastole. Cavity area ranges from about 1 to 12 cm. Pseudoaneurysms more commonly are associated with active prosthetic valve IE, predominantly of the aortic valve. Pseudoaneurysms result from direct extension or metastatic infection. In patients with an infected aortic

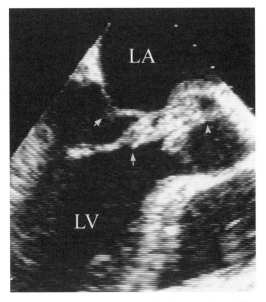

**FIG. 11.4.** Aortic valve infective endocarditis due to *Streptococcus viridans* in a 28-year-old male with an underlying bicuspid aortic valve. Transesophageal echocardiographic long-axis view of the aortic valve demonstrates a large and elongated vegetation of the noncoronary cusp prolapsing into the left ventricle in diastole *(long arrow).* Note an echo-lucency in the body of the vegetation suggestive of an *in situ* abscess formation. Also note the cavitated soft tissue echo-reflectant mass of the posterior aortic annulus and aortic root consistent with an abscess *(arrowhead).* Color and continuous wave Doppler demonstrated severe aortic regurgitation leading to diastolic closure of the mitral valve *(short arrow).* Echocardiographic findings were confirmed at surgery. Abbreviations as in previous figures.

valve, an AR jet can infect and erode the ventricular side of the anterior mitral leaflet and lead to formation of a pseudoaneurysm. Leaflet or intervalvular fibrosa pseudoaneurysms frequently rupture (about 50%). They communicate with the LA and least frequently with the aorta (11,18).

### Fistulas

Extension of the valvular or annular infectious process to the periannular area and

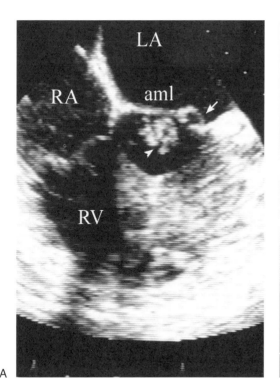
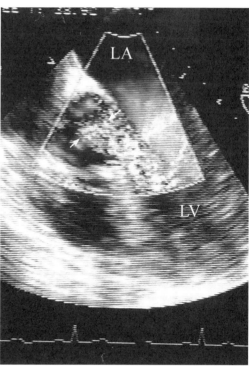

A
B

**FIG. 11.5.** Aortic and metastatic mitral valve infective endocarditis due to *Staphylococcus aureus* in a 57-year-old man with underlying mild aortic stenosis. **A:** Transesophageal echocardiographic four-chamber view tangential to the left ventricle demonstrates a large globular mass with heterogeneous echo-reflectance on the ventricular side and mid portion of the anterior mitral leaflet (aml) *(arrowhead)*. Also note the small pseudoaneurysm at the distal portion of the anterior mitral leaflet *(arrow)*. **B:** Both mitral valve lesions resulted from jet lesions due to severe aortic regurgitation as demonstrated by color Doppler. *Arrows* delineate a large jet width. RA, right atria; RV, right ventricle. (See Color Figure 11.5B.)

aortic–mitral intervalvular fibrosa results in erosion, possible formation of a pseudoaneurysm, and ultimately rupture and communication of LV with LA or aorta with LA or RA. Similarly, extension of the infection to the ventricular septum can lead to the formation of a fistula that communicates the LV with the RV or RA (11). Color Doppler is of important diagnostic value in recognizing this complication.

### Ring Dehiscence

Ring dehiscence appears as a discontinuity between the outer border of the sewing ring and the respective annulus (Fig. 10.6)

(32). Demonstration of a color Doppler jet in this area of discontinuity is of important complementary diagnostic value. An estimate of the extent of ring dehiscence can be made by identifying the circumferential extent of a color Doppler jet (outside the sewing ring) from the transgastric and basal short-axis TEE views of the mitral or aortic valve. Also, careful multiplane color Doppler TEE scanning of the mitral or aortic valve sewing ring from the basilar horizontal views (four- or two-chamber or longitudinal views) helps to assess the extent of dehiscence by defining the angle of persistence of color Doppler through the dehisced area.

## Comparison of Transesophageal Echocardiography and Transthoracic Echocardiography in Diagnosis and Risk Stratification of Infective Endocarditis

### Detection and Characterization of Valve Vegetations

TEE has a significantly higher sensitivity than TTE for detection of native and prosthetic valve vegetations (88% to 100% vs. 33% to 63%, respectively). However, the specificity of both techniques is similarly high (88% to 97% for TEE and 98% to 100% for TTE) (Table 11.6) (12,14,33,34). TEE also is superior to TTE in defining the size, shape, mobility, location, and number of valve vegetations. These characteristics, especially the size and mobility of the vegetation, have important prognostic implications (27,34). Patients with large (>10 mm) and hypermobile vegetations have a higher rate of failure to therapy; a higher incidence of embolism (more common with mitral than with aortic or other valve involvement; odds ratio 2.8); valvular dysfunction or heart failure; valve replacement (odds ratio 2.95); and death (odds ratio 1.55) than patients with sessile or smaller vegetations (20,21,33,34). Patients with a vegetation size ≤5 mm, 6 to 10 mm, and >11 mm have up to 10%, 20% to 40%, and >50% incidence of those complications, respectively.

Although TEE and TTE probably detect tricuspid valve vegetations with equal frequency, TEE defines more accurately the vegetation morphology and associated complications. TEE is valuable for defining the mechanism of TR, detecting chordal or papillary muscle involvement, and determining the extent of leaflet involvement (8,9,15,35). Pulmonary valve IE and that associated with pacemaker or implantable cardiac defibrillators or other right heart catheters are recognized more often by TEE than by TTE. TEE detects vegetations on these devices in about 90% of cases compared to ≤30% by TTE. A lead infection may have a sleevelike appearance rather than distinct vegetation in 25% of cases (Fig. 11.6). Finally, in these patients, a vegetation size defined by TEE as <10 or >10 mm predicts high success and safety rates for percutaneous versus surgical lead extraction, respectively (35,36). Rare cases of infected RA thrombi have been diagnosed by TEE. Because TEE is of superior diagnostic value than TTE, most patients with suspected culture-negative IE should undergo TEE (37).

### Detection of Complications

TEE is superior to TTE for detecting native and prosthetic valve complications such as abscesses, leaflet perforations, leaflet pseudoaneurysms, and fistulas. The sensitivity of TEE for detecting abscesses, leaflet perforations, and pseudoaneurysms ranges from 90% to 100% compared to 22%

**TABLE 11.6.** *Detection of valvular or paravalvular complications by TEE compared to TTE*

| Abnormality | TEE | | TTE | |
|---|---|---|---|---|
| | Sensitivity (%) | Specificity (%) | Sensitivity (%) | Specificity (%) |
| Vegetations* | 83–100 | 93–100 | 17–63 | 83–98 |
| Abscess | 98–100 | — | 22–28 | — |
| Perforation | 95 | 98 | 45 | 98 |
| Pseudoaneurysm | 90 | — | 43 | — |

*Lower transesophageal echocardiography (TEE) sensitivity values apply to prosthetic valves. The reported negative and positive predictive values of TEE for native infective endocarditis are 98%–100% and 95%–98%, respectively. Its negative predictive value for prosthetic valve infective endocarditis is 90%.

TTE, transthoracic echocardiography.

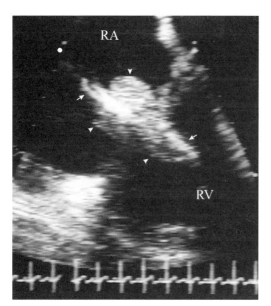

**FIG. 11.6.** Tricuspid valve infective endocarditis associated with a pacemaker infection due to *Staphylococcus aureus.* Transesophageal echocardiographic four-chamber view demonstrates a large mass *(arrowheads)* that extends from the right atrium (RA) to the right ventricle (RV) and is attached to the pacemaker wire *(arrows).* Mild soft tissue thickening of the tricuspid valve, but no valve vegetations, were detected. Associated moderate tricuspid regurgitation was demonstrated by color Doppler. Histopathology of this mass confirmed to be an infective vegetation.

to 45% by TTE. The specificity of both techniques is similarly high (>90%) (Table 11.6) (11,18,29,30,33,38). Similar superiority of TEE compared to TTE has been reported for the detection of bioprosthetic

leaflet perforations (39,40). Because of the infrequency of fistulas due to IE, limited data are available comparing TEE and TTE for the detection of this complication. However, in most series reporting this abnormality, the diagnosis has been made predominantly by TEE.

Shadowing and reverberations from prosthetic materials, especially from mechanical valves in the mitral valve position, decrease the detection rate of prosthetic valve vegetations by TTE. For the same reason, prosthetic MR and less frequently AR (valvular or perivalvular) and other associated complications (i.e., abscesses) are detected infrequently by TTE.

In patients with suspected prosthetic valve endocarditis, TTE provides a complementary assessment of aortic or mitral valve obstruction and AR, and LA and pulmonary artery pressures. In some patients, better or equal characterization of right-sided valves can be accomplished by TTE compared to TEE. In addition, detection of premature mitral valve closure by TTE in the setting of acute AR implies severe regurgitation and markedly elevated LV end-diastolic pressure and heart failure, and indicates the need for urgent surgery (41).

Despite the reported high diagnostic accuracy of TEE in uncomplicated and complicated IE, TEE is not routinely recommended in patients with suspected IE. However, multiple reasons for performing TEE in addition to, or instead of, TTE have been suggested by experts (Table 11.7).

**TABLE 11.7.** *Indications for transesophageal echocardiography in patients with suspected or proven infective endocarditis*

1. Technically limited TTE
2. High clinical suspicion for IE with a negative TTE
3. High clinical suspicion for IE in patients with staphylococcus bacteremia
4. In elderly patients with underlying degenerative valvular heart disease
5. Clinical suspicious for IE and negative blood cultures
6. Clinical suspicious for IE and bacteremia, but negative or inadequate TTE
7. Persistent fever or bacteremia
8. Suspected prosthetic valve endocarditis
9. Suspected valve complications ($\geq$ moderate regurgitation, abscess, perforation, or fistula)

IE, infective endocarditis; TTE, transthoracic echocardiography.

## Role of Echocardiography in Surgical Management of Infective Endocarditis

Echocardiography plays a critical role in identifying patients for whom cardiac surgery is indicated. Currently, eight of nine class I recommendations for valve surgery according to the American College of Cardiology/American Heart Association (ACC/AHA) guidelines for the management of valvular heart disease require information derived from echocardiography (Table 11.8) (32,42–44). In addition, patients with systemic embolism and persistent valve vegetations despite appropriate antibiotic therapy should be considered for surgery (45). Because of the higher diagnostic accuracy of TEE compared to TTE in detecting complications associated with native and prosthetic valve IE, recommendations for valve surgery are based predominantly on TEE data. Furthermore, intraoperative TEE plays an important role in the immediate postoperative assessment of valve replacement or, infrequently, valve repair in patients with IE.

## Echocardiographic Differential Diagnosis

The echocardiographic appearance of infective vegetations overlap with that of other noninfective valve masses, such as valve excrescences, ruptured mitral chordae tendineae, torn bioprosthetic leaflets, Libman-Sacks vegetations, rheumatic valvulitis, thrombotic vegetations (i.e., marantic endocarditis), and papillary fibroelastoma.

Some of these abnormalities may be present in patients with suspected clinical but not echocardiographic evidence of IE (i.e., valve excrescences); may preexist or be caused by IE (ruptured tendineae); or may coexist with infective vegetations (Libman-Sacks vegetations). These facts underscore the importance of clinical and microbiologic data in the diagnosis of IE as well as the need for expert echocardiographic interpretation.

### Valve Excrescences

Valve or Lambl's excrescences are thin (range from 0.6 to 2 mm wide), elongated (4 to 16 mm long), and hypermobile structures seen at the coaptation point of the aortic and mitral valve leaflets and rarely on the right-sided valves. They are seen on the aortic valve prolapsing into the LV outflow tract during diastole (Fig. 11.7). Those on the mitral valve prolapse into the LA during systole. They are detected almost exclusively by TEE and are visible in 35% to 40% of apparently healthy subjects; 45% to 50% of patients undergoing TEE for other reasons than suspected cardioembolism; and 40% of those undergoing TEE for suspected cardioembolism (46). These excrescences persist unchanged over time and are not associated with increased cardioembolic risk. They result from the constant bending and buckling of the leaflets leading to tearing of the subendocardial collagen and elastic fibers with subsequent endothelialization. Valve

---

**TABLE 11.8.** *Class I recommendations for surgery of native or prosthetic valve endocarditis*

1. Acute aortic or mitral regurgitation with heart failure
2. Acute aortic regurgitation with tachycardia and early closure of the mitral valve
3. Valve dysfunction and persistent infection after 7–10 d of appropriate antibiotic therapy
4. Paravalvular regurgitation leak (for prosthetic valve), annular or aortic abscess, sinus or aortic true or false aneurysm, fistula formation, or new-onset conduction disturbances
5. Early prosthetic valve endocarditis
6. Prosthetic valve dysfunction with heart failure
7. Staphylococcal prosthetic endocarditis not responding to antibiotic therapy
8. Prosthetic valve infection with Gram-negative organisms or organisms with a poor response to antibiotics
9. Fungal native or prosthetic valve endocarditis

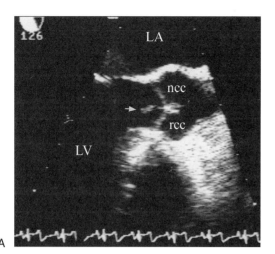
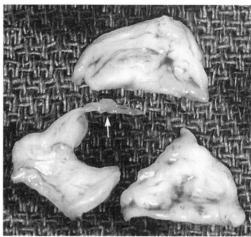

A                                                B

**FIG. 11.7.** Aortic valve excrescence in a noninfected 47-year-old man with chronic symptomatic aortic regurgitation. **A:** Transesophageal echocardiographic long-axis view of the aortic valve demonstrates a distinct elongated mass at the aortic coaptation point prolapsing into the left ventricle during diastole *(arrow)*. Thickening of the aortic valve cusps, especially of the tip portions, was demonstrated. **B:** Diffuse myxomatous thickening of the three aortic valve cusps is noted with a thin and lucent excrescence attached to the tip of the right coronary cusp *(arrow)*. Abbreviations as in previous figures. (See Color Figure 11.7B.)

excrescences have a distribution, leaflet and chamber location, and mobility similar to those of infective vegetations. Nevertheless, infective vegetations are generally >3 mm in diameter; resolve or change in size or appearance over time; and usually are associated with structural and functional valve abnormalities. However, in a patient with suspected IE, it may be difficult to differentiate a valve excrescence from a small or early-stage infective mass.

### Ruptured Chordae Tendineae

A ruptured chordae is an elongated, hypermobile structure that is usually >3 mm thick. It prolapses into the LA during systole and generally is associated with prolapse and myxomatous thickening of the respective leaflet and significant and eccentric MR (Fig. 6.7) (47). Therefore, distinction of a primary or myxomatous ruptured chordae from an infective ruptured chordae can only be made by integrating clinical and echocardiographic data.

### Torn Bioprosthetic Leaflet

The sclerotic degenerative process of a bioprosthetic leaflet can lead to a torn leaflet portion and be associated with significant regurgitation. A torn aortic leaflet portion prolapses into the LV outflow in diastole and that of a mitral valve prolapses into the LA in systole (Fig. 10.8). Unless there are other associated abnormalities of extensive valve infection (i.e., other vegetation, abscess, and fistula), a torn leaflet cannot be clearly differentiated from a primary or associated vegetation (48).

### Libman-Sacks Endocarditis

Libman-Sacks vegetations (characteristic of systemic lupus erythematosus) have similar characteristics to those of infective vegetations. They are located at the leaflet's line of closure but are of heterogeneous echo-reflectance, usually are sessile, and show mobility dependent of leaflet motion (Fig. 11.8) (25). However, they can be elongated and mobile. In addition, infective vegetations can co-

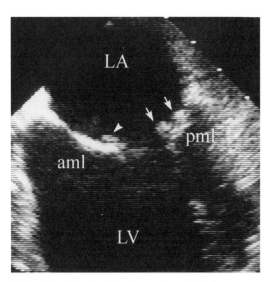

**FIG. 11.8.** Libman-Sacks endocarditis in a non-infected 37-year-old woman with systemic lupus erythematosus. Transesophageal echocardiographic four-chamber view demonstrates a small sessile mass with soft tissue echo-reflectant on the atrial side and distal portion of the anterior mitral leaflet (aml) *(arrowhead)*. Two other sessile masses with similar characteristics were demonstrated on the posterior mitral leaflet (pml) *(arrows)*. Associated thickening of both mitral leaflets and mild mitral regurgitation were noted. Abbreviations as in previous figures.

exist with Libman-Sacks vegetations in the same or different heart valve.

### Rheumatic Valvulitis

Acute rheumatic endocarditis is associated with predominantly mild MR and AR, but moderate to severe lesions are uncommon. Also, valve masses can be seen in at least 25% of these patients. These valve masses are located on the body and tip of the leaflets and are seen predominantly on the mitral valve (>80%). Therefore, in the appropriate geographic locations, it may be difficult to differentiate infective from rheumatic endocarditis (23).

### Nonbacterial Thrombotic Vegetations

NBTVs are seen in patients with malignancies or hypercoagulable states. These masses are associated with underlying mildly thickened or normal leaflets; are found predominantly on the atrial side of the mitral but on the ventricular side of the aortic valve leaflets; and most commonly are located at the closure margins of the leaflets. Therefore, echocardiographically these valve masses are indistinguishable from infective vegetations (49).

### Papillary Fibroelastoma

Papillary fibroelastomas are rare benign cardiac tumors seen predominantly on the aortic (ventricular side) and mitral valves (atrial side). They usually are small (<2 cm), have heterogeneous echo-reflectance, appear frondlike, are attached to the valve by a stalk usually away from the coaptation point, and are hypermobile. The underlying leaflet may be normal or minimally thickened and usually does not cause valve dysfunction (regurgitation). They usually are diagnosed incidentally or when first manifested with systemic embolism (50).

## NATURAL HISTORY AND PROGNOSIS

Unrecognized IE usually results in progressive and significant valve destruction and high morbidity and mortality. After successful medical therapy, 25% to 30% of native valve vegetations resolve; 15% to 20% decrease in size; 35% to 40% persist unchanged in size; and 10% to 15% increase in size. Persistent vegetations commonly become fibrosed or rarely become calcified (51).

In successfully treated IE, relapses (within 6 months of therapy by the same microorganism), recurrences (after 6 months of therapy by different microorganism), and need for valve replacement occur in 3%, 11%, and 20% of patients, respectively (52).

Infective endocarditis caused by *S. aureus, S. epidermidis,* Gram-negative bacilli (*Escherichia coli, Serratia* sp, *P. aeruginosa*), and fungi is associated with worse outcomes.

Infective endocarditis in the elderly (>65 years old) or in patients with renal or heart failure, systemic embolism, or neurologic dysfunction have high mortality (up to 40%) (21).

Patients at highest risk for embolism have recently formed, large (>10 mm), mobile, pedunculated vegetations, especially those attached to the mobile structures of the mitral leaflets. Patients with significant valve dysfunction (regurgitation, abscesses, perforations, fistulas, or pseudoaneurysms) also have a poor prognosis (operative mortality 15% to 30% and overall survival at 1 to 2 years of 50% to 70%) (30).

Native aortic valve IE is generally more severe and of worse prognosis than mitral or right-sided IE. Prosthetic valve IE carries the worst prognosis of all because of the high incidence of associated ring abscesses leading to ring dehiscence and significant paraprosthetic regurgitation, septic embolism, persistent sepsis, and recurrent infection after medical or surgical therapy. Patients with uncomplicated prosthetic valve IE have up to 20% mortality with medical therapy, but up to 80% to 100% mortality if complicated. In these patients, surgical mortality without and

with complications is 10% and up to 50%, respectively (38).

The prognosis of right-sided IE in IVDA is good (4% to 5% mortality rate), but recurrences are frequent (up to 30% of cases). Causes of death include pulmonary disease, LV endocarditis, and AIDS-related complications. Right-sided IE associated with pacemaker wires and catheters is associated with an in-hospital mortality of 5% to 10% and a 12- to 24-month mortality of 25% to 30%.

Despite improvements in medical and surgical therapy, the overall mortality of IE is still high (approximately 20%).

## PREVENTION

Infective endocarditis is associated with significant morbidity and mortality. Therefore, the recognition by a careful history and physical examination or echocardiography of heart disease prone to endocarditis is of importance. In these patients, antibiotic therapy given before a procedure expected to produce bacteremia may prevent the development of IE (53). The antibiotic regimen for dental and oral procedures is directed

**TABLE 11.9.** *Cardiovascular conditions and procedures for which prophylaxis is recommended*

| High-risk cardiovascular conditions | Intermediate-risk cardiovascular conditions |
|---|---|
| Mechanical prosthetic heart valves | PDA, VSD, coarctation of the aorta |
| Bioprosthetic valves (homograft and allograft) | MVP with clinical evidence of MR[a] |
| Previous infective endocarditis | Acquired valvular heart disease |
| Cyanotic congenital heart disease | Mitral or pulmonic valve stenosis |
| Systemic-pulmonary shunts or conduits | Tricuspid valve disease |
| Mitral regurgitation or stenosis | Bicuspid aortic valve |
| Aortic regurgitation or stenosis | Degenerative valvular heart disease |
| | Repaired intracardiac lesions (within 6 mo) |
| | Hypertrophic cardiomyopathy with latent or resting obstruction |
| Bacteremic procedures | |
| Dental procedures associated with bleeding | |
| Tonsillectomy/adenoidectomy | |
| Gastrointestinal or genitourinary surgery | |
| Bronchoscopy with rigid bronchoscope | |
| Esophageal sclerotherapy or dilation | |
| Cystoscopy or urethral dilation | |
| Urethral catheter if urinary tract infection | |
| Incision and drainage of abscess | |

[a]Male patients >45 yr old with mitral valve prolapse (MVP) without mitral regurgitation (MR), but with leaflet thickening (>5 mm) and/or redundancy may be at increased risk for bacterial endocarditis. In addition, about one third of patients with MVP without MR at rest may have exercise or other maneuvers induce MR.
PDA, patent ductus arteriosus; VSD, ventricular septal defect.

against streptococci, which are normal inhabitants of the oral cavity. For genitourinary and lower gastrointestinal procedures, antibiotic prophylaxis is designed to cover enterococci and other Gram-negative organisms. The risk for IE and, therefore, the need and benefit of antibiotic prophylaxis are determined by the interaction of the underlying heart disease and the risk of the procedure to produce significant bacteremia. Underlying heart disease and procedures for which antibiotic prophylaxis is indicated are listed in Table 11.9. However, up to 85% of IE due to *S. viridans* cannot be associated with bacteremic procedures and only 30% to 40% of IE cases due *S. aureus* have an identifiable source.

## SUMMARY

### Diagnostic Value of History, Physical Examination, and Echocardiography

A careful history and physical examination are unquestionably of essential importance for recognition of underlying heart disease, prevention, and early and accurate diagnosis of IE. Indication for echocardiography is based on results of the history, physical examination, and available microbiology results. Clinical data should guide a clinician in the decision to perform TTE or TEE. Of most importance, the diagnosis of IE can be made by clinical and microbiology data independently of echocardiographic findings. Echocardiography alone does not confirm or exclude the diagnosis of IE. Therefore, the integration of clinical data with echocardiographic findings is necessary for accurate diagnosis and risk stratification of IE.

Echocardiography, especially TEE, has definitely contributed to the current earlier and accurate diagnosis of IE. The importance of echocardiography is such that the diagnosis of IE frequently relies on the demonstration of endocardial disease. The presence or absence of valve vegetations (the earliest manifestation of endocarditis) has high positive and negative predictive value for IE. Echocardiography, especially TEE, also has high diagnostic accuracy in the detection or exclusion of valvular complications (i.e., abscesses, leaflet perforation, etc.). Echocardiography not only allows for the diagnosis of IE, but also for the stratification of patients into those with good or poor prognosis. It also helps to determine the need for surgical therapy. Accordingly, the ACC and AHA have established guidelines for the use of echocardiography in patients with suspected or known IE (Table 11.10) (54,55). In four of five class I indications for echocardiography in IE, it is stated that TEE may provide incremental diagnostic value to the information obtained by TTE. Therefore, in the author's opinion and based on the higher diagnostic accuracy of TEE compared to TTE for detection of valve vegetations and associated complications, patients with suspected IE should undergo TEE and, when necessary, a complementary but focused TTE.

---

**TABLE 11.10.** *Class I indications for echocardiography in infective endocarditis of native and prosthetic valves*

1. Detection and characterization of valvular lesions, their hemodynamic severity, and ventricular compensation[a]
2. Detection of vegetations and characterization of lesions in patients with congenital heart disease
3. Detection of abscesses, perforation, or fistulas[a]
4. Reevaluation studies in patients with complex endocarditis (virulent organism, severe hemodynamic lesion, aortic valve involvement, persistent fever or bacteremia, clinical change, or symptomatic deterioration)
5. Patients with highly suspected culture negative infective endocarditis[a]
6. Evaluation of bacteremia without a known source in a patient with a prosthetic valve[a]

[a]Transesophageal echocardiography may provide incremental value in addition to information obtained by transthoracic echocardiography.

## Limitations of History, Physical Examination, and Echocardiography

1. General and cardiovascular symptomatology associated with IE frequently is nonspecific.
2. The most common clinical manifestations of IE (fever and heart murmurs) frequently are nonspecific.
3. In patients with acute and severe valvular dysfunction (MR or AR) and heart failure, regurgitant murmurs may not be audible or may be attenuated.
4. With current earlier detection of IE, more specific and peripheral manifestations of IE (i.e., Osler nodes or Janeway lesions) are uncommon.
5. Echocardiography, including TEE, cannot clearly differentiate an active from a healed vegetation.
6. Echocardiography, including TEE, cannot accurately differentiate an infective vegetation from valve masses seen in patients with malignancies, inflammatory connective tissue diseases (i.e., SLE) with or without antiphospholipid syndrome, rheumatic valvulitis, a noninfective flail portion of a native mitral valve, or a torn bioprosthetic mitral or aortic leaflet.
7. Valvular thickening or calcification, benign leaflet nodules (nodules of Arantii), valve excrescences, suture material around a sewing ring (especially after mitral valve replacement), valve thrombus, or pannus formation on valve structures may mimic vegetations.
8. TTE has limited sensitivity for the detection of native and prosthetic valve vegetations and associated complications (abscesses, perforations, fistulas).
9. TTE is technically difficult or limited in at least 5% to 10% of the general population.

## REFERENCES

1. Bansal RC. Infective endocarditis. Med Clin North Am 1995;79:1205–1240.
2. Spirito P, Rapezzi C, Bellone P, et al. Infective endocarditis in hypertrophic cardiomyopathy: prevalence, incidence, and indications of antibiotic prophylaxis. Circulation 1999;99:2132–2137.
3. Lamas CC, Eykyn SJ. Bicuspid aortic valve—a silent danger: analysis of 50 cases of infective endocarditis. Clin Infect Dis 2000;30:336–341.
4. Robinson DL, Fowler VG, Sexton DJ, et al. Bacterial endocarditis in hemodialysis patients. Am J Kidney Dis 1997;30:521–524.
5. Durack DT, Lukes AS, Bright DK. New criteria for diagnosis of infective endocarditis: utilization of specific echocardiographic findings. Duke Endocarditis Service. Am J Med 1994;96:200–209.
6. Cecchi E, Parrini I, Chinaglia A, et al. New diagnostic criteria for infective endocarditis. A study of sensitivity and specificity. Eur Heart J 1997;18:1149–1156.
7. Lamas CC, Eykyn SJ. Suggested modifications to the Duke criteria for the clinical diagnosis of native valve and prosthetic valve endocarditis: analysis of 118 pathology proven cases. Clin Infect Dis 1997;25:713–719.
8. Hecht SR, Berger M. Right-sided endocarditis in intravenous drug users. Prognostic features in 102 episodes. Ann Intern Med 1992;117:560–566.
9. Laguno M, Miro O, Font C, et al. Pacemaker-related endocarditis. Report of 7 cases and review of the literature. Cardiology 1998;90:244–248.
10. Watanabe G, Haverich A, Speier R, et al. Surgical treatment of active infective endocarditis with paravalvular involvement. J Thorac Cardiovasc Surg 1994;107:171–177.
11. Afridi I, Apostolidou MA, Saad RM, et al. Pseudoaneurysms of the mitral-aortic intervalvular fibrosa: dynamic characterization using transesophageal echocardiographic and Doppler techniques. J Am Coll Cardiol 1995;25:137.
12. Shively BK, Gurule FT, Roldan CA, et al. Diagnostic value of transesophageal compared with transthoracic echocardiography in infective endocarditis. J Am Coll Cardiol 1991;18:391–397.
13. Lindner JR, Case RA, Dent JM, et al. Diagnostic value of echocardiography in suspected endocarditis. An evaluation based on the pretest probability of disease. Circulation 1996;93:730–736.
14. Werner GS, Schulz R, Fuchs JB, et al. Infective endocarditis in the elderly in the era of transesophageal echocardiography: clinical features and prognosis compared with younger patients. Am J Med 1996;100:90–97.
15. Klug D, Lacroix D, Savoye C, et al. Systemic infection related to endocarditis on pacemaker leads. Clinical presentation and management. Circulation 1997;95:2098–2107.
16. Horner SM, Bell JA, Swanton RH. Infected right atrial thrombus—an important but rare complication of central venous lines. Eur Heart J 1993;14:138–140.
17. Rambaldi M, Ambrosone L, Migliaresi S, et al. Infective endocarditis presenting as polyarthritis. Clin Rheumatol 1998;17:518–520.
18. DeCastro S, Cartoni D, d'Amati G, et al. Diagnostic accuracy of transthoracic and multi-plane transesophageal echocardiography for valvular perforation in acute infective endocarditis: correlation with anatomic findings. Clin Infect Dis 2000;30:825–826.
19. Knosalla C, Weng Y, Yankah AC, et al. Surgical treatment of active infective aortic valve endocarditis with

associated peri-annular abscess—11 year results. Eur Heart J 2000;21:490–497.

20. Tischler MD, Vaitkus PT. The ability of vegetation size on echocardiography to predict clinical complications: a meta-analysis. J Am Soc Echocardiogr 1997;10: 562–568.

21. Roder BL, Wandall DA, Espersen F, et al. Neurologic manifestations in Staphylococcus aureus endocarditis: a review of 260 bacteremic cases in non-drug addicts. Am J Med 1997;102:379–386.

22. Shaikholeslami R, Tomlinson CW, Teoh KH, et al. Mycotic aneurysm complicating staphylococcal endocarditis. Can J Cardiol 1999;15:217–222.

23. Vasan RS, Shrivastava S, Vijayakumar M, et al. Echocardiographic evaluation of patients with acute rheumatic fever and rheumatic carditis. Circulation 1996;94:73.

24. Hojnik M, George J, Ziporen L, et al. Heart valve involvement (Libman-Sacks endocarditis) in the antiphospholipid syndrome. Circulation 1996;93:1579.

25. Roldan CA, Shively BK, Crawford MH. An echocardiographic study of valvular heart disease associated with systemic lupus erythematosus. N Engl J Med 1996;335:1424–1430.

26. Heidenreich PA, Masoudi FA, Maini B, et al. Echocardiography in patients with suspected endocarditis: a cost-effectiveness analysis. Am J Med 1999;107: 198–208.

27. Sanfilippo AJ, Picard MH, Newell JB, et al. Echocardiographic assessment of patients with infectious endocarditis: prediction of risk for complications. J Am Coll Cardiol 1991;18:1191–1199.

28. Rohmann S, Erbel R, Gorge G, et al. Clinical relevance of vegetation localization by transoesophageal echocardiography in infective endocarditis. Eur Heart J 1992; 13:446–452.

29. Daniel WG, Mugge A, Martin RP, et al. Improvement in the diagnosis of abscesses associated with endocarditis by transesophageal echocardiography. N Engl J Med 1991;324:795–800.

30. Choussat R, Thomas D, Isnard R, et al. Peri-valvular abscesses associated with endocarditis: clinical features and prognostic factors of overall survival in series of 233 cases. Perivalvular Abscesses French Multi-centre Study. Eur Heart J 1999;20:232–241.

31. Lytle BW, Priest BP, Taylor PC, et al. Surgical treatment of prosthetic valve endocarditis. J Thorac Cardiovasc Surg 1996;111:198–207.

32. David TE. The surgical treatment of patients with prosthetic valve endocarditis. Semin Thorac Cardiovasc Surg 1995;7:47–53.

33. Shapiro SM, Young E, De Guzman S, et al. Transesophageal echocardiography in diagnosis of infective endocarditis. Chest 1994;105:377–382.

34. Job FP, Franke S, Lethen H, et al. Incremental value of biplane and multiplane transesophageal echocardiography for the assessment of active infective endocarditis. Am J Cardiol 1995;75:1033–1037.

35. Victor F, De Place C, Camus C, et al. Pacemaker lead infection: echocardiographic features, management, and outcome. Heart 1999;81:82–87.

36. Jarwe M, Klug D, Beregi JP, et al. Single center experience with femoral extraction of permanent endocardial pacing leads. Pacing Clin Electrophysiol 1999;22: 1202–1209.

37. Rubinstein E, Lang R. Fungal endocarditis. Eur Heart J 1995;16[Suppl B]:84–89.

38. Lengyel M. The impact of transesophageal echocardiography on the management of prosthetic valve endocarditis: experience of 31 cases and review of the literature. J Heart Valve Dis 1997;6:204–211.

39. Sett SS, Hudon MP, Jamieson WR, et al. Prosthetic valve endocarditis: experience with porcine bioprostheses. J Thorac Cardiovasc Surg 1993;105:428–434.

40. Lowry RW, Zoghbi WA, Baker WB, et al. Clinical impact of transesophageal echocardiography in the diagnosis and management of infective endocarditis. Am J Cardiol 1994;73:1089–1091.

41. Cormier B, Vahanian A. Echocardiography and indications for surgery. Eur Heart J 1995;16[Suppl B]:68–71.

42. Acar J, Michel PL, Varenne O, et al. Surgical treatment of infective endocarditis. Eur Heart J 1995;16[Suppl B]:94–98.

43. Yu VL, Fang GD, Keys TF, et al. Prosthetic valve endocarditis: superiority of surgical valve replacement versus medical therapy only. Ann Thorac Sur 1994;58: 1073–1077.

44. Hendren WG, Morris AS, Rosenkranz ER, et al. Mitral valve repair for bacterial endocarditis. J Thorac Cardiovasc Surg 1992;103:124–128.

45. Eishi K, Kawazoe K, Kuriyama Y, et al. Surgical management of infective endocarditis associated with cerebral complications: multi-center retrospective study in Japan. J Thorac Cardiovasc Surg 1995;110:1745–1755.

46. Roldan CA, Shively BK, Crawford MH. Valve excrescences: prevalence, evolution and risk for cardioembolism. J Am Coll Cardiol 1997;30:1308–1314.

47. Shyu KG, Lei MH, Hwang JJ, et al. Morphologic characterization and quantitative assessment of mitral regurgitation with ruptured chordae tendineae by transesophageal echocardiography. Am J Cardiol 1992;70: 1152–1156.

48. Alam M, Serwin JB, Rosman HS, et al. Transesophageal echocardiographic features of normal and dysfunctioning bioprosthetic valves. Am Heart J 1991; 121:1149.

49. Blanchard DG, Ross RS, Dittrich HC. Nonbacterial thrombotic endocarditis. Assessment by transesophageal echocardiography. Chest 1992;102: 954–956.

50. Yee HC, Nwosu JE, Lii AD, et al. Echocardiographic features of papillary fibroelastoma and their consequences and management. Am J Cardiol 1997;80: 811–814.

51. Vuille C, Nidorf M, Weyman AE, et al. Natural history of vegetations during successful medical treatment of endocarditis. Am Heart J 1994;128:1200–1209.

52. Mansur AJ, Dal Bo CMR, Fukushima JT, et al. Relapses, recurrences, valve replacements, and mortality during long-term follow-up after infective endocarditis. Am Heart J 2001;141:78–86.

53. Dajani AS, Taubert KA, Wilson W, et al. Prevention of bacterial endocarditis. Recommendations by the American Heart Association. JAMA 1997;277:1794–1801.

54. Cheitlin MD, Alpert JS, Armstrong WF, et al. ACC/AHA guidelines for the clinical application of echocardiography. Circulation 1997;95:1686–1744.

55. Bonow RO, Carabello B, De Leon AC, et al. ACC/AHA guidelines for the management of patients with valvular heart disease. J Am Coll Cardiol 1998;32:1486–1588.

# 12

# The Patient with Suspected Systemic Embolism

Gerald A. Charlton

*Department of Internal Medicine, University of New Mexico School of Medicine; and Department of
Internal Medicine, Veterans Affairs Medical Center, Albuquerque, New Mexico*

## INTRODUCTION

Acute neurologic ischemic syndromes and suspected peripheral emboli account for a substantial number of referrals to the echocardiography laboratory. In 1997, stroke accounted for approximately 160,000 deaths in the United States, making it the third leading cause of death. There are about 600,000 patients with new or recurrent strokes every year, and approximately 14% of patients who survive a first stroke or transient ischemic attack (TIA) will have a recurrence within 1 year (1). Stroke prevalence ranges from 1.1% to 2.2% for men and from 0.8% to 1.9% for women, and the prevalence increases with increasing age. Similar epidemiologic data regarding other peripheral emboli are limited.

The precise etiology of an acute neurologic ischemic syndrome often is difficult to definitively identify in an individual patient. Possibilities include intrinsic local vascular disease and penetrating artery disease (lacunar infarcts), atheromatous emboli from proximal vessels, including the ascending aorta, and emboli of cardiac origin. It has

been estimated that a cardioembolic mechanism may be responsible for approximately 20% of ischemic strokes, with another 30% to 40% being labeled as "cryptogenic," many of which may have an underlying cardiac etiology (Fig. 12.1).

Even the definition of a cardioembolic event is not straightforward. It was defined in 1989 by the Cerebral Embolism Task Force as the "presence of a potential cardioembolic source in the absence of cerebrovascular disease in a patient with a nonlacunar stroke" (2). Obviously, there is no "gold standard" by which to make this diagnosis.

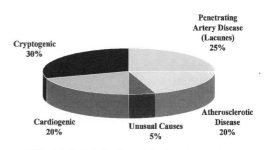

**FIG. 12.1.** Etiologies of ischemic strokes.

More difficult than finding an abnormality on an echocardiogram that may represent a potential source of embolus is deciding how such findings should alter therapy in an effort to reduce the risk of a recurrent event. Data are lacking on the optimal therapy for many of the abnormalities identified on echocardiography that have been associated with strokes and systemic embolization. Therefore, the utility of routine echocardiograms in the workup of patients with acute neurologic syndromes remains undefined.

## HISTORY

Certain aspects of a patient's clinical course increase the likelihood that cardioemboli may be the etiology of a systemic embolus. For cerebrovascular accidents or TIAs, these include sudden or abrupt onset of symptoms, findings consistent with middle or anterior cerebral circulation ischemia, and multiple events in different territories.

According to the National Institute of Neurological Disorders and Stroke (NINDS) Stroke Data Bank, patients with a cardioembolic source were more likely to have sudden onset of symptoms, other systemic emboli, decreased level of consciousness, aphasia, visual field defects, hemineglect, or large or multiple defects on neuroimaging (3).

As we will see later in the discussion on the use of echocardiography in this patient group, a history of cardiovascular disease has a significant influence on the utility and findings on echocardiography. These historic elements include a history of atrial fibrillation, hypertension, myocardial infarction, congestive heart failure, and valvular heart disease.

## PHYSICAL EXAMINATION

Systemic emboli can present with a multitude of manifestations, depending on the vascular territory involved.

Cerebral emboli (stroke or TIA) typically present with a focal neurologic deficit, which varies according to the particular cerebral artery territory involved. Occlusion of an ophthalmic artery leads to total or partial monocular blindness. Emboli involving the anterior cerebral artery cause contralateral weakness, predominantly of the leg. Occlusion of the anterior branch of the middle cerebral artery predominantly leads to contralateral motor and sensory loss of the face, hand, and arm, and nonfluent (Broca) aphasia, whereas occlusion of the posterior branch leads to contralateral hemisensory loss, homonymous hemianopsia, and fluent (Wernicke) aphasia. Vertebral artery strokes may present with binocular visual loss, quadriparesis, altered consciousness, ipsilateral cranial nerve or contralateral limb abnormalities, dysarthria, diplopia, vertigo, and ataxia.

Acute limb ischemia from a systemic embolus leads to severe limb pain, paresthesias, motor dysfunction, and loss of distal pulses. Of all noncerebral arterial emboli, approximately 60% are to the leg and 20% to the arm (4).

Emboli may cause visceral artery occlusion and can lead to mesenteric artery ischemia with symptoms of severe abdominal pain with or without peritoneal signs. Splenic infarction may present with left upper quadrant or left shoulder pain and a left pleural effusion. Infarction of a renal artery causes flank pain and gross or microscopic hematuria.

As is true for the history, findings on physical examination should focus on uncovering or quantifying cardiovascular abnormalities in patients suspected of having suffered a cardioembolic event. These include findings such as hypertension, the irregularly irregular rhythm of atrial fibrillation, the third heart sound and double apical impulse of a left ventricular aneurysm, or the diastolic murmur of mitral stenosis. Clinical signs and symptoms of endocarditis include fever, a new or changing murmur, fatigue, and a high erythrocyte sedimentation rate. Obviously, none of these findings is sufficiently sensitive or specific for a cardiac source of embolism, but rather increases the likelihood of finding a substrate for intracardiac thrombus with the potential for embolization.

## ECHOCARDIOGRAPHY

Echocardiography, either by transthoracic echocardiography (TTE) or transesophageal echocardiography (TEE), commonly is utilized in the evaluation of patients with suspected emboli of cardiac origin. The purpose of echocardiography in stroke patients is threefold: (i) detection of cardiac sources of cerebral emboli, (ii) selection of appropriate therapy, and (iii) prevention of recurrent strokes (5).

Long-term stroke recurrence rates range from approximately 4% to 14% per year (6). These numbers are based on studies such as those from Framingham (5-year recurrence 42% for men, 24% for women) and the Mayo Clinic (5-year recurrence 29%). Recurrent events are generally due to the same cause as the initial stroke or TIA, with lacunar strokes having the lowest likelihood of recurrence, atheromatous strokes the highest, and cardioembolic strokes intermediate.

In a scientific statement on secondary prevention in patients with prior stroke or TIA, the American Heart Association (AHA) divided cardioembolic stroke patients into two groups (6). First are patients with a definite source for cardioemboli (atrial fibrillation, left ventricular thrombus, and prosthetic heart valves), each of which should be treated with oral anticoagulation unless contraindicated. All other subtypes of embolic stroke are grouped under the category of "possible sources" and should be treated with antiplatelet agents. Studies are under way to evaluate oral anticoagulation in some subsets of this group. These recommendations are important in that they stress that the optimal therapy for many possible causes of cardiac embolism has not yet been determined.

Abnormalities sought on echocardiographic evaluation can be subdivided into abnormal intracardiac masses, abnormalities that may predispose to development of intracardiac thrombi, and abnormalities that may serve as potential sources for systemic embolism (7). Intracardiac masses include left atrial and left ventricular thrombi, cardiac tumors, and vegetations. Abnormalities that may predispose to development of intracardiac thrombi include left ventricular aneurysms, rheumatic mitral stenosis, spontaneous echo contrast (SEC), and atrial fibrillation. Much attention has been focused on other abnormalities that may serve as potential sources of emboli, such as patent foramen ovale (PFO) and atrial septal aneurysms. The optimal treatment for these conditions is unknown or unproved.

It has been demonstrated for years that echocardiography can be used to help identify possible sources of emboli. In 1983, Come et al. (8) reported on 280 patients who underwent TTE as part of their workup for ischemic stroke. Thirty-five percent had an abnormality that "might" be associated with a source of emboli. These findings included left atrial enlargement, rheumatic mitral valve disease, prosthetic heart valves, left ventricular aneurysm, and left ventricular dysfunction. Four percent (11 patients) had abnormalities classified as "possible or probable" sources of emboli, including intracardiac thrombi, left atrial myxomas, and valvular vegetations. As has been borne out in subsequent studies, the probability of finding an abnormality on echocardiography that may be associated with cardiac emboli was much higher for patients with clinical evidence of heart disease. Of patients with clinical evidence of heart disease, 47% had possible sources for emboli on echocardiography versus 14% in those without heart disease. All 11 patients with possible or probable sources of emboli had clinical heart disease.

When compared to control subjects without a history of emboli, many identifiable abnormalities are more prevalent in patients with suspected emboli, such as left atrial thrombus, atrial septal aneurysm, PFO, SEC, and aortic atheroma (9). Similarly, patients identified as having a "cryptogenic" cause for their stroke also have an increased prevalence of these findings.

### Specific Lesions Associated with Systemic Embolization

#### *Left Ventricular Thrombus*

Thrombi in the left ventricle usually are associated with a segment of dyskinetic myocardium and aneurysm formation, especially in the apical region (Fig. 12.2). This is most commonly secondary to a prior myocardial infarction, although ventricular thrombi also can be seen in the setting of dilated cardiomyopathy with severely depressed left ventricular systolic function. Both TTE and TEE have a similar sensitivity of approximately 85% to 95%, although apical thrombi may be better seen with TTE from the apex, especially with harmonic imaging and/or myocardial contrast agents (Fig. 12.3A–B). In some patients, TTE is limited secondary to poor echocardiographic windows, chronic lung disease, or obesity. Such patients may require TEE to help identify and define an intraventricular thrombus.

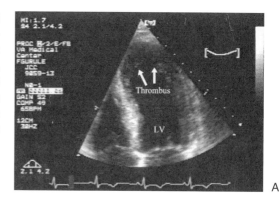
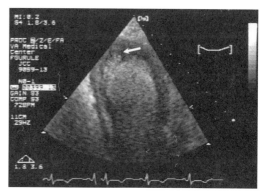

**FIG. 12.3. A:** Noncontrast apical view of the left ventricle (LV) obtained using harmonic imaging. It is difficult to discern if there is thrombus present in the apex. **B:** Contrast-enhanced apical view of the LV, with evidence of contrast infiltrating an apical thrombus.

#### *Left Atrial Mass*

Masses found in the left atrium include thrombi, especially in the left atrial appendage, which are associated with atrial fibrillation or mitral stenosis (Fig. 12.4). Multiplanc probes improve the ability to identify the left atrial appendage, usually at around 30 to 40 degrees of rotation from the basilar short-axis view of the aortic valve. Because the appendage has pectinate muscles, care must be taken to identify thrombi as irregularly shaped masses, separate and distinct from the underlying myocardium (see Figure 2.8).

Tumors can be found in the left atrium. The most common primary cardiac tumor is a myxoma, usually found in the left atrium and most commonly attached to the atrial septum

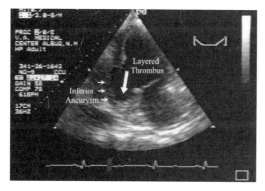

**FIG. 12.2.** Large inferior wall left ventricular aneurysm with associated layered thrombus.

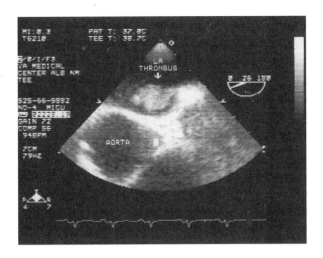

**FIG. 12.4.** Thrombus attached to the anterolateral wall of the left atrium (LA), as seen by transesophageal echocardiography.

by a stalk. Many of these tumors can be visualized on TTE, but some may require TEE to completely define and identify suspected left atrial masses.

SEC or "smoke" can be found in the left atrium, especially in patients with atrial fibrillation or low cardiac output (Fig. 12.5). This phenomenon is thought to be caused by slow blood flow and rouleau formation by the red blood cells. SEC is associated with the presence of left atrial thrombi and increased thromboembolic risk (10).

TEE has been reported to have a sensitivity of >95% for atrial masses, due to the close proximity of the probe to the left atrium and the use of higher-frequency transducers. TTE

has much lower sensitivity, ranging from approximately 40% to 60%, and is dependent on the size of the mass.

### Valvular Abnormality

Abnormalities of the aortic and mitral valves associated with systemic emboli include vegetations from infective endocarditis (Fig. 12.6A–B) as well as those associated with nonbacterial thrombotic endocarditis. Valvular vegetations have been identified using M-mode echocardiography, but two-dimensional echocardiography is the preferred method. Vegetations usually appear to have a lower level of reflectance than the normal underlying

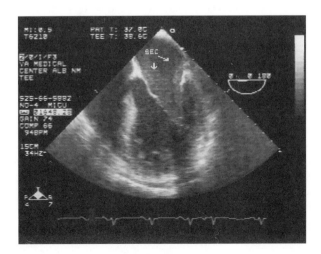

**FIG. 12.5.** Left atrial spontaneous echo contrast (SEC) seen by transesophageal echocardiography.

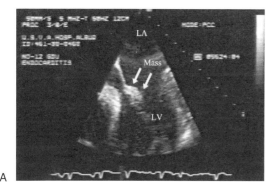

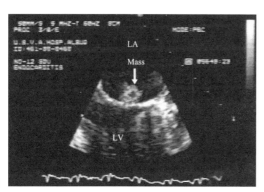

**FIG. 12.6. A:** Vegetation on the anterior mitral valve leaflet during diastole. **B:** Same vegetation seen in **A**, imaged during systole.

valve tissue and are seen on the upstream side of the valve (on the atrial side of the mitral valve and the ventricular side of the aortic valve). They usually are lobulated, mobile, and amorphous (11). TEE is the preferred method to evaluate for evidence of endocarditis, with reported sensitivity and specificity of well over 95% compared with TTE, which has a similar specificity but much lower sensitivity of approximately 45% to 60% (12). TEE also is more sensitive in the evaluation of possible complications of endocarditis, such as abscess formation, which has therapeutic implications.

Prosthetic heart valves, especially mechanical valves, are another potential source for systemic emboli. TEE is more sensitive than TTE for valvular vegetations, especially small ones, although aortic valve imaging sometimes is problematic even from the transesophageal approach due to acoustic shadowing from the prosthetic valve itself.

Another potential source of emboli are Lambl's excrescences or fibrin strands. These fine strands can be found on the aortic, mitral, and tricuspid valves, usually near the coaptation point (see Figure 2.9). In 1997, Roldan et al. (13) demonstrated that these strands are not more prevalent in patients with stroke compared with controls, do not appear to significantly change when imaged serially over time, and do not appear to be associated with future cardioembolic events.

### Aortic Atheroma

Atheromatous material in the aorta can serve as a potential source of thrombi, fibrinous material, and cholesterol emboli. Such emboli may occur spontaneously, or they may be secondary to manipulation, such as during cardiac catheterization or surgery. Aortic atheromas can be divided into simple atheromas, which are smooth and protrude into the lumen <4 to 5 mm, and complex atheromas, which are >4 to 5 mm thick, appear irregular, and may demonstrate evidence of ulceration or mobile debris. Mobile atheromas appear to be strongly associated with systemic embolization (Fig. 12.7). TEE is required to make this diagnosis by echocardiography. It is performed by advancing the probe into the stomach, rotating the probe 180 degrees, and slowly withdrawing the probe while imaging in the transverse plan. Longitudinal imaging may be performed to help characterize any abnormal plaques found on transverse imaging. As the aortic arch is ap-

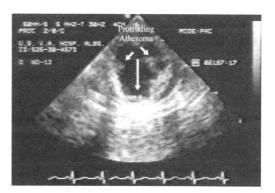

**FIG. 12.7.** Protruding and mobile atheroma in the descending aorta.

proached, a change in the imaging plane will be noted. A significant portion of the arch may be imaged by using omniplane transducers.

### Patent Foramen Ovale

PFO can be found in up to 10% to 15% of the normal population. Its prevalence appears to be much higher in patients with stroke, especially cryptogenic strokes, with rates up to 50% (9). Abnormal right to left shunting through a PFO can occur only when the right atrial pressure exceeds the left atrial pressure, which can occur transiently during straining or the Valsalva maneuver, or when the right heart pressures are chronically elevated, as can be seen in cor pulmonale or any cause of pulmonary hypertension. This abnormal right to left shunting may lead to paradoxic embolization of a venous thomboembolus into the arterial circulation.

The diagnosis can be made by both TTE and TEE, using either color flow Doppler and/or agitated saline contrast. Saline contrast studies are performed by drawing up a small amount of sterile saline into a syringe connected to a three-way stopcock. The saline is agitated by brisk injection from one syringe to another attached to the stopcock, then rapidly injected into a peripheral vein. This results in opacification of the right atrium and right ventricle; the two-dimensional image then is observed for evidence of abnormal right to left communication, defined as passage of more than three microbubbles into the left atrium within the first three cardiac cycles after complete opacification of the right atrium (Fig. 12.8). If negative, the study can be repeated while the patient performs a Valsalva maneuver, which causes a transient increase in right atrial pressure. Imaging is performed from either the apical four-chamber view or subcostal view when using TTE. TEE imaging is done directly over the thin fossa ovalis.

TEE is very sensitive for finding PFOs; TTE is less sensitive, especially for small PFOs. Once a PFO has been identified, the optimal treatment is controversial, ranging from no therapy to antiplatelet therapy to anticoagulant therapy and finally to surgical closure.

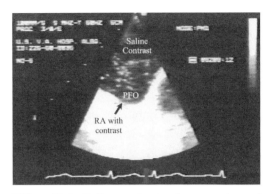

**FIG. 12.8.** Saline-contrast transesophageal echocardiogram of a small patent foramen ovale (PFO).

### Atrial Septal Aneurysm

An atrial septal aneurysm is redundant tissue in the intraatrial septum, in the region of the fossa ovalis. To meet criteria for this diagnosis, the septum must be hypermobile with a base >15 mm in size and with total excursion (into the right and left atria) of the redundant tissue exceeding 11 mm (Fig. 12.9). It is found in 1% to 5% of the normal population, but has been found in up to 22% of patients with a cryptogenic stroke. These aneurysms may be associated with tiny strands of fibrin or thrombus and frequently are associated with a PFO.

Atrial septal aneurysms are seen best on TTE using the subcostal or apical four-chamber views, and in the four-chamber view using

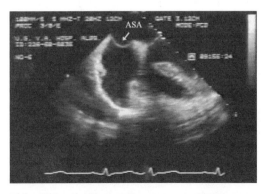

**FIG. 12.9.** Atrial septal aneurysm (ASA) seen on transesophageal echocardiographic four-chamber view.

the transverse plan from the mid esophagus on TEE.

### Transthoracic Versus Transesophageal Echocardiography

Many of the abnormalities being sought on echocardiography for evaluation of suspected cardiac emboli can be imaged adequately from the transthoracic approach. Recent advances, such as harmonic imaging and multiple-frequency transducers, have improved image resolution. Findings such as mitral stenosis, dilated cardiomyopathy, and left ventricular thrombus usually can be diagnosed from a high-quality, standard TTE.

However, many possible sources of emboli are better imaged using the transesophageal approach. Although TEE is a safe procedure, it is invasive and requires sedation of the patient to be performed comfortably. It also requires nursing support for patient monitoring during and after the study, as well as direct physician input during the acquisition of the images. Abnormalities best visualized using TEE include the left atrial appendage thrombus, aortic atheroma, atrial septal aneurysms, left atrial SEC, PFO, and valvular vegetations and excrescences. Regarding intracardiac masses or thrombi, pooled data suggest that, overall, no more than 11% of patients with stroke will have an intracardiac mass on TEE compared with 4% by TTE (5). When patients with and patients without clinical heart disease were analyzed, masses were more prevalent in the patients with heart disease by both TEE and TTE.

Pearson et al. (14) compared the utility of TTE versus TEE in a group of patients with unexplained stroke. They found that 57% of these patients had an abnormality that was a possible source for emboli on TEE versus only 15% by TTE. TEE was significantly better than TTE at demonstrating atrial septal aneurysm with PFO, left atrial thrombus or tumor, and left atrial SEC. Again, the echocardiogram found more possible sources of emboli in patients with known heart disease. In patients without clinical heart disease, the only abnormality for which TEE was better than TTE was atrial septal aneurysm associated with PFO.

### THERAPEUTIC IMPLICATIONS

There are very few series in the literature that look at recurrence rates of neurologic events for patients with specific cardiovascular abnormalities. Additionally, there are no randomized clinical trials using echocardiography to help guide therapy with patient outcome as the primary endpoint. Therapeutic trials that evaluate oral anticoagulation versus various platelet inhibitors, for entities such as atrial septal aneurysm, SEC, PFO, and aortic atheroma, are needed.

A recently published multicenter study attempted to evaluate the effect of echocardiography, specifically TEE, on the treatment and outcome in patients with unexplained cerebral ischemia. The STEPS (Significance of Transesophageal Echocardiography in the Prevention of recurrent Stroke) trial performed TEE in 242 patients with unexplained cerebral ischemia (15). Treatment was at the discretion of the patient's physician, who did have knowledge of the TEE results.

Sixty-one percent of the patients had an abnormal echocardiogram, with findings such as abnormal left ventricular function, PFO, intracardiac thrombus, atrial septal aneurysm, aortic plaque, and SEC. Additionally, 22% of the subjects were in atrial fibrillation at the time of the study. At the discretion of the treating physician, 132 subjects were treated with aspirin and 110 received warfarin. The warfarin-treated group was older, had lower ejection fractions, and had more atrial fibrillation than the aspirin-treated group, yet those treated with warfarin had a significantly lower incidence of recurrent events at 1 year (13% vs. 5%; p<0.02). There was no difference in the prevalence of any of the abnormalities found by TEE when comparing those who suffered a recurrent stroke to those who did not. There was a suggestion that patients with left ventricular enlargement or aortic plaque had fewer recurrent events when treated with warfarin, but no other lesion-specific differences in treatment were found.

**TABLE 12.1.** *Indications for echocardiography in patients with neurologic events or other vascular occlusive events*

| Clinical scenario | Class |
|---|---|
| Patients of any age with abrupt occlusion of a major peripheral or visceral artery | I |
| Younger patients (typically <45 yr) with cerebrovascular events | I |
| Older patients (typically >45 yr) with neurologic events without evidence of cerebrovascular disease or other obvious cause | I |
| Patients for whom a clinical therapeutic decision (anticoagulation, etc.) will depend on the results of echocardiography | I |

Data from reference 9.

## SUMMARY AND AVAILABLE GUIDELINES

The appropriate use of echocardiography in the evaluation of patients with suspected cardioemboli remains controversial. There are many possible options, including the following:

No routine echocardiograms
Routine TTE
Routine TEE
Routine TTE followed by TEE if findings are noncontributory
Selective TTE or TEE in patients with cardiac disease who would not otherwise receive anticoagulation

There are currently two guidelines in the literature addressing the issue of echocardiography in stroke/systemic embolism. The first, published in 1997 by the American College of Cardiology (ACC)/AHA (9), is a summary of appropriate application of echocardiography in the clinical setting. Section XI, "Neurological Disease and Other Cardioembolic Disease," reviews the prevalence of cardiac abnormalities found on echocardiography and lists recommendations for the use of echocardiography in patients with neurologic events or other vascular events (Table 12.1). No distinction is made between using TTE versus TEE.

The second guideline comes from the Canadian Task Force on Preventive Health Care (5). This document stresses the importance of evaluating the effectiveness of treatment, or lack thereof, for cardiac sources of emboli in relation to the performance of echocardiography in secondary prevention of stroke. Unlike the ACC/AHA guidelines, this document addresses the differences between TTE and TEE (Table 12.2).

Evaluation for a cardiac source of embolism is a frequent indication for referral to

**TABLE 12.2.** *Recommendations of the Canadian Task Force on Preventive Health Care for screening potential cardioembolic sources in patients with stroke*

| Maneuver | Level of evidence | Recommendation |
|---|---|---|
| Patients with clinical cardiac disease and no preexisting indications for anticoagulation | Case-control and cross-sectional studies | Fair evidence to recommend echocardiography in this group. Transesophageal echocardiography preferred initial screening test. |
| Patients with preexisting indications for anticoagulation or contraindications for anticoagulation | Case-control and cross-sectional studies | Fair evidence to recommend against echocardiography in this patient group |
| Patients without clinical cardiac disease | Case-control and cross-sectional studies | Insufficient evidence to recommend for or against echocardiography in this group |

Data from reference 5.

**TABLE 12.3.** *Sources of emboli*

| Definite | Probable | Possible |
|---|---|---|
| Left ventricular thrombus | Left ventricular aneurysm | Atrial septal aneurysm |
| Left atrial thrombus | Spontaneous echo contrast | Patent foramen ovale |
| Vegetation | Aortic atheroma | |
| Cardiac tumor | | |
| Atrial fibrillation | | |

the echocardiography laboratory. With echocardiography, especially TEE, many abnormalities that may be potential or definite sources for emboli can be found (Table 12.3).

Conversely, what to do with the information once a potential source has been found remains controversial. Some abnormalities, such as an intracardiac thrombus, have a recommended and accepted therapy, i.e., oral anticoagulation. For other abnormalities, such as aortic atheroma and atrial septal aneurysm, the best therapy remains to be elucidated in randomized clinical trials.

## REFERENCES

1. American Heart Association. 2000 heart and stroke statistical update. Dallas: American Heart Association, 1999.
2. Cerebral Embolism Task Force. Cardiogenic brain embolism. The second report of the Cerebral Embolism Task Force. Arch Neurol 1989;46:727–743.
3. NINDS Stroke Data Bank.
4. Abbott WM, Maloney RD, McCabe CC, et al. Arterial embolism: a 44-year perspective. Am J Surg 1982;143:460.
5. Kapral MK, Silver FL, with the Canadian Task Force on Preventive Health Care. Preventive health care, 1999 update: 2. Echocardiography for the detection of a cardiac source of embolus in patients with stroke. Can Med Assoc J 1999;161:989–996.
6. Wolf PA, Clagett P, Easton D, et al. Preventing ischemic stroke in patients with prior stroke and transient ischemic attack: a statement for healthcare professionals from the Stroke Council of the American Heart Association. Stroke 1999;30:1991–1994.
7. Otto CM. Textbook of clinical echocardiography. Philadelphia: WB Saunders, 2000.
8. Come PC, Riley MF, Bivas NK. Roles of echocardiography and arrhythmia monitoring in the evaluation of patients with suspected systemic embolism. Ann Neurol 1983;13:527–531.
9. American College of Cardiology/American Heart Association Task Force on Practice Guidelines (Committee on Clinical Application of Echocardiography). ACC/AHA guidelines for the clinical application of echocardiography. Circulation 1997;95:1686–1744.
10. Daniel WG, Nellessen U, Schroder E, et al. Left atrial spontaneous echo contrast in mitral valve disease: an indicator for an increased thromboembolic risk. J Am Coll Cardiol 1988;11:1204–1211.
11. Redberg RF. Echocardiographic evaluation of the patient with a systemic embolic event. In: Otto CM, ed. The practice of clinical echocardiography. Philadelphia: WB Saunders, 1997:629–648.
12. Shively BK, Gurule FT, Roldan CA, et al. Diagnostic value of transesophageal compared with transthoracic echocardiography in infective endocarditis. J Am Coll Cardiol 1991;18:391–397.
13. Roldan CA, Shively BK, Crawford MH. Valve excrescences: prevalence, evolution and risk for cardioembolism. J Am Coll Cardiol 1997;30:1308–1314.
14. Pearson AC, Labovitz AJ, Tatineni S, et al. Superiority of transesophageal echocardiography in detecting cardiac source of embolism in patients with cerebral ischemia of uncertain etiology. J Am Coll Cardiol 1991;17:66–72.
15. Labovitz AJ, for the STEPS Investigators. Transesophageal echocardiography and unexplained cerebral ischemia: a multicenter follow-up study. Am Heart J 1999;137:1082–1087.

# 13

# The Patient with Congenital Heart Disease

Phoebe A. Ashley and *M. Beth Goens

*Department of Internal Medicine, University of New Mexico School of Medicine; and Department of Internal Medicine, Veterans Affairs Medical Center, Albuquerque, New Mexico; *Department of Pediatrics, University of New Mexico School of Medicine; and Department of Pediatrics, University of New Mexico Health Sciences Center, Albuquerque, New Mexico*

Abnormalities of the heart and great vessels that are present from birth are termed congenital heart diseases. The most common congenital heart diseases, atrial septal defect (ASD), ventricular septal defect (VSD), patent ductus arteriosus (PDA), and coarctation of the aorta will be discussed.

## ATRIAL SEPTAL DEFECT

### Definition and Etiology

Three clinically significant ASDs are the primum, secundum, and sinoseptal defects (Fig. 13.1). A fourth form, a probe patent fora-

men ovale, occurs in up to 25% of people and is not considered a pathologic occurrence.

A primum defect is caused by failure of the endocardial cushions to meet the atrial septum. It is always associated with a cleft in the anterior leaflet of the mitral valve. This type of defect lies posteroinferior to the aortic root. Ostium primum defects account for approximately 20% of ASDs (1).

Sinoseptal defects include sinus venosus-type defects and unroofed coronary sinus. Superior vena cava (SVC) sinus venosus defects are the most common sinoseptal defects, accounting for about 10% of all ASDs. They occur at the most superior portion of the atrial

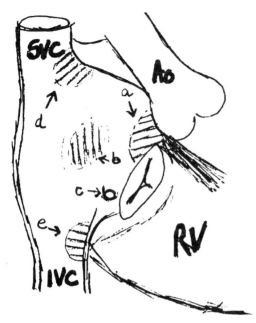

**FIG. 13.1.** Schematic representation of the right atrial side of the atrial septum. Letters and arrows indicate the location of the different types of atrial septal defects (ASD). **a:** Primum ASD located just behind the aorta (AO). **b:** Secundum ASD at the fossa ovalis. **c:** Coronary sinus ostium. This is either dilated or atretic in unroofed coronary sinus. If it is atretic, the left to right shunt is via retrograde flow in the left superior vena cava (SVC) through the innominate vein to the right SVC and right atrium. **d:** SVC sinus venosus ASD. **e:** Inferior vena cava (IVC) sinus venosus ASD. RV, right ventricle.

septum at the junction of the SVC with the right atrium (RA). There is nearly always anomalous drainage of the right upper and, commonly, middle pulmonary veins into the SVC. Inferior vena cava (IVC) sinus venous defects are accompanied by anomalous drainage of the right lower pulmonary vein. These defects are found inferior to the fossa ovalis at the IVC–RA junction. An unroofed coronary sinus is a defect between the LA and the coronary sinus that allows flow from the left atrium (LA) to the RA. These defects often are accompanied by persistence of the left SVC (Raghib Anomaly). Both the IVC sinus venosus and the unroofed coronary sinus are rare defects.

The most common ASD is the secundum defect. It is caused by a deficient septum primum that does not cover the ostium secundum. These defects are located centrally in the septum and can be multiple, the so-called fenestrated atrial septum.

### Pathophysiology

All types of ASD have the same hemodynamic consequences. There is left to right shunting across the defect with volume overload of the right ventricle (RV) and pulmonary vascular bed. The volume of the shunt is dependent upon the size of the defect and the relative compliance of the RV and left ventricle (LV) in diastole. RV volume overload causes diastolic flattening of the interventricular septum toward the LV. LV preload is decreased and cardiac output may be mildly diminished. Pulmonary blood flow will increase with subsequent enlargement of the pulmonary arteries and veins. The RV may pump 15 L/min through the pulmonary circulation compared to the 5 L/min output of the LV as in a 3:1 pulmonary to systemic flow ratio ($Q_p/Q_s$). There may be flow-related pulmonary hypertension, although usually pulmonary artery systolic pressure does not rise beyond 35 to 40 mm Hg in children. The torrential flow may result in a modest gradient (up to 40 mm Hg) across the RV outflow tract (in the absence of anatomic outflow obstruction) and in prolonged RV ejection time.

### Size of the Defect

In adults, if the defect is <1 cm² in area, it does not permit significant shunting, and LA pressure remains greater than RA pressure. Atrial defects of 2 to 3 cm² or larger result in a low-resistance shunt with near equalization of mean atrial pressures.

### Pulmonary Vascular Disease

The pulmonary arteriolar circulation in patients with large ASDs undergoes medial hypertrophy over time, but the intimal proliferation and small vessel occlusion of pulmonary vascular occlusive disease usually do not occur before the second decade of life. Over time, the continued volume overload of the pulmonary vascular bed leads to increases in pulmonary resistance. Consequently, the RV is confronted with an increasing pressure load that gradually replaces the previous volume load. With increased RV pressures, the degree of left to right shunting decreases, RV compliance decreases, and a dominant right to left shunt across the defect may occur. At this stage, there are irreversible morphologic changes in the pulmonary vessels, and pulmonary pressure equals or exceeds systemic arterial pressure. The development of right to left shunting, pulmonary hypertension, and cyanosis is classified as the Eisenmenger reaction.

### Incidence

ASDs account for approximately 7% of congenital heart lesions in children (Table 13.1). However, about 25% of patients in adult congenital heart disease clinics have ASDs, with a female predominance of 2:1 (2). The exact incidence is difficult to determine because children usually are asymptomatic and the ASD can be undiagnosed until adult life. Smaller secundum ASDs close spontaneously, usually in the first 2 years of life. Therefore, prevalence varies with the age of the population studied.

### History

Children with an ASD usually are asymptomatic. The exception is when there is LV cardiomyopathy or left-sided obstruction such as mitral stenosis, aortic stenosis, or coarctation of the aorta. These lesions cause increased LV diastolic pressure and encourage larger left to right shunts at the atrial level. The increased pulmonary blood flow may be the cause of a more protracted course of bronchiolitis or other lower respiratory tract infections. Adults with an ASD are asymptomatic until the third or fourth decade of life, but women may become symptomatic when they become pregnant at any age. Symptoms and signs include exercise intolerance, dyspnea on exertion, atrial arrhythmias, and pulmonary hypertension.

**TABLE 13.1.** *Relative frequency of congenital heart disease*

| Lesion | Percentage of all lesions |
| --- | --- |
| Ventricular septal defect | 25–30 |
| Atrial septal defect | 6–8 |
| Patent ductus arteriosus | 6–8 |
| Coarctation of the aorta | 5–7 |
| Tetralogy of fallot | 5–7 |
| Pulmonic valve stenosis | 5–7 |
| Aortic valve stenosis | 4–7 |
| Transposition of the great arteries | 3–5 |
| Hypoplastic left ventricle | 1–3 |
| Hypoplastic right ventricle | 1–3 |
| Truncus arteriosus | 1–2 |
| Total anomalous pulmonary venous return | 1–2 |
| Tricuspid atresia | 1–2 |
| Single ventricle | 1–2 |
| Double-outlet right ventricle | 1–2 |
| Others | 5–10 |

*Note:* The table excludes patent ductus arteriosus in the preterm neonate, bicuspid aortic valve, peripheral pulmonic stenosis, and mitral valve prolapse.

Adapted from Behrman RE, Kliegman RM, Arvin AM, et al. Nelson textbook of pediatrics, 15th ed. Philadelphia: WB Saunders, 1996:1286.

It is unusual to find a truly asymptomatic patient with an ASD after the age of 40 years unless the shunt is small (<1.2:1). About 15% of patients develop pulmonary hypertension and progressive pulmonary vascular obstructive disease between 20 and 40 years of age. Once this occurs, it can be rapidly progressive, causing a reversal of the shunt with arterial oxygen desaturation and eventual death. Late surgical closure of the ASD may not stop the progression of the pulmonary vascular obstructive disease. Large ASDs cause RA enlargement and eventually chronic atrial arrhythmias. The onset of LV disease of any cause (e.g., coronary artery disease, hypertension) may cause a secondary rise in LA pressure with a resultant increase in left to right shunting.

A patient with an ASD may be diagnosed with a "functional" systolic murmur for years until he becomes symptomatic. Thus, it is important for clinicians to keep ASD in mind when evaluating any adult with a pulmonic ejection murmur.

## Physical Examination

### General Appearance

In patients with a large left to right shunt, the left chest may bulge anteriorly due to the chronically dilated and hypertrophied RV. ASDs have been associated with rare disorders such as the Holt-Oram syndrome (absence of the thumbs and other bony defects of the hand and arm), Ehlers-Danlos syndrome (hyperplastic skin, kyphoscoliosis, hyperextensible joints), and Marfan syndrome. Patients with severe pulmonary hypertension and Eisenmenger syndrome will be cyanotic, and the distal phalanges will be clubbed.

### Arterial Pulse and Blood Pressure

There are no diagnostic abnormalities of the pulse contour or systemic blood pressure in patients with an ASD. In patients >40 years of age, the prevalence of atrial fibrillation is 20% to 30%. These patients will have an irregular pulse.

### Jugular Venous Pulse

Although the mean venous pressure is rarely elevated, the RA V wave characteristically is accentuated in patients with a large left to right shunt. The height of the RA V wave peak is roughly proportional to the size of the left to right shunt. The absence of a large V wave, however, does not rule out an ASD.

### Palpation

Chronic diastolic volume overload produces an enlarged and hyperdynamic RV. This results in a parasternal systolic impulse that is easily palpable at the left lower sternal border. The most common parasternal impulse has increased amplitude and normal duration (hyperdynamic motion) with retraction during late systole. This brief outward impulse may be subtle and felt only in held expiration, or it may be prominent, producing a forceful parasternal motion, depending upon the magnitude of the atrial shunt. To bring out the RV impulse, ask the patient to stop breathing at maximal inspiration and palpate the subxiphoid area with the fingers directed upwards. Large shunts can result in a sustained RV lift or heave, even in the absence of pulmonary hypertension. When a sustained parasternal heave is detected, the presence of pulmonary hypertension should be strongly suspected. Occasionally, a large left to right shunt will be associated with normal (impalpable) RV activity. In general, the more prominent the parasternal activity (amplitude and duration), the larger the left to right shunt.

Because the LV is normal in an uncomplicated ASD, palpable LV movement usually is minimal or absent. The RV may displace the LV posteriorly, further decreasing the likelihood of a palpable LV impulse.

Palpation of the upper left sternal region may reveal a lift or impulse in the second or third left intercostal space. This is caused by an enlarged RV outflow tract and dilated central pulmonary artery transmitting a large volume of blood during systole. Gentle palpation with the ball of the hand is best for detection of this subtle buzzing sensation. Such a finding suggests pulmonic stenosis that may be either functional or anatomic.

A palpable pulmonic valve component ($P_2$) in subjects with ASDs suggests the presence of pulmonary hypertension. Nevertheless, palpable pulmonary artery activity and an increased $P_2$ in the second or third left interspace can be seen with large left to right shunts and normal pulmonary artery pressure.

### Auscultation

#### Heart Sounds

The major characteristic of the first heart sound ($S_1$) in a subject with an ASD is increased amplitude of the second major component ($T_1$). Audible splitting of $S_1$ is common in adults. The classic second heart sound ($S_2$) in ASD is widely split in both expiration and inspiration, with little or no detectable respiratory variation. Splitting of $S_2$ tends to widen with age and typically is more prominent in adults than children. In fact, infants and young children with ASDs can have normal splitting of $S_2$. The combination of a large RV stroke volume and increased capacitance of the pulmonary arterial bed accounts for the wide splitting of $S_2$. Because the RA and LA communicate with one another, the stroke volume of each chamber varies in the same way throughout the respiratory cycle. Patients with pulmonary hypertension and RV failure from any cause may have narrowed, fixed splitting of $S_2$.

There are conflicting views as to whether a third heart sound ($S_3$) or fourth heart sound ($S_4$) may be commonly associated with an ASD in the absence of congestive heart failure. A physiologic $S_3$ may be heard in normal young children.

#### Opening Snap

The opening snap relates to atrial hypertension and rapid, torrential flow across the tricuspid valve and occurs at the point of maximum opening of the tricuspid leaflets. An opening snap suggests a pulmonary to systemic flow $\geq 2:1$. The opening snap of the tricuspid valve in an ASD is soft and lower pitched than the typical mitral valve opening snap. It is located at the lower left sternal border and may increase in intensity during inspiration.

#### Pulmonic Ejection Sound

An ejection click or sound may be present in as many as 50% of subjects with ASDs. The sound is best heard at the upper left sternal border (second to third left interspace) and is detected more easily during inspiration. It is softer and not as high in frequency as the pulmonic ejection sound of pulmonic stenosis. It is more likely to be present in patients with pulmonary hypertension.

#### Systolic Murmur

No audible sound is created by the low-pressure shunt flow across the atrial defect itself. The characteristic murmur is a *pulmonic ejection murmur* related to increased flow across the pulmonic valve. The murmur often is described as scratchy or superficial; it is rarely greater than grade 3/6 intensity. It is best heard at the upper left sternal border, in the second to fourth left intercostal spaces adjacent to the sternum. It may radiate into the lung fields in young children, but this radiation in adults suggests branch pulmonary artery stenosis.

The murmur has a crescendo-decrescendo shape. Typically there is a short, silent period after $S_1$ (during isovolumic contraction), followed by the murmur, which ends well before $S_2$. Generally, shorter murmurs accompany smaller shunts. A longer murmur suggests RV volume overload or associated pulmonic stenosis. If the intensity of the murmur is grade 4/6, there is associated pulmonic stenosis with an ejection sound.

#### Diastolic Murmur

In patients with large shunts and torrential flow across the tricuspid valve, a functional

RV filling murmur may be heard. This murmur is heard when the $Q_P/Q_S$ is >2:1. It begins early in diastole and is best heard at the lower left sternal border, in the fourth to fifth interspace. It has a crescendo-decrescendo shape and is described as a scratchy, superficial, rublike sound. Some have described it as "an absence of silence." It may simulate a loud $S_3$ when brief.

When LA pressure is abnormally elevated, a pressure differential across the atrial septum can exist, and the resultant flow across the defect may cause sufficient turbulence to produce a murmur. It is found when a small ASD coexists with either mitral stenosis (*Lutembacher syndrome*) or mitral regurgitation with elevated LA pressure.

## Echocardiography

The interatrial septum is a thin muscular membrane between the atria. The septum stretches from the posteromedial margin of the aortic root to the common posterior atrial wall and from the mid portion of the superior atrial border to the upper margin of the interventricular septum. In the mid portion of the septum is an oval depression, the fossa ovalis, which is the remnant of the fetal foramen ovale.

Direct visualization of the interatrial septum is the most accurate method to diagnose and localize these lesions. However, the diagnosis is suspected based upon indirect echocardiographic findings, such as RV dilation or flattening of the interventricular septum during diastole (paradoxic septal motion). These signs are indicative of volume overload. RV volume overload out of proportion to the size of the ASD suggests partial anomalous pulmonary venous return.

The goals of echocardiography in ASD are (i) identification of the precise location of the defect; (ii) demonstration of the pulmonary venous connections; (iii) exclusion of additional associated lesions; (iv) assessment of chamber size (dilation) and wall thickness (hypertrophy); (v) calculation of the magnitude of the left to right shunt (pulmonary blood flow); and (vi) estimation of pulmonary arterial pressure (3).

### M-Mode Echocardiography

Abnormal ventricular septal motion is appreciated on M-mode echocardiography of the ventricles from a parasternal view. M-mode echocardiography shows the RV dilation; however, because of the oblique angle of the M-mode cursor to the LV, this measurement can be difficult to reproduce.

### Two-Dimensional Echocardiography

Two-dimensional echocardiography has the advantage of showing other chambers for size comparison as well as demonstrating the entire septum as it flattens in diastole. During systole, the transseptal gradient is restored and the septum appears more rounded. RV dilation out of proportion to the size of the ASD suggests the presence of anomalous pulmonary venous return. All four pulmonary veins ideally should be visualized entering the LA in light of the common association (9% of secundum and 100% of sinus venosus defects) of anomalous pulmonary venous return in patients with ASDs (4).

Defects in the interatrial septum can be visualized directly using a variety of views: parasternal short-axis view at the aortic level; right parasternal long- and short-axis views; and subcostal long- and short-axis views. The diagnosis of an ASD should be based upon imaging the defect in multiple planes and systematic sweeps of the ultrasound beam. The subcostal window is particularly useful when imaging children, and the right parasternal window often is a useful alternative in older patients.

Defects appear as areas of focal dropout or as discontinuities in the normal band of echoes arising from the interatrial septum. The edges of a true defect usually are more echogenic and produce the *T-artifact* (5). The T-artifact gives the edges of a defect a broadened appearance, forming the image of a T, clearly marking the edges of a true defect and distinguishing it from echocardiographic dropout because of thinning of the septum in the fossa ovalis. Fig. 13.2 demonstrates the problem of imaging parallel to the septum from the apical four-chamber view. The false dropout in the area of the thin fossa ovalis gives the appearance of an ostium secundum defect. Note the absence of RV dilation in this patient with an intact atrial septum.

The apical four-chamber view can be useful in identifying ostium primum defects because the atrioventricular valves are at the same level and perpendicular to the imaging plane. Absence of tissue in the most anterior, inferior portion of the interatrial septum (at the level of insertion of the atrioventricular valves) is diagnostic and serves to differentiate an ostium primum defect from an ostium secundum defect. The presence of any atrial

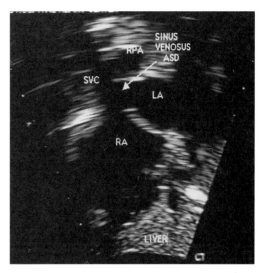

FIG. 13.3. Subcostal short-axis view of a sinus venosus atrial septal defect. This view is obtained by sweeping the patient's right atrium from the standard superior vena cava/inferior vena cava view. RPA, right pulmonary artery.

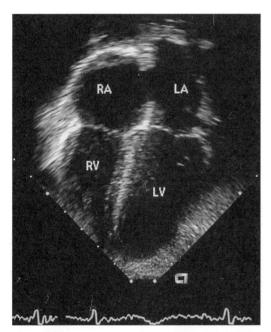

FIG. 13.2. Apical four-chamber view showing artifactual dropout in the region of the fossa ovalis. This shows the importance of imaging the atrial septum perpendicular to the ultrasound beam. This patient's atrial septum actually is intact, as was evident from the subcostal views. Note the lack of right ventricular dilation. Color Doppler can be helpful in this situation. LA, left atrium; LV, left ventricle; RA, right atrium; RV, right ventricle.

septal tissue above the base of the atrioventricular valves excludes the diagnosis of a primum defect. If an ostium primum defect is identified, the size of the cleft in the anterior leaflet of the mitral valve should be assessed. There can be chordal attachments of the anterior leaflet to the interventricular septum causing LV outflow obstruction.

Sinus venosus defects are best identified from the subcostal short-axis or right parasternal view. The transducer is positioned such that the SVC and IVC are aligned, then a rightward sweep is performed to identify the defect. The area of dropout is identified at the entry of the SVC or less commonly the IVC (Fig. 13.3).

### Contrast Echocardiography

Intravenous saline contrast echocardiography is sensitive in detecting a shunt at the atrial level. Right to left shunting is seen as the presence of contrast echoes in the LA. Left to right shunting is seen as a negative jet of blood interrupting the contrast echoes in the RA. Almost all patients with an interatrial communication demonstrate some right to left shunting. Right to left shunting during saline contrast studies may be enhanced by the Valsalva maneuver or by coughing.

### *Doppler Echocardiography*

Pulsed and color Doppler flow mapping from a subcostal approach may help to identify an ASD, confirm the presence of shunt flow (when two-dimensional imaging is incomplete), and differentiate artifactual echo dropout from a true ASD. Two-dimensional echocardiography and pulsed Doppler ultrasound can be used to estimate the magnitude of left to right shunting by calculating the pulmonary to systemic flow ratio ($Q_p/Q_s$).

### *Pulsed Wave Doppler*

Pulsed Doppler can be used to estimate pulmonary and systemic blood flow in patients with intracardiac shunts by measuring stroke volume at two intracardiac sites. The site for $Q_P$ analysis should be where the full pulmonary blood flow crosses. The site for $Q_S$ analysis should be where the full systemic blood flow crosses. Typically the pulmonary artery and LV outflow tract are chosen.

$$Q_p = CSA_{PA} \times VTI_{PA}$$

$$Q_s = CSA_{LVOT} \times VTI_{LVOT}$$

$$Q_p/Q_s = \frac{CSA_{PA} \times VTI_{PA}}{CSA_{LVOT} \times VTI_{LVOT}}$$

$Q_P$ = pulmonic volume flow

$Q_S$ = systemic volume flow

$CSA_{PA}$ = cross-sectional area of the pulmonary artery = $\pi(d/2)^2$

$CSA_{LVOT}$ = cross-sectional area of the LV outflow tract = $\pi(d/2)^2$

$VTI$ = velocity time integral (area under the Doppler envelope)

It is important to recognize that there are many limitations to the estimation of the $Q_P/Q_S$ ratio by Doppler. To use this equation, one must assume that laminar flow through a rigid tube is occurring. However, cardiac flow is not truly laminar, and the pulmonary artery is more distensible than the LV outflow tract. A VSD itself can disturb flow in the LV and RV outflow tracts.

### *Color Doppler*

Color Doppler techniques enhance detection of small septal shunts and provide accurate alignment of the cursor for pulsed wave Doppler interrogation. The presence of high flow at the level of the SVC suggests the presence of a sinus venosus ASD. All four pulmonary veins should be identified entering the LA. Imaging from the suprasternal notch in the horizontal plane demonstrates the pulmonary veins in the "crab view." If the color scale is decreased to approximately 30 cm/s, low-velocity flows are more easily identified. Any venous flow away from the heart is likely anomalous pulmonary venous return and warrants further investigation. Evaluation of the innominate vein and coronary sinus, as well as determination of the presence or absence of a left SVC, should be performed.

Visualization of the pulmonary veins can be very difficult in adults and older children because of the distance of the veins from the transthoracic window. In these cases, TEE should be performed preoperatively.

### *Transesophageal Echocardiography*

TEE is useful because the transducer is close to the atrial septum and the scan plane is oriented perpendicular to the septum. The four-chamber view, at approximately 30 cm, offers optimal visualization of the atrioventricular valves, subvalvular apparatus, and LV outflow tract. This view is used to detect the presence of a patent foramen ovale. During a systemic venous saline injection, echogenic microbubbles can be seen in the LA. Color Doppler flow imaging also may visualize an ASD or patent foramen ovale. As the probe is withdrawn using the horizontal plane, the short axis of the base of the heart comes into view. In this view, the aortic valve, aortic root, proximal ascending aorta, proximal coronary and pulmonary arteries, and pulmonary veins can be visualized.

The vertical plane image at approximately 25 cm with rotation to the patient's right provides visualization of the atrial septum, IVC, SVC, and anterior and septal leaflets of the tricuspid valve. This view also is helpful for identifying a patent foramen ovale. Rotation to the patient's left shows the left pulmonary veins and LA appendage.

Using a biplane probe, both the vertical and horizontal planes are useful in identifying a secundum ASD. The vertical plane generally is more effective for identifying a sinus venosus defect; the horizontal plane is best to identify a primum ASD (6). Visualization of the more anterior cardiac structures is limited with TEE imaging. Omniplane TEE probes allow optimization of the image plane between the horizontal and vertical planes.

## VENTRICULAR SEPTAL DEFECT

### Definition

A VSD is a communication between the ventricles. These defects vary in size, amount of pulmonary blood flow, and clinical presentation. This chapter will deal only with the isolated VSD. Endocardial cushion or atrioventricular septal defects will not be discussed in detail.

### Etiology

VSDs are classified based upon their location in the septum. A variety of names have been used to identify the types of VSDs. Table 13.2 summarizes the synonyms used for each kind of defect. The ventricular septum can be divided into three main anatomic and developmental components: inlet septum or atrioventricular septum; muscular or sinus septum; and conoventricular septum (Fig. 13.4A–B).

Inlet defects, also termed endocardial cushion defects, are located beneath the septal leaflet of the tricuspid valve. These defects may be classified further based upon their association with or without atrioventricular valve abnormalities. These abnormalities range from two separate annuli of the tricuspid and mitral valves with only a cleft in the anterior leaflet of the mitral valve to a common annulus for both atrioventricular valves. Inlet defects account for approximately 8% to 10% of VSDs (7).

Muscular defects are located in the mid or apical portions of the interventricular septum. Mid-muscular defects are subdivided further into anterior or posterior defects based upon

**TABLE 13.2.** *Terminology used to describe ventricular septal defects*

| Our terminology | Alternative terminology |
|---|---|
| I. Inlet | Atrioventricular canal, endocardial cushion defect, type III defect |
| II. Muscular | Trabecular, swiss cheese septum, type IV defect |
|   1. Anterior | |
|   2. Posterior | |
|   3. Apical | |
| III. Conoventricular | |
|   1. Paramembranous | 1. Perimembranous, membranous, infracristal, type II defect |
|   2. Subpulmonary | 2. Supracristal, doubly committed subarterial, infundibular, conal, outlet, type I defect |
|   (The terms conus and infundibulum are synonymous) | (Intracristal or junctional describe defects located at the junction between the paramembranous septum and the crista supraventricularis) |
|   3. Malaligned | 3. Malaligned |
|     A. Anterior |   A. Tetralogy of Fallot-like |
|     B. Posterior |   B. (Can be associated with subaortic stenosis, coarctation, or interruption of the aorta) |

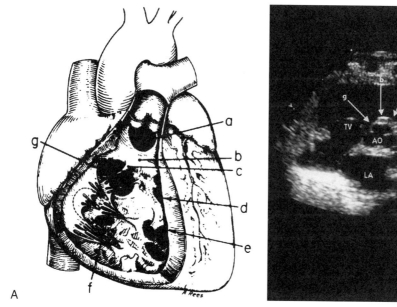

**FIG. 13.4. A:** Location of ventricular septal defects (VSD) viewed from the right ventricular side. **a:** Subpulmonary; **b:** crista supraventricularis; **c:** papillary muscle of the conus; **d:** anterior muscular VSD; **e:** apical muscular VSD; **f:** inlet VSD; **g:** paramembranous VSD. **B:** Parasternal short-axis image showing the conoventricular septum as a crescent shape anterior to the aortic valve. Lettering as in panel **A**. **a:** Subpulmonary; **b:** crista supraventricularis; **g:** paramembranous VSD. AO, aorta; LA, left atrium; MPA, main pulmonary artery; TV, tricuspid valve.

their relationship to the moderator band. Muscular defects are bounded entirely by muscular septum and often are multiple. They are found in 5% to 20% of patients with VSD, and they are the most likely to close spontaneously early in life.

Conoventricular defects account for 75% of VSDs (4,8). These defects can be divided into paramembranous, subpulmonary, and malaligned. The conoventricular septum includes the membranous septum, the conal septum, and the area that lies between these regions. When viewed in cross section, it is the crescent-shaped area of the septum that is anterior and just below the aortic valve, curving between the tricuspid and pulmonary valves (Fig. 13.4B). Defects adjacent to the tricuspid valve are termed paramembranous, and those adjacent to the pulmonary valve are termed subpulmonary. Large VSDs often extend into more than one area of the septum. For example, one might have a large para-

membranous defect with inlet extension. In paramembranous defects with conal extension, the conal septum may be hypoplastic, malaligned, or both. These defects may be associated with outflow tract obstruction. Anterior malalignment of the conal septum narrows the RV outflow, resulting in tetralogy of Fallot. Posterior malalignment narrows the LV outflow tract, causing subaortic stenosis and often coarctation or interruption of the aortic arch.

In conoventricular septal defects, the muscular support below the aortic valve may be deficient, which allows the right coronary cusp to prolapse into the defect and cause significant aortic regurgitation. Surgical closure of the VSD when aortic regurgitation is still mild usually halts progression and prevents the need for aortic valve replacement. Aortic valve prolapse is most likely to occur with subpulmonary VSDs; however, it can occur with paramembranous defects as well. In the non-Asian population, paramembranous defects are the most common; hence, aortic valve prolapse with paramembranous defects will be seen most commonly. However, in Asian populations, subpulmonary defects associated with prolapse of the aortic valve constitute up to 30% of VSDs (7).

## Prevalence and Incidence

A VSD is the most common congenital cardiac anomaly, representing 20% to 25% of all *isolated* congenital cardiovascular defects (Table 13.1). VSDs are found in about two per 1,000 live births and occur equally in females and males. VSDs often are found in association with more complex congenital lesions. When isolated and complex forms are considered together, the total incidence of VSD approaches 50% of all congenital cardiac lesions. Muscular and paramembranous defects close spontaneously; inlet and subpulmonary defects do not. The rate of spontaneous closure of muscular defects can be as high as 80%; for paramembranous defects, the rate can be 35%, depending upon the size of the defect (7).

## Pathophysiology

The hemodynamic consequences of a VSD relate both to the *size* of the defect and the *relative resistance to flow between the pulmonary and systemic vascular beds.* The location of the defect in the ventricular septum is of less importance. Small defects limit flow and restrict pressure equalization between the ventricles. The left to right shunt is small ($Q_p/Q_s$ <1.5) and RV pressure is normal or minimally elevated. Moderate-size defects are generally less than or equal to half the cross-sectional area of the aortic orifice and offer resistance to pressure but usually little resistance to flow. RV pressure remains less than LV pressure but is above normal. Large defects are equal to or greater in size than the area of the aortic orifice. They offer no resistance to flow with equalization of ventricular pressures. The magnitude of the left to right shunt depends entirely on the relative pulmonary and systemic vascular resistances.

High pulmonary blood flow can lead to pulmonary vascular changes and increased right heart pressures. As the shunt of blood from left to right decreases, RV compliance decreases and eventually the shunt reverses, causing cyanosis. Development of right to left shunting and cyanosis is termed Eisenmenger syndrome.

## History

The clinical state of the patient depends upon the patient's age, surgical history, size of the defect, and pulmonary vascular resistance. Small to moderate defects may close completely or reduce in size over time. Spontaneous closure occurs by age 3 years in 45% of patients. Some patients do not experience spontaneous closure until after the age of 8 to 10 years (9). Patients with small defects are asymptomatic and their life expectancy is normal. They do require endocarditis prophylaxis for any procedure likely to cause transient bacteremia (10,11).

Patients with elevated pulmonary artery pressures and pulmonary to systemic flow ratios ($Q_P/Q_S$) >1.5:1 should have surgical repair before 1 year of age. Patients with nonrestrictive defects can develop Eisenmenger complex by young adult life. Irreversible changes in pulmonary vascular resistance can occur as early as the first year of life and often have occurred by the end of the first decade of life.

## Symptoms

Exercise intolerance and fatigue are associated with moderate left to right shunts. Patients with large defects experience dyspnea, exercise intolerance, and respiratory infections. In patients with conoventricular defects, symptoms may develop secondary to aortic regurgitation due to aortic cusp prolapse. Eisenmenger patients experience cyanosis, markedly reduced exercise capacity, breathlessness, hemoptysis, angina, and palpitations secondary to atrial and ventricular arrhythmias.

## Physical Examination

### General Appearance

Small to moderate VSDs produce no change in the general appearance of a patient. Infants and children with large left to right shunts have congestive heart failure and may be underweight. These patients have "quiet tachypnea" with a rapid respiratory rate into the 60s to 80s without retraction or respiratory distress. A bulge in the left chest area reflects cardiomegaly produced by LV volume load. In Eisenmenger complex, the lips and nail beds are dusky or overtly cyanotic. Clubbing of the distal phalanges is present. End-stage patients will be weak and easily fatigued; pedal edema and ascites may be present if RV failure occurs.

### Arterial Pulse

The arterial waveform usually is normal. If the left to right shunt is large, there may be a brisk upstroke resulting in a carotid pulse with a rapid rate of rise and normal pulse pressure. In the presence of congestive heart failure, the pulse volume is reduced and the contour remains normal.

### Jugular Venous Pulse

Venous pulse pressure and contour are normal in the majority of patients with a VSD. In congestive heart failure, the mean pressure is elevated and the A and V waves are accentuated. In the Eisenmenger complex, the A wave is prominent.

### Palpation

LV impulse is normal to hyperdynamic because of LV volume overload and may be displaced lateral to the mid-clavicular line. The apical impulse may be increased in amplitude but is not sustained unless LV failure occurs.

As pulmonary vascular resistance increases, there will be the RV impulse of RV hypertrophy and sometimes the palpable $P_2$ of pulmonary hypertension. A systolic thrill at the lower left sternal border (third or fourth left interspace) is common in restrictive VSDs. Subpulmonary defects produce a more superior thrill, which may be palpable at the suprasternal notch.

### Auscultation

#### First and Second Heart Sounds

$S_1$ is increased in large left to right shunts. VSD murmurs can obscure $S_1$ because flow across the defect begins with isovolumic contraction (hence, the name $S_1$ coincident murmur). The loud (grade 3 or 4) holosystolic murmur also may obscure detection of an aortic valve component ($A_2$) and even $P_2$. $A_2$ is commonly "lost" in the murmur and only $P_2$ can be heard. Careful auscultation at sites away from maximal murmur intensity may be helpful in identifying both components of $S_2$.

Respiratory motion of $S_2$ is normal, although the maximal $A_2$–$P_2$ interval during inspiration may be wide if the shunt is large. RV dysfunction results in wide $S_2$ splitting, whereas elevated pulmonary vascular resistance narrows the $S_2$ split. In the Eisenmenger complex, $S_2$ may be closely split or single, with no respiratory variation. When $P_2$ is very loud, it may be helpful to listen several centimeters away from the pulmonic area in an effort to hear both components of $S_2$. A *normal* splitting interval with a loud $P_2$ in the absence of conduction delay on the electrocardiogram suggests that pulmonary vascular resistance is not yet maximally elevated and that the VSD is still operable.

#### Third Heart Sound

The presence of an $S_3$ roughly correlates with the magnitude of left to right shunting. It is a sign of an excessive volume of blood returning to the left heart across the mitral valve. An LV $S_3$ in conjunction with signs of pulmonary hypertension suggests hyperkinetic pulmonary hypertension and implies that the defect is still operable. As pulmonary vascular resistance increases and left to right flow decreases, the $S_3$ will disappear.

### Ejection Sound

With long-standing pulmonary hypertension and a large, tense pulmonary artery, a pulmonic ejection click or sound may be heard. This is a high-frequency sound just after $S_1$ that is best heard at the second or third left interspace. It may decrease with inspiration. The presence of a pulmonic ejection click is common in patients with Eisenmenger complex.

### Murmurs

*Systolic Murmur.* The hallmark of the VSD is a loud holosystolic murmur at the lower left sternal border. Classically described as a mixed-frequency, even-shaped murmur extending from $S_1$ to $S_2$, the VSD murmur may have mid-systolic accentuation. In small muscular defects, the murmur may be decrescendo and end well before $S_2$, as left to right shunting ceases in late systole. In the presence of congestive heart failure, the systolic murmur may be short.

When significant pulmonary hypertension is present, the systolic murmur shortens and may become decrescendo in shape. Both hyperkinetic pulmonary hypertension (high flow) and a nonreactive pulmonary vascular bed can result in a shortened systolic murmur. A holosystolic murmur at the lower sternal edge in the presence of severe pulmonary hypertension may represent tricuspid regurgitation. Careful attention to respiratory variation will resolve this differential.

If the defect begins to close, usually in early childhood, the systolic murmur will decrease in length and eventually may disappear. In this setting, it is imperative to carefully listen for the murmur of aortic regurgitation. If aortic regurgitation is present, it suggests that the aortic cusp has prolapsed across the defect functionally, making the defect smaller.

*Intensity.* The VSD murmur can range from soft to loud, but it usually is prominent. Auscultation is best using the diaphragm of the stethoscope. Small defects produce the loudest murmurs, and the classic "maladie de Roger" is a small shunt with an extremely loud murmur. These murmurs are usually of grade 4/6 intensity or louder.

In the presence of congestive heart failure or pulmonary hypertension, the murmur may be soft. As left to right shunting decreases and right to left flow dominates, the murmur may completely disappear.

*Location and Radiation Patterns.* The maximal intensity of paramembranous and inlet VSD murmurs is at the third or fourth left interspace adjacent to the sternum or xiphoid area. It often radiates widely and may be heard to the right of the sternum or mid way between the sternum and the apex. A subpulmonary defect should be suspected when the maximal murmur intensity is more superior, at the first or second interspace. Subpulmonary defect murmurs may radiate into the neck and beneath the left clavicle but do not radiate well to the lower sternal edge. Apical muscular VSDs are heard near the apex.

*Diastolic Murmur.* An early to mid-diastolic murmur or "flow rumble" is an important finding. Such a murmur signifies a large volume of blood traversing the mitral valve and indicates a pulmonary to systolic flow ratio >2:1. This murmur typically follows a loud $S_3$ and has a brief duration, ending well before late diastole. It is best heard at the apex with the patient in the left lateral decubitus position. It may be audible only when light pressure is used in placing the bell of the stethoscope on the chest. When the patient is in the upright position, this murmur may not be heard or may become softer. The murmur is low frequency and rumbling in quality, similar to the diastolic murmur of mitral stenosis; however, no opening snap is present, and the murmur is not audible in late diastole. Mild exercise may increase the intensity of the mid-diastolic murmur. The murmur does not increase with inspiration.

The disappearance of a mid-diastolic murmur is an indication of decreasing left to right shunting due to either development of increased pulmonary vascular resistance and pulmonary hypertension or spontaneous narrowing of the defect.

### Aortic Regurgitation

An unusual but important complication of VSDs is aortic regurgitation. Aortic regurgitation may be seen in either paramembranous or subpulmonary defects. Typically the right coronary cusp is involved. There may be thickening and distortion of the valve leaflets or overt prolapse of an entire cusp. Occasionally, the aortic leaflet may herniate and obliterate the VSD. Associated aortic regurgitation may not be discovered until late childhood. The aortic regurgitation is progressive and may be quite severe. Its hemodynamic importance ultimately may outweigh the consequences of the VSD itself. The murmur of aortic regurgitation is a faint blowing diastolic murmur or a loud, medium-frequency rough regurgitant murmur.

### Echocardiography

#### M-Mode Echocardiography

Early M-mode echocardiography was useful for indirect assessment of the hemodynamic effects of left to right shunting. LV and LA dilation can be identified; however, neither LA size nor the ratio of the diameter of the LA to the aortic root is reliably correlated to measured pulmonary blood flow. M-mode findings of septal discontinuity are unreliable except for very large defects.

#### Two-Dimensional Echocardiography

VSDs typically occur along the fusion lines between the different anatomic areas of the septum. Imaging of VSDs should be performed from multiple imaging planes. All views, including the subcostal views, are successful in identifying VSDs in infants and children, whereas the parasternal and apical views are more useful in adults. In adults, successful visualization of isolated VSDs ranges from 74% to 88% in prospective studies and from 88% to 100% in patients known to have a VSD (12).

The parasternal long-axis view images the septum along its longitudinal axis, traversing predominantly the infundibular and muscular portions of the septum. Because the septum does not lie in a single plane, only portions of these regions are imaged. By sweeping the plane anteriorly and to the left, a parasternal long-axis view through the conal septum and RV outflow tract can be obtained. The paramembranous and inlet septum are imaged as the ultrasound plane is swept posteriorly and to the right.

The parasternal short-axis view can be used to image portions of the conoventricular, muscular, and atrioventricular septa. With the ultrasound beam directed at the base of the heart, the membranous septum is located to the patient's right, beneath the septal leaflet of the tricuspid valve and the conal septum is to the patient's left, adjacent to the pulmonary valve (Fig. 13.4B). The parasternal short-axis view through the two atrioventricular valves allows visualization of the inlet defects (located posteriorly between the atrioventricular valves) as well as mid-muscular and anterior muscular defects (located leftward). At the level of the papillary muscles, posterior, mid, and anterior muscular defects are visible. Inferior to this view, defects in the apical muscular septum may be identified. Because the septum is imaged perpendicular to the scan plane in the parasternal short-axis views, the resolution for imaging relatively small muscular VSDs is maximized.

The standard apical four-chamber view provides a posterior projection through both the atrioventricular valves and the muscular portions of the ventricular septum. Inlet defects are visualized in the superior one third of the septum; mid-muscular defects are visualized in the middle half of the septum; and apical defects are visualized in the remaining portion of the septum, distal to the moderator band. In this view, extension of conoventricular defects and muscular defects toward the atrioventricular valves can be determined. The coronary sinus also is visible in this view. Additionally, the apical four-chamber view provides information concerning the chordal attachments of the atrioventricular valves. It is imperative to distinguish between a straddling valve, where some of the chordal attachments cross through the defect and insert into the opposite ventricle, and an overriding valve, where the valve annulus partially overrides the septal defect. Four different relationships may exist between the atrioventricular valve and the septal defect (5): (i) the valve can override the defect without straddling; (ii) the valve can override and straddle the defect; (iii) the valve can straddle the defect without overriding it; and (iv) the valve can neither override nor straddle the defect.

In the subcostal four-chamber view, thorough evaluation of the entire ventricular septum can be performed as the ultrasound plane is swept from a posterior to anterior position. Subcostal short-axis views are best for identifying anterior muscular VSDs and assessing malalignment of the conal septum.

### Contrast Echocardiography

As with ASDs, contrast studies have been used to evaluate the hemodynamic effects of VSDs by both M-mode and two-dimensional techniques. Contrast is needed more often with ASDs because there is low-velocity flow across the defect. With VSDs, the flow velocity usually is high and there is good visualization of the defect with color Doppler, which limits the need for contrast studies.

### Doppler Echocardiography

Color Doppler flow mapping and pulsed Doppler interrogation greatly increase the sensitivity, specificity, and physiologic assessment of VSDs. Doppler analysis provides estimation of the pulmonary and systemic

blood flows, pressure gradient across the VSD, and diastolic filling patterns of the ventricles.

### Color Doppler

Color flow mapping is an important tool for identifying small VSDs that can be missed by two-dimensional imaging. Figure 13.5 demonstrates multiple small VSDs. The direction of the flow, size of the defect, and additional shunts are easily identified with color Doppler. Color Doppler also is useful for identifying residual defects in patients who have undergone surgical closure of a VSD.

### Continuous Wave Doppler

Continuous wave Doppler usually is necessary for restrictive VSDs because the systolic velocities are generally high, often exceeding the Nyquist limit of pulsed wave Doppler. In the setting of a large defect with systemic RV pressure, systolic velocities may be low (<2.5 m/s) or undetectable. When there is elevated LV diastolic pressures (e.g., LV dysfunction), the diastolic left to right velocity is accentuated. Diastolic left to right flow ceases if there is elevated RV diastolic pressure.

Continuous wave Doppler can be used to estimate RV systolic pressure in patients with a VSD. If the systemic blood pressure is known, RV systolic pressure can be estimated using the modified Bernoulli equation:

RV systolic pressure
$$= \text{systolic arm blood pressure} - 4(\text{peak velocity of VSD jet})^2$$

RV systolic pressure also can be estimated from the peak velocity of the tricuspid regurgitant (TR) jet:

RV systolic pressure
$$= 4(\text{TR peak velocity})^2 + \text{RA pressure}$$

RA pressure can be estimated from the jugular venous distention or the IVC dynamics (in the subcostal view), or it can be measured from a central venous catheter. Good correlation has been found between Doppler

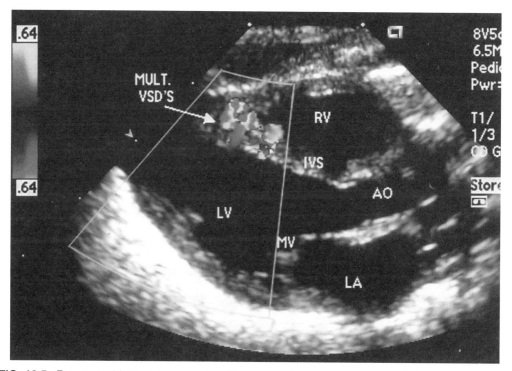

**FIG. 13.5.** Parasternal long-axis view of multiple muscular ventricular septal defects in a newborn baby. These defects will likely close spontaneously. Note the lack of left atrial or left ventricular dilation and the minimal turbulence by color Doppler. The left to right shunt volume is small because pulmonary vascular resistance has not yet fallen. AO, aorta; IVS, interventricular septum; MV, mitral valve; RV, right ventricle. (See Color Figure 13.5.)

and cardiac catheterization measurements of RV systolic pressure.

### Pulsed Wave Doppler

As with ASDs, pulsed Doppler has been used to estimate pulmonary and systemic blood flow in patients with VSDs (see ASD, pulse wave Doppler). However, the LV outflow tract may not be a suitable site for Doppler analysis because of the turbulence caused by the proximity of the defect. An alternative site to the LV outflow tract for evaluation of $Q_s$ is the mitral valve annulus. However, because the mitral annulus is elliptical in shape, $\pi r^2$ does not describe the valve area well.

Pulsed wave Doppler techniques are useful in assessing diastolic filling in patients with VSDs. A variety of abnormalities have been identified that demonstrate late diastolic ven-

tricular filling due to impaired ventricular relaxation. This is characterized by decreased E/A velocity ratio, increased deceleration time, and increased isovolumic relaxation time (IVRT; $A_2$ to mitral valve opening). Diastolic shunt flow often demonstrates a biphasic pattern similar to atrioventricular inflow, with a first peak early in diastole and a second peak late in diastole, following atrial contraction.

### Transesophageal Echocardiography

The ventricular septum is identified in the four-chamber horizontal view with the probe in the mid esophagus. From this position, a gradual sweep of the septum is performed with the transducer slightly retroflexed; this reveals the posterior structures. The transducer then is slowly flexed to visualize the more anterior structures. Slowly withdrawing the transducer in the flexed position provides an *en face* view of the aortic valve and the conoventricular septum.

Longitudinal sweeps are performed by rotating the transducer from the patient's right to the left with the probe at the mid-esophageal level (approximately 30 cm in adults). The longitudinal image of the RV outflow tract is helpful in identifying malalignment of the conal septum. It also is a useful position to identify residual VSDs or RV outflow tract obstruction during postoperative study.

## PATENT DUCTUS ARTERIOSUS

### Definition and Etiology

The ductus arteriosus is an arterial vascular structure between the aorta and the pulmonary artery. A PDA is necessary in the fetal circulation to allow diversion of RV output away from the unexpanded lungs and into the descending aorta. The PDA constricts physiologically in response to oxygen and the withdrawal of placental prostaglandins in the first hours to days of life.

### Prevalence

Persistent patency beyond the newborn period occurs in about 1 of 1,500 to 2,500 live, term-gestation births. A PDA is more common in premature infants and in children born at high altitude (13). It can be associated with maternal rubella infection during the first trimester of pregnancy. It is more common in females than males by a ratio of 2:1.

### History

Most patients with a PDA outside of infancy are asymptomatic. However, PDA can be the cause of congestive heart failure, pulmonary hypertension, and endocarditis. A large PDA can cause pulmonary vascular obstructive disease as early as 1 to 2 years of age. John et al. (14) reported a large series of adults with PDA. Of 600 patients with a patent ductus arteriosus at one hospital during the years 1967 to 1979, 131 patients were >14 years and 62 underwent cardiac catheterization. Of those patients undergoing catheterization, 50% had a $Q_P/Q_S$ ratio >1.5:1 and 33% had a ratio >3:1. Thirty of the 62 patients had mean pulmonary artery pressure >50 mm Hg and 18 patients had pulmonary vascular resistance >5 Woods units. Infective endocarditis has been estimated to have an incidence of 0.45% per year (15,16), and this is the rationale for closing even very small PDAs. Rarely, a PDA can be aneurysmal or be associated with dissection or rupture. In adults, histology has shown atheromatous changes in the ductus and sclerosis of the aorta. Calcification of the ductus can be seen on chest radiographs.

### Physical Examination

#### General Appearance

There is no particular body habitus associated with PDA. If the patient is in congestive heart failure, some or all of the typical heart failure signs will be present. If pulmonary vascular obstructive disease develops and the shunt across the PDA becomes right to left, there is differential cyanosis with lower oxygen saturations in the lower extremities (postductal) compared to the upper extremities.

#### Arterial Pulse

Patients with a large PDA have bounding pulses and a wide pulse pressure. Systemic diastolic pressure is low because of runoff from the aorta into the low-resistance pulmonary artery. Systolic arterial pressure may be slightly lower than normal.

#### Jugular Venous Pulse

No abnormalities of jugular venous pulse are present unless there is congestive heart failure, in which case the mean venous pressure may be elevated.

## Palpation

There is typically a prominent and laterally displaced LV apical impulse when there is sufficient shunt flow to produce LV volume overload. If elevated pulmonary vascular resistance is present, an RV impulse will be felt at the lower left sternal border.

## Auscultation

### Heart Sounds

There are no abnormalities of $S_1$ or $S_2$ in most patients with a PDA. Occasionally, the heart sounds can be obscured by the murmur at the upper sternal border but should be audible at the apex. As pulmonary vascular resistance increases, $P_2$ increases in intensity and $S_2$ becomes narrowly split, no longer obscured by the murmur at the upper left sternal border. If there is a very large left to right shunt, there may be paradoxic splitting of $S_2$ with $P_2$ occurring before $A_2$. An $S_3$ may occur if the patient is in congestive heart failure.

### Murmur

The classic PDA murmur is described as machinery-like and is continuous. It peaks in intensity around $S_2$; thus, it is crescendo in systole and decrescendo in diastole. The systolic component is described as "shaking dice" with multiple clicks. The murmur is best heard at the left infraclavicular area (second left intercostal space). If auscultation is only performed along the sternal borders and at the apex, a small PDA murmur can be missed.

Auscultation at the apex is important. If the PDA shunt is large, a diastolic flow rumble will be heard at the apex. The increased volume of flow across the mitral valve causes the rumble, as also is heard with large VSDs. LV volume overload can cause dilation of the mitral annulus and resultant mitral regurgitation with a high-pitched, holosystolic murmur at the apex.

With pulmonary hypertension, the systolic component of the murmur will be of lower frequency. The diastolic component shortens as pulmonary diastolic pressure increases and may become inaudible. A high-pitched, diastolic decrescendo murmur of pulmonary regurgitation may be present with severe pulmonary hypertension, and the ductal murmur may be absent.

## Echocardiography

### M-Mode Echocardiography

M-mode echocardiography will show LA and LV enlargement if there is a large left to right shunt at the ductus. In most cases, the M-mode echocardiogram will be normal. RV hypertrophy and systolic flattening of the interventricular septum will be present if there is pulmonary hypertension.

### Two-Dimensional Echocardiography

Transthoracic imaging of the ductus arteriosus is obtained from a high left parasternal window with the plane of the sector rotated clockwise from the typical long-axis view. This gives the so-called, "three-legged pant" view of the right pulmonary artery, left pulmonary artery, and ductus (Fig. 13.6). The ductus inserts into the proximal left pulmonary artery. In older children and adults, the lungs can obscure this view, so a typical left parasternal view with superior and leftward angulation may be used.

The long-axis, suprasternal notch view with angulation toward the left pulmonary artery can better define the ductal insertion into the descending aorta and aortic isthmus. Again, lung interference can be a problem in adults. The length and width of the ductus should be measured, and the lateral resolution of the echocardiogram should be used, if possible. Constriction of the ductus at either the pulmonary (most common) or aortic end should be noted. This information is helpful when planning for coil or device closure of the ductus by cardiac catheterization.

If surgery is planned, it is particularly important to determine the aortic arch anatomy

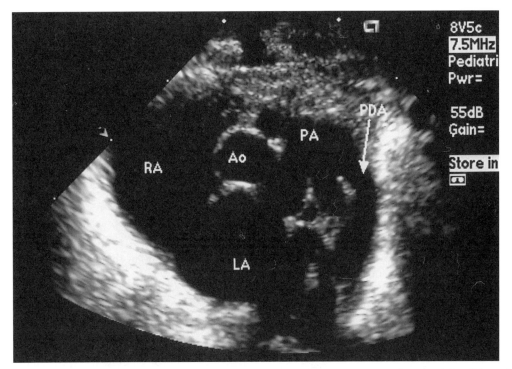

**FIG. 13.6.** High parasternal short-axis view showing the "three-legged pants" view of the right pulmonary artery, left pulmonary artery, and patent ductus arteriosus (PDA). The aortic arch is out of the plane and the left atrium is dilated. AO, aorta; PA, pulmonary artery.

and branching. Ligation of the PDA usually is accomplished via left thoracotomy or, more recently, left thoracoscopy. No echocardiographer wants to be known for missing a right aortic arch preoperatively! Arch anatomy is visualized from the suprasternal notch view by following each branch off of the aortic arch. A short-axis sweep from this position will show the first branch going to the right and dividing into the subclavian and right carotid arteries. If the first branch goes to the left, a right or double aortic arch may be present. Most patients with a right aortic arch have a left ductus arteriosus, although occasionally a right ductus entering the right pulmonary artery is seen. Bilateral ductus are rare.

Finally, two-dimensional imaging of the intracardiac anatomy from the standard views is done to evaluate LV volume overload and exclude other congenital cardiac defects.

### *Doppler Echocardiography*

#### *Color Doppler*

Because the ductus arteriosus can be difficult to image due to lung interference, the use of color Doppler has been invaluable in the diagnosis. The retrograde flow into the pulmonary artery is hard to miss. Typically, there is a red Doppler jet hugging the anterior and leftward wall of the main pulmonary artery. The normal antegrade pulmonary blood flow provides an obvious blue background in systole. The size of the color Doppler envelope does not necessarily predict the size of the ductus; it is more dependent on relative resistance in the systemic and pulmonary vascular beds. When there is pulmonary hypertension and bidirectional shunting, it is important to separate the ductal flow from both the left pulmonary artery flow and the descending aorta flow. Normal pulsation of these closely related structures can give the false impression of blue, right to left flow in the ductus. Right to left flow in a ductus throughout the cardiac cycle is unusual and is seen only when there is pulmonary vascular resistance exceeding systemic vascular resistance or when there is critical coarctation of the aorta.

### Pulse and Continuous Wave Doppler

Continuous wave Doppler can be used to estimate pulmonary artery pressure. The modified Bernoulli equation ($4V^2$ = gradient in mm Hg) is used along with systolic blood pressure. This can be inaccurate when the ductus is long and tortuous or when it is very small. The Bernoulli equation is based on laminar flow through a straight tube. Aortic flow is perpendicular or even antiparallel to ductal flow. Keeping these limitations in mind, the equation is especially useful when a high gradient is obtained consistent with normal pulmonary artery pressure.

### Transesophageal Echocardiography

It can be difficult to adequately image a ductus arteriosus by TEE because the left bronchus lies between the esophagus and ductus arteriosus. However, TEE may be helpful if there is aneurysm of the ductus at the aortic end. A small ductal diverticulum at the aortic end is not abnormal after spontaneous constriction of the ductus. TEE images may delineate thrombus within or dissection of a large ductal aneurysm.

In summary, PDA is a common congenital heart disease in children. Most PDA lesions that escape detection in childhood will be small in the adult. Large PDA lesions cause pulmonary vascular obstructive disease if not treated. The indication for closure of small PDA is to prevent bacterial endocarditis. Transcatheter techniques are now commonly used for closure. Echocardiographic definition of PDA size and morphology is important to guide the choice of closure technique.

## COARCTATION OF THE AORTA

### Definition

Coarctation of the aorta is a narrowing of the aortic arch that almost always is located just distal to the left subclavian artery and opposite to the insertion of the ductus ligamentum. It is typically a shelf of media protruding into the lumen of the aorta from the posterior and lateral aspect of the aortic wall. With time there is increasing thickness of the intima as well; thus, coarctation of the aorta is a progressive lesion.

### Prevalence

Coarctation of the aorta occurs in about one of 2,000 live births. It is more common in males than females by a ratio of >2:1. It is commonly associated with other cardiac defects, with only one third of uncomplicated coarctations being truly isolated (4). Aortic and mitral valve abnormalities are the most common associated defects. The presence of multiple left-sided obstructive lesions is termed Shone syndrome. Left-sided obstructive lesions, including coarctation, may have a higher recurrence rate in some families than other congenital heart disease. If a woman has coarctation of the aorta, the risk to her offspring may be as high as 12% for some form of left-sided obstruction ranging in severity from bicommissural aortic valve to hypoplastic left heart syndrome (17). Coarctation of the aorta is often seen in patients with Turner syndrome (45,X). Only isolated coarctation will be discussed here.

### Natural History

The natural history of unoperated coarctation of the aorta has been described from clinical and autopsy series (18,19). The average age at death in the autopsy series was 34 years; 90% of the deaths occurred by age 58 years. The causes of death in patients <30 years of age were cerebrovascular events (especially berry aneurysm rupture), aortic dissection or rupture, and bacterial endocarditis. After 30 years of age, congestive heart failure was the most common cause of death.

Women with coarctation are particularly at risk for aortic dissection during late pregnancy, labor, and the early postpartum period. Medical treatment of hypertension during pregnancy theoretically can compromise uterine and fetal perfusion. Angiotensin-converting enzyme inhibitors are teratogenic during pregnancy, and maternal beta-blocker treatment can result in hypoglycemia in the newborn.

Older children with isolated coarctation usually are asymptomatic and are identified because of hypertension or diminished femoral pulses noted on physical examination. In many pediatric practices, routine physical examinations do not include evaluation of blood pressure until the children are about 5 years of age because of the difficulty obtaining accurate blood pressures in toddlers and infants. Essential hypertension is rare in children before adolescence. Renal parenchymal disease causes 60% to 80% of hypertension in children, followed by coarctation of the aorta, which causes 5% to 15% (20).

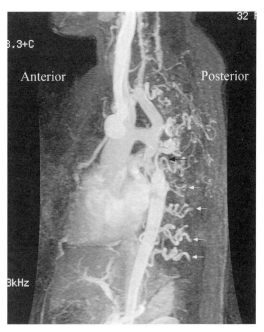

**FIG. 13.7.** Magnetic resonance image of severe coarctation of the aorta in a 32-year-old woman. The *black arrow* indicates the region of coarctation. The aorta is actually interrupted. The vessel that appears to bridge the proximal and distal ends of the interruption is the left pulmonary artery. The *white arrows* indicate the prominent collateral vessels.

## Pathophysiology

Coarctation of the aorta is a progressive disease. The posterior coarctation "shelf" is mainly heaped up media in infancy, but with time the turbulence of flow causes intimal thickening as well. As the aortic lumen narrows, most patients will develop collateral vessels that supplement lower body blood flow. These vessels arise from the subclavian, mammary, and intercostal arteries (Fig. 13.7). As the vessels dilate, they cause the classic rib notching noted by chest radiograph along the ribs. The collateral vessels also may lower the hypertension in the upper body but never completely eliminate it.

## History

Initially, infants with critical coarctation have pallor and poor feeding. Poor urine output and cardiogenic shock can develop in a matter of hours as the ductus arteriosus closes. Cases of critical coarctation often are associated with aortic arch hypoplasia and hypoplasia of other left-sided structures, such as the aortic valve, subaortic area, and mitral valve. At birth, arm and leg blood pressures are obtained in most nurseries. However, a blood pressure gradient may not be evident until after the ductus arteriosus closes.

Patients <40 years of age usually are asymptomatic. Lower extremity coolness or cramping with exercise is rarely reported. Patients >40 years of age often develop congestive heart failure. Regardless of the patient's age, central nervous system symptoms should be investigated because of the risk of cerebral aneurysm.

## Physical Examination

### General Appearance

The general appearance of the patient with coarctation of the aorta is normal. There are occasional references to a well-developed upper body and thinner lower body, but this finding is inconsistent. It may be that the male body habitus is being described because there is such a male predominance in coarctation incidence. In females with short stature, a shield-shaped chest, and webbed neck, Turner syndrome may be present.

In infants, if there is a significant coarctation so that the ductus arteriosus is supplying a good part of the lower body blood flow, then pulse oximetry saturations measured in the toe will be lower than in the hand. An oxygen saturation difference of >3% between upper and lower extremities warrants further investigation. The first step should be to repeat the physical examination, including four extremity blood pressures and saturations. If the discrepancy persists, an echocardiogram should be performed. In older children and adults who did not have a critical coarctation initially, the ductus arteriosus has usually closed.

### Blood Pressure and Arterial Pulse

Even in the presence of collateral vessels, the hallmark of coarctation is blood pressure discrepancy proximal and distal to the obstruction. Rarely, the left subclavian artery can be involved in the coarctation, so blood pressure measurements in the right arm and either leg are recommended. The exception would be in the patient with a left aortic arch and aberrant right subclavian artery. In this case, the right subclavian arises distal to the coarctation, so the blood pressure in the right arm would be similar to the legs. Very rarely,

both subclavian arteries can arise distal to the coarctation.

The pulse pressure is widened proximal to the coarctation because systolic pressure is significantly more elevated than diastolic pressure. Pulse pressure is narrow distal to the coarctation, with a low systolic and near normal diastolic pressure. The systolic gradient across a coarctation is more informative than the mean blood pressure gradient.

The classic physical examination findings of coarctation of the aorta are bounding carotid pulses and diminished or absent femoral pulses. In mild coarctation, the femoral pulses may be present, but there will be a distinct lag in peak pulse when the radial or brachial and femoral pulses are felt simultaneously. The feet may be cooler than the hands, but capillary refill usually is normal in patients after infancy.

### Jugular Venous Pulse

There are no characteristic abnormalities of jugular venous pulse with coarctation of the aorta.

### Palpation

Newborns with coarctation have RV hypertrophy and, therefore, will have a prominent RV impulse at the left lower sternal border and at the xiphoid process. In adults, the LV apical impulse is normally placed but may be sustained because of LV hypertrophy. A suprasternal notch thrill sometimes is present, even in the absence of aortic stenosis. If there is congestive heart failure, the apical impulse is diminished in intensity and laterally displaced.

### Auscultation

#### Heart Sounds

$S_1$ is normal or increased in patients with coarctation of the aorta. $S_2$ is physiologically split in patients with coarctation of the aorta. $A_2$ can be increased and "snappy" because of hypertension. Because a bicuspid aortic valve is common in patients with coarctation, there often is an early systolic ejection click at the upper right sternal border. An S$_4$ may be present at the apex.

### Murmur

Flow across the coarctation is heard as a low-intensity murmur that peaks in early to mid systole and spills into diastole. It can be heard at the left infraclavicular area; at the upper left back, medial to the scapula; and often in the axilla. A continuous murmur of collateral flow often is heard over the lung fields in older children and adults. In the infant or adult with LV failure, a murmur may not be heard because there is less flow across the obstruction when cardiac output is low.

Associated auscultatory findings can include an aortic stenosis or regurgitation murmur and a mitral stenosis or regurgitation murmur. Aortic murmurs are caused by the increased incidence of bicuspid aortic valve. Mitral valve murmurs are caused by abnormalities such as parachute mitral valve, double orifice mitral valve, and a small mitral annulus.

## Echocardiography

### M-Mode Echocardiography

The coarctation itself is not visible with M-mode echocardiography. LV wall thickness and fractional shortening is determined by M-mode imaging. From the parasternal short-axis view, the cursor position can be set between the papillary muscles of the mitral valve and at the tips of the mitral valve leaflets. The aortic valve leaflets may appear eccentric on M-mode echocardiography, but two-dimensional imaging gives a more accurate view of aortic valve morphology. Aortic annulus and root measurements should be obtained from two-dimensional rather than M-mode imaging. It is difficult to position the M-mode cursor perpendicular to both walls of the aorta, so M-mode imaging gives an oblique measurement of the aortic root. Aortic root and ascending aortic dilation is a common finding in patients with bicuspid aortic valve. Whether the degree of root dilation is predictive of aortic dissection as it is in Marfan syndrome is unknown but is under study.

### Two-Dimensional Echocardiography

Suprasternal notch and high left parasternal views are best for imaging coarctation in children. The transducer can be rotated counterclockwise from the usual long-axis plane of the aortic arch to image a longer segment of the proximal descending aorta. A pillow should be placed behind the patient's shoulders to optimize neck extension and allow the transducer to be positioned nearly parallel to the long axis of the body. Lung interference often is encountered in adults.

The branches of the aortic arch should be defined by following their course. The innominate artery should be about twice the caliber as the left carotid and subclavian arteries, and it should branch into the right subclavian and carotid arteries. If the first branch is not the largest, suspect an aberrant origin of the right subclavian artery from the descending aorta. If the first branch heads to the left, then a right aortic arch with mirror image branching is likely.

The length and diameter of the aortic arch segments should be measured (Fig. 13.8). If there is transverse arch hypoplasia, the incidence of recurrent coarctation at long-term follow-up is high. Good preoperative visualization of the entire aortic arch may help the surgeon with clamp placement. The distance from the subclavian artery to the coarctation is important if a subclavian flap repair is planned. This was once the favored repair in young infants; however, coarctation resection with end-to-end anastomosis is more common today. The descending aorta at the diaphragm

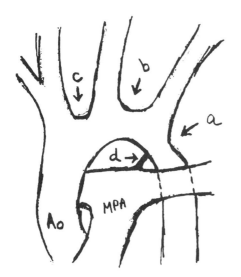

**FIG. 13.8.** Schematic representation of the aortic arch. **a:** Isthmus; **b:** distal transverse arch between the left common carotid artery and left subclavian artery; **c:** proximal transverse arch between the innominate artery and left common carotid artery; **d:** ductus ligamentum. AO, aorta; MPA, main pulmonary artery.

should be imaged and will lack pulsatility in coarctation.

A complete cardiac echocardiogram should be performed in cases of apparent isolated coarctation. Left SVC to the coronary sinus can be associated with coarctation. Any left-sided obstructive lesion may be found, including cor triatriatum; supravalvular or valvular mitral stenosis; and subaortic or valvular aortic stenosis. In newborns, RV hypertrophy is prominent. In older children and adults, LV hypertrophy may be present. In newborns, it is especially important to image the ductus arteriosus. If it is patent, the severity of the coarctation may be underestimated. Echocardiography is useful in monitoring ductal patency when prostaglandins are used to maintain patency prior to coarctation repair. Finally, in all patients, LV function should be assessed.

### Doppler Echocardiography

In the adult with poor two-dimensional windows, the Doppler echocardiogram can be diagnostic. Figures 13.9 and 13.10 show

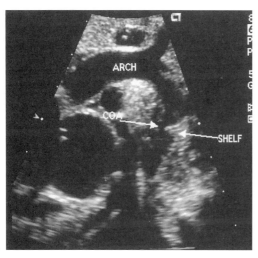

A

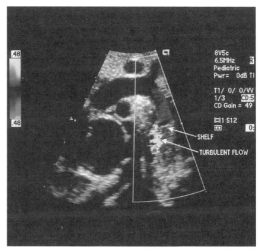

B

**FIG. 13.9.** Two-dimensional and Doppler images of the aorta and a coarctation. **A:** Suprasternal notch view demonstrating a discrete posterior aortic shelf. **B:** Turbulence of flow begins at the shelf. (See Color Figure 13.9B.)

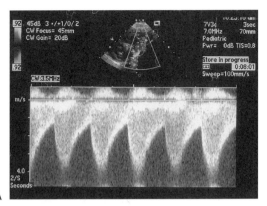
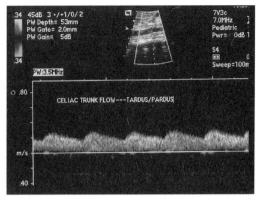

A

B

**FIG. 13.10. A:** Continuous wave Doppler at the level of the coarctation. Note the classic Doppler findings of coarctation: delayed upstroke, antegrade diastolic flow, and high peak velocity. **B:** Pulse wave Doppler of the celiac trunk demonstrates slow system upstroke, antegrade diastolic flow, and lack of pulsation.

the classic color and continuous wave Doppler patterns of coarctation. Turbulence of color Doppler begins at the coarctation shelf. There is continuous antegrade flow in diastole distal to the coarctation. Interrogation of the celiac trunk from a subcostal view shows a slow, blunted upstroke and decreased peak velocity.

### Transesophageal Echocardiography

TEE may be helpful if transthoracic windows are inadequate. However, the area of a coarctation may be obscured because of the proximity of the left bronchus. Magnetic resonance imaging and angiography have the advantage of giving better definition of collateral vessels in older patients who have poor transthoracic echocardiographic windows.

### Exercise Echocardiography

Exercise echocardiography has been used mainly in the postoperative patient with per-

sistent systemic hypertension. Often, a pressure gradient can be documented during exercise when none exists at rest. Unless a clear obstruction can be seen on imaging studies, it is unclear whether balloon dilation or surgical augmentation of the aortic arch will abolish this exercise gradient. It is not uncommon for resting or exercise-induced hypertension to persist after coarctation repair, especially if the repair is done after infancy. This is thought to be caused by abnormal systemic arterial wall compliance and is treated medically unless an obvious obstruction is seen.

### SUMMARY AND GUIDELINES

Tables 13.3 and 13.4 summarize the role and limitations of physical examination and echocardiography in diagnosing the congenital heart defects discussed in this chapter. Table 13.5 summarizes the American College of Cardiology/American Heart Association indications for echocardiography in patients with congenital heart disease.

**TABLE 13.3.** *Physical and echocardiographic findings and recommendations in congenital heart disease*

| | Atrial septal defect | Ventricular septal defect | Patent ductus arteriosus | Coarctation of the aorta |
|---|---|---|---|---|
| Small (mild) | 1. ASD area <1 cm², $Q_p/Q_s$ <1.5, no RV dilation.<br>2. Asymptomatic.<br>3. May be at risk for systemic thromboemboli.<br>4. Consider surgery or device closure if stroke or arrhythmia. | 1. Area <1/2 aortic annulus area, $Q_p/Q_s$ <1.5, no LA or LV dilation.<br>2. Asymptomatic.<br>3. Need SBE prophylaxis.<br>4. No intervention. | 1. Restrictive by Doppler, normal pulmonary artery pressure, no LA dilation.<br>2. Asymptomatic.<br>3. Need SBE prophylaxis.<br>4. Risk of closure is lower than risk of SBE.<br>5. Coil or device closure in catheterization laboratory. | 1. Systolic BP gradient between arms and legs <10 mm Hg; no LVH.<br>2. Asymptomatic.<br>3. At risk for increased BP gradient and abnormal BP response to exercise.<br>4. Need SBE prophylaxis.<br>5. Medical treatment of hypertension. |
| Moderate | 1. ASD area 1–3 cm² or $Q_p/Q_s$ 1.5–2, RV volume overload.<br>2. Asymptomatic or mild exercise intolerance, especially with pregnancy.<br>3. At risk for atrial arrhythmias, systemic thromboemboli.<br>4. Recommend surgical or device closure at diagnosis (if >2–4 yr old). Surgery necessary for primum or sinoseptal ASDs. | 1. Area 1/2 to 1× the size of aortic annulus, RV pressure < LV pressure, $Q_p/Q_s$ 1.5–2, some LA and LV dilation.<br>2. Asymptomatic or mild exercise intolerance.<br>3. Need SBE prophylaxis.<br>4. Recommend surgical closure if >6 mo old and pulmonary hypertension.<br>5. Consider catheterization to define pulmonary artery pressure and resistance. | 1. Restrictive by Doppler but LA/LV dilated, PDA ~ size of branch pulmonary artery.<br>2. Asymptomatic.<br>3. Recommend surgical or device closure (device if <3–4 mm in diameter). | 1. Systolic BP gradient between arms and legs >20 mm Hg.<br>2. Asymptomatic but hypertensive in upper body.<br>3. Recommend surgical repair.<br>4. Balloon dilation if recurrent coarctation late postoperative. |

| | | | | |
|---|---|---|---|---|
| Large (severe) | 1. ASD area >3 cm², $Q_p/Q_s$ >3, RV volume overload.<br>2. Fatigue, dyspnea on exertion; commonly palpitations.<br>3. Lower respiratory tract infections common.<br>4. At risk for stroke, atrial arrhythmias, RV failure, and pulmonary hypertension.<br>5. Surgical closure. Device closure only possible if there is adequate atrial septum around all edges of defect. | 1. VSD area > aortic valve area, $Q_p/Q_s$ >3.<br>2. Tachypnea, poor growth, fatigue.<br>3. Lower respiratory tract infections common.<br>4. Rare to reach adolescence without developing elevated pulmonary vascular resistance.<br>5. Preoperative catheterization with shunt calculations in room air and on 100% oxygen + nitric oxide to determine operative mortality.<br>6. Surgical closure. Fenestrated VSD patch can be used in cases of high but reactive pulmonary resistance. | 1. PDA >20–30 mm.<br>2. Tachypnea, poor growth in infants, pulmonary hypertension in older children and adults.<br>3. Lower respiratory tract infections common.<br>4. Surgical closure if pulmonary vascular resistance permits; may need preoperative catheterization as with VSD. | 1. Absent femoral pulses, catheter gradient >50 mm Hg (Doppler gradient often overestimates); LVH.<br>2. Generally asymptomatic but may have exercise induced angina; at risk for sudden death.<br>3. Surgical repair. Preoperative angiography or magnetic resonance imaging can help to define collateral circulation. |
| Pulmonary hypertension with Eisenmenger (pulmonary vascular obstructive disease) | 1. Any size ASD with right to left shunting and, therefore, systemic hypoxemia. With small ASD may actually be primary pulmonary hypertension with incidental ASD.<br>2. Fatigue, cyanosis, clubbing, hemoptysis.<br>3. Prominent right ventricular impulse, palpable $P_2$, jugular venous distention.<br>4. May have murmur of tricuspid or pulmonary regurgitation that is high pitched. | 1. Moderate to large VSD untreated into second decade of life but can occur in first year of life in small percentage of patients.<br>2. Symptoms/physical examination like ASD with Eisenmenger syndrome plus can have mitral or aortic regurgitation.<br>3. No murmur from VSD.<br>4. Inoperable. | 1. Differential cyanosis with blue lower body.<br>2. Symptoms/physical examination like ASD/VSD. Lose ductal murmur, loud $P_2$, aortic or pulmonary regurgitation.<br>3. High operative mortality (>30%) but improvement in PVR has been reported in survivors. | N/A |

ASD, atrial septal defect; BP, blood pressure; LA, left atrium; LV, left ventricle; LVH, left ventricular hypertrophy; PDA, patent ductus arteriosus; PVR, pulmonary vascular resistance; SBE, subacute bacterial endocarditis; RV, right ventricle; VSD, ventricular septal defect.

**TABLE 13.4.** *Limitations of physical examination and echocardiography in congenital heart disease*

| | ASD | VSD | PDA | Coarctation of the aorta |
|---|---|---|---|---|
| Physical examination | 1. Physical examination findings are subtle until late.<br>2. Fixed splitting of $S_2$ is commonly missed in childhood because it is quite variable with heart rate.<br>3. There is no murmur associated with the ASD itself.<br>4. Elevated jugular venous pulse and liver enlargement are easily recognized; however, they are late findings. | 1. Recognition of a loud $P_2$ may be difficult in some patients.<br>2. Aortic regurgitation is imperative to exclude when restriction of the VSD develops.<br>3. In children, the clinical findings of congestive heart failure are more subtle. There is no peripheral edema and there is a quiet tachypnea. | 1. Recognition of pulmonary hypertension may be difficult.<br>2. Auscultation in the classic "aortic, pulmonary, tricuspid, and mitral" positions can miss a small PDA. | 1. It may be difficult to identify a brachial-femoral arterial delay in adults.<br>2. It may be difficult to auscultate an aortic click.<br>3. Collateral blood flow may not be recognized during examination of the back.<br>4. An inclusive differential diagnosis of hypertension must be entertained in all patients. |
| TTE and TEE | 1. False dropout of the septum may lead to inaccurate diagnoses. (The probe must be perpendicular to the interatrial septum to identify an ASD.)<br>2. During contrast studies, inadequate opacification of the right atrium with saline may miss small ASDs. A negative contrast effect has low specificity.<br>3. Doppler $Q_p/Q_s$ estimate assumes laminar flow through a rigid tube, similar pulmonary artery and aortic compliances, and adequate measurement of the outflow tract.<br>4. Pulmonary venous return is difficult to define in adult patients. | 1. False dropout of the septum may lead to inaccurate diagnoses. (The probe must be perpendicular to the interventricular septum to identify a VSD.)<br>2. As with ASDs, many assumptions are made when using the $Q_p/Q_s$ shunt ratio. A VSD may significantly affect the turbulence of flow and alter the ratio calculation.<br>3. The size of the VSD can be underestimated when the aortic valve prolapses into the VSD. | 1. Estimation of $Q_p/Q_s$ from the mitral and tricuspid annuli is imprecise because the annuli are not circular, giving rise to false calculations.<br>2. On TTE images, the lung obscures visualization of a PDA.<br>3. On TEE images, the left bronchus lies between the ductus and the esophagus and produces an air artifact. | 1. The coarctation gradient may be overestimated due to acceleration of flow around the aortic arch.<br>2. Patients with persistent hypertension may have a gradient only on exercise.<br>3. On TTE images, the left pulmonary artery crosses and shadows the coarctation.<br>4. With TEE it is difficult to obtain Doppler image of the coarctation from the esophagus because the interrogation angle is perpendicular to the direction of blood flow. |

ASD, atrial septal defect; TEE, transesophageal echocardiography; TTE, transthoracic echocardiography; VSD, ventricular septal defect.

**TABLE 13.5.** *Indications for echocardiography in congenital heart disease*

| | Class I indications | Class II indications |
|---|---|---|
| ASD, VSD, PDA, or COA in the infant, child, or adolescent | 1. Pathologic murmur or other abnormal cardiac finding.<br>2. Cardiomegaly on chest radiograph.<br>3. Patients with a known cardiac defect to assess timing of medical or surgical treatment.<br>4. Immediate preoperative evaluation for cardiac surgery of a patient with known CHD to guide surgical management and to inform the patient and family of the risks of surgery *(can be intraoperative TEE)*.<br>5. Patient with known CHD and change in physical findings.<br>6. Postoperative CHD with suspected residual abnormality *(can be intraoperative TEE)*. Evaluation for ventricular function, thrombosis, infection, and pericardial effusion.<br>7. Presence of a genetic syndrome with high association of CHD or multiple affected family members (e.g., Down, Marfan, Turner, hypertrophic cardiomyopathy).<br>8. *To direct interventional catheterization procedures such as atrial septostomy, valvuloplasties, and ASD or VSD device closures.* | 1. Failure to thrive in absence of definite abnormal clinical findings. |
| ASD, VSD, PDA, or COA in the adult | 1. Patients with suspected CHD by physical examination, electrocardiography or chest radiography.<br>2. Patients with known CHD when there is a change in clinical findings.<br>3. Patients with known CHD when there is uncertainty in the original diagnosis or when the anatomy or hemodynamics are unclear.<br>4. Periodic echocardiograms in patients with known CHD to evaluate ventricular function and atrioventricular valve regurgitation (especially single ventricle after Fontan, transposition with right ventricle pumping to systemic circulation, palliative shunts, coarctation).<br>5. Patients with known CHD for whom following pulmonary artery pressure is important (moderate VSD, ASD, PDA).<br>6. Follow-up after surgical treatment of CHD if there is a change in clinical status or if ventricular function and pulmonary artery pressure need to be followed.<br>7. To direct interventional catheterization procedures, such as valvuloplasty, and ASD or VSD device closure. | 1. Follow-up every 1–2 yr in patients with known hemodynamically significant CHD without evident changes in clinical condition. |

Modified from Cheitlin MD, Alpert JS, Armstrong WF, et al. ACC/AHA guidelines for the clinical application of echocardiography: a report of the American College of Cardiology/American Heart Association Task Force on Practice Guidelines (Committee on Clinical Application of Echocardiography 1997,95:1686–1744). Additions to the ACC/AHA guidelines made by the chapter authors are in italics.

ASD, atrial septal defect; CHD, congenital heart disease; COA, coarctation of the aorta; PDA, patent ductus arteriosus; TEE, transesophageal echocardiography; VSD, ventricular septal defect.

# REFERENCES

1. Graham TP. Medical and surgical advances in the care of adults with congenital heart disease. ACC Symposium, San Diego, California, 1993.
2. Ryan T. Atrial septal defect in the adult. ACC Curr J Rev 1996;39–42.
3. Silverman NH. Pediatric echocardiography. Baltimore: Williams & Wilkins, 1993:109–122.
4. Fyler DC, ed. Nadas' pediatric cardiology. Philadelphia: Hanley Belfus, 1992.
5. Snider AR, Serwer GA, Ritter SB. Echocardiography in pediatric heart disease, 2nd ed. St. Louis: Mosby-Year Book, 1997.
6. Marelli AJ, Child JS, Perloff JK. Transesophageal echocardiography in congenital heart disease in the adult. Cardiol Clin 1993;11:505–520.
7. Gumbiner CH, Takao A. Ventricular septal defect. In: Garson A, Bricker JT, Fisher DJ, et al., eds. The science and practice of pediatric cardiology, 2nd ed. Baltimore: Williams & Wilkins, 1998:1119–1140.
8. Van Praagh R, Geva T, Kreutzer J. Ventricular septal defects: how shall we describe, name and classify them? J Am Coll Cardiol 1989;14:1298–1299.
9. Braunwald E, ed. Braunwald heart disease: a textbook of cardiovascular medicine, 5th ed. Philadelphia: WB Saunders, 1997.
10. Kidd L, Driscoll DJ, Gersony WM, et al. Second natural

history study of congenital heart defects results of treatment of patients with ventricular septal defects. Circulation 1993;87[Suppl I]:I-38–I-51.

11. Morris CD, Reller MD, Menashe VD. Thirty-year incidence of infective endocarditis after surgery for congenital heart defect. JAMA 1998;279:599–603.

12. Weyman AE, ed. Principles and practice of echocardiography, 2nd ed. Philadelphia: Lea & Febiger, 1994.

13. Miao CY, Zuberbuhler JS, Zuberbuhler JR. Prevalence of congenital cardiac anomalies at high altitude. J Am Coll Cardiol 1988;12:224–228.

14. John S, Muralidharan S, Jairaj PS, et al. The adult ductus. Review of surgical experience with 131 patients. J Thorac Cardiovasc Surg 1981;82:314–319.

15. Fisher RG, Moodie DS, Sterba R, et al. Patent ductus arteriosus in adults—long-term follow-up: nonsurgical versus surgical treatment. J Am Coll Cardiol 1986;8:280–284.

16. Jones JC. Twenty five years' experience with the surgery of patent ductus arteriosus. J Thorac Cardiovasc Surg 1965;50:149–165.

17. Allan LD, Crawford DC, Chita SK, et al. Familial recurrence of congenital heart disease in a prospective series of mothers referred for fetal echocardiography. Am J Cardiol 1986;58:334–337.

18. Liberthson RR, Pennington DG, Jacobs ML, et al. Coarctation of the aorta: review of 234 patients and clarification of management problems. Am J Cardiol 1979;43:835–840.

19. Campbell M, Baylis JH. The course and prognosis of coarctation of the aorta. Br Heart J 1956;18:475.

20. DeSwiet M. The epidemiology of hypertension in children. Br Med Bull 1986;42:172–175.

# 14

# The Pregnant Patient

Robert A. Taylor

*Department of Internal Medicine, University of New Mexico School of Medicine; and Staff
Cardiologist, Department of Internal Medicine, University of New Mexico Health Sciences Center,
Albuquerque, New Mexico*

## INTRODUCTION

The pregnant patient illustrates the manner in which changing physiology can affect the physical as well as the echocardiographic examination. As women progress through pregnancy, both obvious and subtle changes to the physical appearance and auscultative examination occur. Changes in the cardiovascular system during the gravid period influence and alter the manifestations and magnitude of both valvular and nonvalvular cardiac findings previously demonstrated on physical examination or echocardiography. New physical examination and echocardiographic findings often are found in women without structural heart disease. The normal physiologic changes of pregnancy must be kept in mind when approaching the physical diagnosis and echocardiographic examination of the preg-

nant patient in order to distinguish between what is expected and what is unexpected (or what is pathologic vs. nonpathologic). This is especially important in the patient with known cardiac abnormalities.

## PHYSIOLOGY

### Normal Physiology

#### Pregnancy

Significant hemodynamic changes are seen as a woman progresses through the first trimester toward term (Fig. 14.1). The overall blood volume begins to increase due to augmented salt and water reabsorption (1,2). Expansion of blood volume is found as early as 6 weeks, peaks at the mid portion of the second trimester, and may be doubled (1,2). Con-

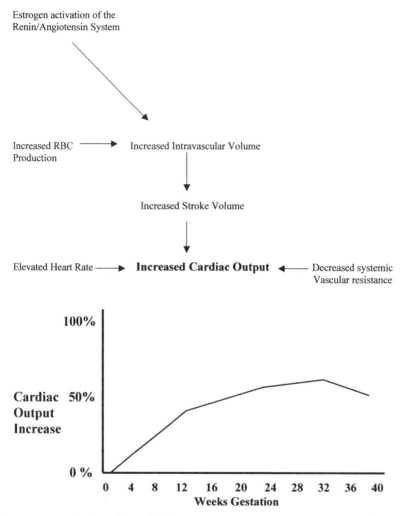

**FIG. 14.1.** Time course of hemodynamic changes associated with pregnancy. RBC, red blood cell.

currently, a decrease in systemic and pulmonary vascular resistance occurs, contributing to augmentation of cardiac stroke volume (1–3). The increased blood volume in the maternal circulation concomitant with increased cardiac output and workload may produce changes in the physical examination and exacerbate symptoms in women with intracardiac abnormalities. Additionally, a decrease in systemic and pulmonary vascular resistance may influence the physical and echocardiogram examination. For example, blood flow across stenotic aortic or mitral valves is increased during pregnancy, augmenting their

auscultatory and Doppler ultrasound manifestations.

The enlarging fetus and uterus have a direct effect on the pregnant woman. As the gravid uterus increases in size, it may physically impinge on the inferior vena cava, decreasing the venous return (3). This venocaval compression may cause an increase in the femoral venous pressure (4). These mechanical effects may produce peripheral edema. Placing the supine patient in the left lateral decubitus position lessens the venocaval compression. This maneuver moves the gravid uterus away from the right-sided inferior vena cava, relieving caval compression and improving the venous return to the right cardiac chambers.

The pregnant state places an additional stress on the maternal respiratory system. The demand on the mother to keep up with the fetus' rising oxygen requirements stimulates an increase in the resting minute ventilation. This is accomplished by an increase in maternal resting tidal volume and respiratory rate (5).

### *Labor*

Maternal hemodynamics change again with the onset of active labor. With each contraction, there is approximately an additional 500 mL of blood entering the maternal circulation due to constriction of the uterine vasculature (6). Circulating catecholamines, in part stimulated by pain and anxiety, elevate heart rate and blood pressure, augmenting an already elevated cardiac output.

### *After Delivery*

In the immediate postpartum period, venous return increases with removal of the venocaval impingement. At the same time, there is movement of blood from the placenta to the maternal circulation, compensating for the blood loss during delivery. Both augment cardiac preload and cause a brief rise in cardiac output. Increased preload and cardiac output may induce hemodynamic decompen-sation in patients with stenotic valvular disease, severe pulmonary hypertension, cardiomyopathy, or Eisenmenger syndrome. The overall hemodynamics return to baseline within the first month after delivery (7). There is generally little adverse hemodynamic consequence in normal women or in those with regurgitant valvular disease during the postpartum period. Patients with left to right shunts also do well.

### Pathophysiology in Patients with Heart Disease

Some conditions are in particular adversely affected by the physiologic changes of pregnancy and are at high risk for decompensation (Table 14.1). Increased cardiac and respiratory work may further elevate pulmonary artery pressures in women with pulmonary hypertension. These changes are most significant during the second trimester and during delivery. Worsening pulmonary hypertension may precipitate right heart failure or, in the extreme, cause the susceptible patient to develop right to left shunting.

A shunt may occur through a preexisting left to right heart connection, or blood in the right atrium may flow through the foramen ovale that has opened as a consequence of the high right-sided pressures. In similar fashion, patients with Eisenmenger syndrome may develop an increased right to left shunt. This may precipitate a worsening of symptoms and

**TABLE 14.1.** *Cardiovascular diseases at high risk for complications during pregnancy*

| Condition | Complication |
| --- | --- |
| Pulmonary hypertension | Increased pulmonary pressures, right to left shunt, fetal and maternal death |
| Eisenmenger syndrome | Increased shunt, desaturation, hemodynamic decompensation, fetal growth retardation, fetal and maternal death |
| Marfan syndrome | Aortic dissection or rupture |
| Coarctation of the aorta | Aortic dissection or rupture, severe hypertension |
| Hypertrophic cardiomyopathy | Congestive heart failure, arrhythmias, chest pain |
| Dilated cardiomyopathy | Congestive heart failure |
| Complex congenital heart disease with cyanosis | Desaturation, congestive heart failure, arrhythmias, endocarditis, fetal and maternal death |
| Severe valvular stenosis | Increased valvular gradient, hemodynamic decompensation |
| Bioprosthetic valves | Valve deterioration, regurgitation, stenosis |
| Mechanical prosthetic valve pannus | Thromboembolic phenomena, thrombus, stenosis or regurgitation |

alter the physical examination (e.g., increased cyanosis) and echocardiographic findings.

Pregnancy increases the risk of complications in those with mechanical and bioprosthetic valves. It appears to hasten the deterioration of bioprosthetic heart valves (8,9). Women with mechanical heart valves are at risk due to an increased incidence of thromboembolic phenomena, valve thrombosis, and pannus ingrowth (10).

### Cardiovascular Disease and Pregnancy

Specific abnormalities related to the pregnancy may occur in the cardiovascular system and may manifest as symptoms and/or changes in the physical or echocardiographic examination. These conditions require early recognition by the clinician because they increase the mortality and morbidity of the mother and fetus. The hypertensive syndromes of pregnancy, peripartum cardiomyopathy, and aortic dissection are included in this category.

Peripartum cardiomyopathy, also referred to as pregnancy-induced cardiomyopathy, is a form of dilated cardiomyopathy observed in gravid women without prior history of left ventricular (LV) dysfunction. Onset occurs in the 6th to 8th month of pregnancy and extends into the fifth month postpartum. This form of cardiomyopathy occurs in approximately one of every 10,000 term pregnancies and has no obvious etiology (11).

Pregnancy-related hypertensive syndromes are seen more commonly than peripartum cardiomyopathy, occurring in approximately 5% of all pregnancies (12). These entities include gestational hypertension (or pregnancy-induced hypertension), preeclampsia, and eclampsia. The hypertension associated with these syndromes usually occurs toward the end of pregnancy, at the time of delivery, or shortly thereafter. Elevation of systemic vascular resistance associated with hypertension may cause symptoms and alter the physical examination of previously healthy women, or it may adversely affect existing cardiac abnormalities, causing new or more pronounced symptoms or physical examination findings.

Women are at risk of aortic dissection during pregnancy, especially when concomitant aortic disease such as coarctation of the aorta or Marfan syndrome is present. Approximately one half of the aortic dissections seen in women <40 years old occur during pregnancy (13). This is believed to be secondary to the increased cardiac output as well as hormonal influences on aortic wall connective tissue. The incidence is elevated even in the absence of overt aortic disease. One series found up to 63% dissections in young pregnant women without evidence of Marfan syndrome, coarctation, or bicuspid aortic valve (14). The risk for dissection is greatest during the third trimester.

Some women with silent undiagnosed cardiac disease initially will become symptomatic during pregnancy (e.g., rheumatic mitral stenosis). Evaluation of the symptoms with careful physical examination often will provide the proper diagnosis. Echocardiography is useful in confirming the diagnosis or in making the diagnosis whether the physical examination is classic or nondiagnostic. Most cardiovascular processes unmasked by the physiology of pregnancy can be diagnosed accurately by history, physical examination, and echocardiography without the need for invasive studies.

Women who have undergone complete correction of congenital or acquired heart disease usually tolerate pregnancy well and have minimal need for intervention. If they are asymptomatic, they only need periodic assessment for changes in their status. If symptomatic, they require further evaluation with echocardiography. Others who have been partially corrected may have more difficulty during the physiologic changes of pregnancy.

### HISTORY

### Symptoms During Normal Pregnancy

Several physiologic alterations occur during pregnancy that prepare the woman's body for the growing fetus. Associated symptoms of seeming cardiac nature may be experienced in normal women during this time and are summarized in Table 14.2. These symptoms

**TABLE 14.2.** *Common cardiac symptoms during normal pregnancy*

Dyspnea on exertion
Resting breathlessness
Fatigue
Peripheral edema
Orthopnea
Paroxysmal nocturnal dyspnea
Palpitations
Rarely syncope

in and of themselves should not be considered diagnostic of cardiovascular disease unless accompanied by abnormal physical examination findings.

Hormonal changes can lead to complaints of flushing as well as lightheadedness. Some normal women may even experience brief episodes of syncope. Hormonal activation causes blood volume expansion, which commonly leads to symptoms of bloating and peripheral edema. Benign arrhythmias may present as palpitations. These usually represent premature beats of ventricular origin (15).

With increasing fetal size, there is progressive elevation of the diaphragm with diminished expansion of the lungs during breathing. This leads to a decrease in total lung capacity, especially the functional residual capacity. Increase in oxygen consumption due to the metabolic needs of the mother and fetus is compensated for by an increase in minute ventilation. An elevated respiratory rate and tidal volume achieve this. The increased respiratory rate along with a reduced residual capacity may cause symptoms of breathlessness. There often is worsening of these symptoms in the supine position and during late pregnancy, when the fetus is near full size. Pregnant women may complain of decreased exercise tolerance (a consequence of the decreased total lung capacity and increased body weight).

### Symptoms in the Pregnant Patient with Heart Disease

Although mild symptoms of dyspnea are common during pregnancy, moderate to ex-

treme difficulty in breathing may signify underlying cardiac pathology. In particular, associated symptoms of orthopnea, paroxysmal nocturnal dyspnea, and more than trace peripheral edema may suggest pulmonary congestion due to LV dysfunction. The diagnosis usually can be made by physical examination and can be quantitated further by echocardiography. Symptoms of cyanosis, such as a bluish tint of the lips and distal digits, are clearly an ominous sign that requires careful evaluation by physical examination. If underlying complex cardiac anomalies are suspected, echocardiography is the procedure of choice to define more clearly the intracardiac anatomy.

During pregnancy, valvular disease, either previously diagnosed or silent, may develop new or worsening manifestations. The expanded intravascular volume and enhanced cardiac output can exacerbate flow-limiting intracardiac lesions, such as aortic or mitral stenosis. In such cases, the patient may experience symptoms of easy fatigability, dyspnea on exertion, angina, orthopnea, or paroxysmal nocturnal dyspnea. Patients with severe valve stenosis may develop overt hemodynamic decompensation. This becomes a clinical problem particularly at the time of delivery, when the increased cardiac output, preload, and blood pressure may exert their greatest effect. Consequently, these factors combine to create the most significant elevation in the transvalvular gradient. Women who had been tolerating pregnancy well may become quite symptomatic during this portion of the pregnancy. Some may develop fulminant congestive heart failure.

Regurgitant valvular disease usually is well tolerated by most women during pregnancy. The reduced systemic and pulmonary resistance decreases the postvalvular pressure gradient and usually diminishes the degree of regurgitation. Therefore, the murmurs of mitral or aortic regurgitation, for example, may diminish or even disappear during pregnancy. A shortened diastole from the elevated heart rate additionally decreases the hemodynamic consequences of regurgitant lesions. Consequently, subjective worsening of the symptoms of valvular regurgitation is rarely seen unless there is an increase in the blood pressure (pregnancy-induced hypertension) or an insult to the valvular apparatus, such as superimposed acute endocarditis.

Women with atrial or ventricular septal defects tend to tolerate pregnancy well as long as they do not have significant pulmonary hypertension. This usually is the case since pulmonary hypertension is uncommon during the childbearing years. An increase in the pulmonary capillary pressure may be seen with atrial septal defect or ventricular septal defect, causing mild symptoms of pulmonary congestion such as dyspnea on exertion, orthopnea, or paroxysmal nocturnal dyspnea. Overt congestive heart failure, however, is rare.

The hemodynamic changes of pregnancy in the patient with pulmonary hypertension (with or without Eisenmenger syndrome) may produce cyanosis and/or deterioration with worsened hypoxemia. As the patient desaturates, the pulmonary pressures rise, accentuating the right to left shunting. This vicious cycle may be terminal. Patients with pulmonary hypertension without cyanosis may complain of fatigue and difficulty in breathing. There may be an increase in right heart failure with worsening peripheral edema. Women who have Eisenmenger physiology and/or pulmonary hypertension are at high risk of death, especially during the third trimester and during the time of delivery. Because of this high risk, it is generally recommended that these women do not become pregnant.

The pregnant patient may present acutely with aortic dissection. This is especially prevalent in women with Marfan syndrome and coarctation of the aorta who should be counseled against becoming pregnant. Symptoms include sudden onset of chest pain often described as tearing. Significant dissection or rupture may present with complete cardiac arrest. In some patients, the dissection may migrate proximally to the aortic cusps, causing aortic regurgitation or pericardial effusion with or without cardiac tamponade. Both may present with dyspnea and hemodynamic decompensation.

## PHYSICAL EXAMINATION

### General Appearance

Patients should be examined for signs of cyanosis. Peripheral cyanosis of the distal fingers and toes is seen in patients with cardiomyopathy and low cardiac output. Central cyanosis of the lips and gums suggests a right to left intracardiac shunt. The vitals signs and physical examination change predictably during the gravid period due to the normal hemodynamic and metabolic changes in the pregnant patient (Table 14.3).

**TABLE 14.3.** *Normal physical examination findings during pregnancy*

Elevated heart rate
Increased pulse pressure
Mild elevation of the jugular venous pulse with prominent a and v waves
Brisk carotid pulses
Enlarged PMI
Leftward and superior displacement of PMI
Louder $S_1$
Split $S_2$ with louder $P_2$
$S_3$
Systolic flow murmur
Mammary soufflé
Mild lower extremity edema

PMI, point of maximal impulse.

## Heart Rate and Blood Pressure

Increased metabolic demands and augmented blood volume with a relative anemia result in a mild increase in heart rate. A widened pulse pressure is seen as a consequence of a greater decrease in the diastolic compared to systolic blood pressure due to decreased systemic vascular resistance. The blood pressure falls during the first and second trimester, later rising slowly toward prepregnancy levels as the patient progresses toward term (3). The patient with gestational hypertension typically will experience elevation of the blood pressure in the third trimester and in the postpartum period. The definition of gestational hypertension is a rise in systolic or diastolic blood pressure of ≥30/15 mm Hg, respectively, or an absolute level >140/90 mm Hg (12).

## Jugular Venous Pulse

Examination of the neck veins may demonstrate a modest increase in the jugular venous pulse amplitude due to increased intravascular blood volume with associated increased prominence of the A and V waves. Because the jugular venous pulse is only marginally elevated, any significant elevation of the jugular venous pressure should signal the examiner to look for pathologic explanations for the elevation of right heart pressures, such as right-sided heart failure or pulmonary hypertension. A pronounced V wave suggests the diagnosis of tricuspid regurgitation.

## Arterial Pulse

Palpation of the carotid artery upstroke demonstrates brisk pulses due to elevated cardiac output. It should be remembered that pregnancy is a hyperkinetic state. Any condition associated with increased stroke volume and decreased peripheral resistance may produce abnormalities of the arterial pulse that can simulate aortic regurgitation.

## Lungs

With increasing fetal size, there is progressive elevation of the diaphragm with decreased excursion of the lungs as measured by percussion before and after full inspiration. The basilar breath tones may be diminished, with associated dullness to percussion. Women presenting with peripartum cardiomyopathy and congestive failure may have pulmonary interstitial edema producing basilar rales on auscultation. More significant fluid overload may include pleural effusions, which will cause dullness to percussion and decreased resonance at the site of the effusion.

## Precordial Palpation

Palpation of the precordium usually demonstrates a mildly displaced and increased apical impulse. Displacement of the point of maximal impulse or LV apex beat is to the left and superior (15). The apical pulse continues to shift leftward and superiorly, reaching its final displacement as the gravid uterus reaches term. Patients with peripartum cardiomyopathy may manifest more significant displacement of the apex impulse that may be difficult to distinguish from normal. The point of maximal impulse or LV apex beat in cases of cardiomyopathy is enlarged and sustained due to LV chamber dilation and dysfunction.

## Cardiac Auscultation

Auscultation of the heart during pregnancy demonstrates specific changes.

### *First and Second Heart Sounds*

There is usually an increase in the amplitude of the first heart sound ($S_1$) and the pulmonic valve component ($P_2$) of the second heart sound ($S_2$) (16). As a consequence of increased blood volume flowing across the pulmonic valve, there often is wide although not fixed splitting of the $S_2$ (15). Fixed splitting of the $S_2$ should raise the suspicion of an atrial septal defect. Patients with pulmonary hypertension will have a very prominent $P_2$.

### Third and Fourth Heart Sounds

Although a fourth heart sound ($S_4$) is not attributable to normal changes during pregnancy, as many as 84% of normal pregnant women may manifest a third heart sound ($S_3$) (15). *Practical Point: The finding of an $S_3$ in the absence of other symptoms or signs of heart failure should not alarm the examiner.* However, symptoms of congestive heart failure in the context of an audible $S_3$ should lead to further evaluation of LV dysfunction.

### Heart Murmurs

Systolic flow murmurs resulting from increased blood flow across the semilunar valves (especially of the pulmonary outflow) are common and found in >90% of pregnant women (17). The intensity of flow murmurs during pregnancy should be no more than grade 2/6. Systolic murmurs of greater magnitude require further evaluation to rule out outflow tract obstruction, such as pulmonary or aortic stenosis.

Diastolic murmurs should never be considered a normal finding during pregnancy (15). Mammary flow murmurs best heard in the left sternal border during diastole are not uncommonly heard during auscultation of the heart. These sounds, called mammary soufflé, are caused by increased blood flow through the internal mammary artery during pregnancy and may mimic the presence of a diastolic valvular murmur (15).

Changes may occur in previously documented cardiac physical examination findings (Table 14.4). The increased volume state may lessen or even abolish the click and murmur of mitral valve prolapse and the murmur of hypertrophic obstructive cardiomyopathy. The murmurs of aortic, tricuspid, pulmonic, and mitral stenosis are increased in amplitude as the higher blood volume flowing across the valves augments the transvalvular gradients. The decrease in systemic vascular resistance often diminishes the intensity of the murmurs of aortic and mitral regurgitation.

### Peripheral Manifestations

Examination of the lower extremities often demonstrates pedal edema, which may begin to occur early in pregnancy. The edema is due to the effects of increased estrogen levels, with salt and fluid retention resulting in increased intravascular volume. Pedal edema usually is mild (1 to 2+). However, as the pregnancy progresses, compression of the inferior vena cava by the gravid uterus, especially in the supine position, can lead to an increase in the femoral venous pressure. This may lead to further worsening of the peripheral edema. More generalized edema is not consistent with normal pregnancy and suggests possible preeclampsia. The peripheral pulses of the lower extremities should be normal.

## ECHOCARDIOGRAPHY

### Echocardiography During Normal Pregnancy

Many of the normal changes that occur with pregnancy can be seen during echocardiographic evaluation of the heart (Table 14.5). These include chamber dilation, increased stroke volume, enhanced ejection fraction, and mild valvular alterations. However, these changes seen during pregnancy have no pathologic significance in the vast majority of women; consequently, routine echocardiography cannot be recommended

**TABLE 14.4.** *Auscultatory changes in pregnant women with heart disease*

Decrease in regurgitant murmurs
Increase in stenotic murmurs
Decrease in murmur of hypertrophic cardiomyopathy
Decrease in the murmur and click of mitral valve prolapse
Decreased murmur of ventricular septal defect
Increased murmur of atrial septal defect
Increased signs of pulmonary hypertension

**TABLE 14.5.** *Normal echocardiographic parameters during pregnancy at term or third trimester*

| Parameter | Technique | Mean ± SD |
|---|---|---|
| LVEDD (mm) | M-mode | 47 ± 4 |
| LV wall thickness (mm) | M-mode | 10 ± 1 |
| LV mass (gm) | M-mode | 186 ± 39 |
| FS (%) | M-mode | 40 ± 7 |
| EF (%) | 2-D | 60 ± 4 |
| LA (mm) | 2-D | 38 ± 4 |
| RV (mm) | 2-D | 20 ± 1 |
| Mitral annulus (mm) | 2-D | 24 ± 5 |
| Tricuspid annulus (mm) | 2-D | 27 ± 3 |
| Aortic root (mm) | M-mode | 30 ± 12 |

2-D, two-dimensional; EF, ejection fraction; FS, fractional shortening; LA, left atrium; LV, left ventricle; LVEDD, left ventricular end-diastolic diameter; RV, right ventricle.

in women having an uncomplicated pregnancy.

The enhanced cardiac output and stroke volume can be measured by echocardiography through either two-dimensional (2-D) echocardiographic measurements of LV volumes or by Doppler ultrasound to calculate stroke volume and cardiac output by standard methods.

The small increases in overall myocardial thickness and dilation of the left and right ventricular cavity dimensions can be documented by 2-D and M-mode echocardiography. Echocardiography also can be used to calculate LV mass. Although the overall LV mass increases, LV hypertrophy as measured by end-diastolic wall thickness should not occur in normal pregnancy. Although the right ventricular mass probably increases as well, there is no established method to calculate this parameter. The left and right atrial dimensions also may be increased. In general, the chamber dilation seen during pregnancy is minimal and more evident in the right-sided cardiac chambers.

The mild dilation of the cardiac chambers may cause a slight dilation in the annular rings of the cardiac valves (18). Increase in the annular dimension may interfere with the dynamics of the valvular apparatus, leading to mild regurgitation. Consequently, it is not uncommon to observe mild regurgitant jets on color flow Doppler across any of the heart valves, generally not associated with an audible murmur. It is uncommon to find any more than mild regurgitant jets in pregnancy.

Echocardiography may be necessary to distinguish the existence of diastolic valvular abnormalities from mammary soufflé when diastolic sounds are appreciated during auscultation of the heart and the diagnosis is unclear.

Small pericardial effusions may be found during echocardiographic examination in up to 40% of pregnant women (19). Effusions tend to occur most frequently during the latter portions of the pregnancy; they usually are small and without consequence. When found, effusions most often represent an incidental finding.

**Echocardiography in Patients with Known or Suspected Heart Disease**

Echocardiography is necessary to evaluate higher risk patients or symptomatic patients in whom the history and physical examination suggest a cardiac pathology. Women with known mild to moderate valvular heart disease may need echocardiographic evaluation if symptoms suggest progression of valve pathology during pregnancy. Patients with complex intracardiac lesions, moderate to severe obstructive or regurgitant valvular disease, Eisenmenger syndrome, Marfan syndrome, or pulmonary hypertension should have echocardiographic evaluation at baseline and during the second trimester (the period when the effects of hemodynamic changes will be at their greatest). Symptomatic patients should be evaluated immediately.

Echocardiography is necessary to evaluate systolic ejection murmurs of grade 3/6 or greater intensity, new or worsened diastolic murmurs, or physical examination findings suggesting an undiagnosed atrial or ventricular septal defect. The magnitude of intracardiac shunting ($Q_p/Q_s$ ratio) in patients with an atrial septal defect, ventricular septal defect, or patent ductus arteriosus can be defined accurately by Doppler echocardiography (see chapter 13).

Dilation and dysfunction of the LV must be evaluated in the patient with suspected or known peripartum cardiomyopathy. When the pregnant patient presents with symptoms and physical findings of LV dysfunction, echocardiographic quantification of LV function is necessary to rule out the presence of peripartum cardiomyopathy. LV function can be estimated by 2-D echocardiography and can be quantified by several methods, such as the shortening fraction, ejection fraction measured by the simplified Simpson method, or acoustic quantification on echocardiographic machines with the appropriate software to perform these calculations.

Any new valvular regurgitation of moderate or severe degree should be considered pathologic and requires further evaluation to explain its etiology. It should be noted that just as the auscultatory findings of previously noted regurgitation is lessened during pregnancy, the echocardiographic manifestations of mitral or aortic regurgitation usually are diminished. Both are reflections of decreased pulmonary and systemic vascular resistance.

Echocardiographic evaluation is necessary for patients with known valvular stenotic lesions, especially if symptomatic. The magnitude of the gradient across the cardiac valves by Doppler is influenced by the hemodynamic changes of pregnancy. There is increased transvalvular flow, which increases the measured mean and peak gradients across the heart valves. However, overall calculated valve area should not be influenced.

The modified Bernoulli equation can be utilized to measure the right ventricular and pulmonary artery pressures. The right atrial pressure is estimated from observing the inferior vena cava dynamics during respiration. The right atrial pressure in considered >10 mm Hg if there is dilation of the inferior vena cava and shows <50% collapse with normal inspiration (20,21). These measurements are of particular importance when evaluating the patient with pulmonary hypertension; a pulmonary artery pressure >50 mm Hg places a patient at significant risk of complications (22). In general, chronic systolic pulmonary artery pressures >50 mm Hg are a relative contraindication for pregnancy because of the high rate of maternal and fetal mortality.

Echocardiography aids in the evaluation of women with Marfan syndrome who become pregnant. The risk of complication from aortic dissection, aortic rupture, and aortic regurgitation are high in these patients. This is especially the case when the aortic root diameter is found to be >40 mm (23). In such instances, termination of the pregnancy may be recommended. In those women continuing with their pregnancy, it may be necessary to evaluate for dissection or aortic regurgitation based on symptoms and physical examination findings. The ascending aorta can be evaluated proximally in the parasternal long-axis view to measure the cross-sectional diameter at the valvular, sinus, and tubular levels. Two-dimensional echocardiography from the suprasternal notch can image the distal ascending aorta and arch. The aortic root abnormalities found in Marfan syndrome also may be seen in the descending aorta. Therefore, transesophageal echocardiography (TEE) may be necessary in most patients to evaluate for aortic dissection. TEE can be performed safely in the pregnant patient and carries the same indications of TEE as in nonpregnant patients.

Echocardiography may be an invaluable asset in evaluating women with prosthetic heart valves, who are at increased risk of complication during pregnancy. When symptoms and physical findings suggest valve deterioration with either valvular regurgitation or obstruction, echocardiography can diagnose the abnormality and grade its severity. Mechanical valves can be evaluated for thrombosis or pannus ingrowth if the clinical manifestations of peripheral embolism or obstruction occur. TEE is superior to precordial echocardiography in these conditions. Echocardiography also can measure the prosthetic valve gradient to rule out stenosis. When the technical quality of transthoracic echocardiography is not adequate to make the diagnosis, TEE permits greater definition and visualization of the desired structures.

## SUMMARY

Normal changes of the physical and echocardiographic examination need to be anticipated during the course of a normal pregnancy (Tables 14.2–14.5). However, significant alteration occurs in the patient with cardiac abnormalities. By appreciating the normal variations, one can better understand the findings on physical examination and echocardiography, which will allow timely and precise diagnosis of heart disease in a pregnant woman. This is of great importance, as the results can have a lasting impact on the well-being of both the mother and fetus. By knowing the hemodynamic changes that occur

in pregnancy, one can better distinguish normal from abnormal symptoms and findings on the physical examination or echocardiography, thus preventing the pregnant patient with underlying cardiovascular disease from not being recognized and timely managed.

Close evaluation of symptoms and the physical examination is necessary for risk assessment at the beginning of the pregnancy. Echocardiography can be useful in these cases to support the physical examination findings and to add information to the overall evaluation. Echocardiography can be used to measure right-sided pressures, image structural abnormalities, and identify and quantify intracardiac shunts. The physical and echocardiographic examination can help to optimize management of the patient during the course of pregnancy. Periodic reevaluation occasionally is necessary to assess the patient's tolerance to the hemodynamic changes (especially in mid pregnancy and at delivery). Although currently there are no guidelines for echocardiography in the pregnant patient, proposed recommendations are listed in Table 14.6.

**TABLE 14.6.** *Recommendations for performing echocardiography in the pregnant patient*

| Condition | Echocardiography |
| --- | --- |
| Known or suspected ≥ mild valvular regurgitation | Murmur intensity worsens or symptoms occur |
| Known or suspected mild aortic or mitral stenosis | Murmur intensity worsens or symptoms occur |
| Mitral stenosis with refractory heart failure | Valvuloplasty under echocardiographic guidance |
| Symptomatic severe pulmonic stenosis | Valvuloplasty under echocardiographic guidance |
| Known or suspected moderate or severe regurgitation | Beginning and mid pregnancy, and if symptoms occur |
| Known or suspected moderate or severe aortic or mitral stenosis | Beginning and mid pregnancy, and if symptoms occur |
| New murmur suggestive of atrial or ventricular septal defect or patent ductus arteriosus | Indicated |
| Systolic ejection murmur III/VI or greater | Indicated |
| New diastolic murmur (any grade) | Indicated |
| Old diastolic murmur | Symptoms occur or murmur intensity increases |
| Symptoms or physical findings suggestive of cardiomyopathy | Indicated |
| History of cyanotic congenital disease | Initial and with symptoms |
| History of corrected congenital disease | If symptoms occur |
| History or clinically suspected pulmonary hypertension | Baseline echocardiogram and with symptoms |
| History of or clinically suspected Marfan disease or coarctation | Baseline echocardiogram, third trimester, and if symptoms occur (transesophageal echocardiogram may be needed) |
| History of valve replacement | If symptoms or physical findings of valve regurgitation, stenosis, or thromboembolism occur |

# REFERENCES

1. Longo LD. Maternal blood volume and cardiac output during pregnancy: a hypothesis of endocrinologic control. Am J Physiol 1983;245:R720.
2. Metcalfe J, Ureland K. Maternal cardiovascular adjustments to pregnancy. Prog Cardiovasc Dis 1974;16: 363–374.
3. Elkayam U, Gleicherm N. Hemodynamics and cardiac function during normal pregnancy and the puerperium. In: Elkayam U, Gleicherm N, eds. Cardiac problems in pregnancy: diagnosis and management of maternal and fetal disease, 2nd ed. New York: Alan R. Liss, 1990:5.
4. Lee W, Shah PK, Amim DK, et al. Hemodynamics monitoring of cardiac patients during normal pregnancy and the puerperium. In: Elkayam U, Gleicherm N, eds. Cardiac problems in pregnancy: diagnosis and management of maternal and fetal disease, 2nd ed. New York: Alan R. Liss, 1990:61.
5. Cunningham FG, MacDonald PC, Grant, NF, et al. Williams obstetrics, 20th ed. Stamford, Conn; Appleton and Lange 1997:210.
6. Robson SC, Dunlop W, Boys RJ, et al. Cardiac output during labour. BMJ 1987;295:1169.
7. McAnulty JH, Morton MJ, Ueland K. The heart and pregnancy. Curr Probl Cardiol 1988;3:589–665.
8. Badduke BR, Jameieson WR, Miyagshima RT, et al. Pregnancy and childbearing in a population with biologic valvular prostheses. J Thorac Cardiovasc Surg 1991;102:179–186.
9. Sbarouni E, Oakley CM. Outcome of pregnancy in women with valve prostheses. Br Heart J 1994;71: 196–201.
10. Hanania G, Thomas D, Michel PL, et al. Pregnancy and prosthetic heart valves: a French cooperative retrospective study of 1555 cases. Eur Heart J 1994;15:1651–1659.
11. Elkayam U. Pregnancy and cardiovascular disease. In: Braunwald E, ed. Heart disease: a textbook of cardiovascular disease. Philadelphia: WB Saunders, 1997:1851.
12. Kaplan NM. Clinical hypertension, 4th ed. Baltimore: Williams & Wilkins, 1986:345.
13. Snir E, Levinsky L, et al. Dissecting aortic aneurysm in pregnant women without Marfan disease. Surg Gynecol Obstet 1988;167:463–465.
14. Konishi IY, Tatsuta N, et al. Dissecting aneurysm during pregnancy and the puerperium. Jpn Circ J 1980;44: 726–733.
15. Harvey WP. Alterations of the cardiac physical examination in normal pregnancy. Clin Obst Gynecol 1975; 18:51–63.
16. Elkayam U, Gleicher N. The evaluation of the cardiac patient. In: Gleicher N, ed. Principles and practice of medical therapy in pregnancy, 2nd ed. Norwalk: Appleton and Lange, 1992:759.
17. Cutforth R, MacDonald CB. Heart sounds and murmurs in pregnancy. Am Heart J 1966;71:741–747.
18. Sadaniantz A, Kocceril AG, Emaus SP, et al. Cardiovascular changes in pregnancy evaluated by two-dimensional and Doppler echocardiography. J Am Soc Echocardiogr 1992;5:253–258.
19. Enein M, Aziz A, Zima A, et al. Echocardiography of the pericardium during pregnancy. Obstet Gynecol 987; 69:851.
20. Gullace G, Savoia MT. Echocardiographic assessment of the inferior vena cava as an index of right-sided cardiac function. Am J Cardiol 1990;66:493.
21. Kircher BJ, Himmelman RB, Schiller NB. Non-invasive estimation of the right atrial pressure based on two-dimensional echographic measurements of the inferior vena cava during measured inspiration. J Am Coll Cardiol 1988;11:557.
22. Sugishita Y, Ito I, Ozeki K, et al. Pregnancy in cardiac patients: possible influence of volume overload by pregnancy on pulmonary circulation. Jpn Heart J 1986;50: 376–383.
23. Pyeritz RE. Maternal and fetal complications of pregnancy in the Marfan syndrome. Am J Med 1981;71: 784–790.

# 15

# The Patient with Pericardial Disease

David Spodick and *Carlos A. Roldan

*Department of Medicine, University of Massachusetts Medical School; and Department of
Cardiovascular Medicine, Saint Vincent Hospital at Worcester Medical Center, Worcester,
Massachusetts; *Department of Internal Medicine, University of New Mexico School of Medicine;
and Department of Internal Medicine, Veterans Affairs Medical Center, Albuquerque, New Mexico*

## INTRODUCTION

The major pericardial conditions to be distinguished by physical examination and echocardiography include acute, noneffusive ("clinically dry") pericarditis; pericardial effusion without and with cardiac tamponade; and constrictive pericarditis without and with effusive-constrictive elements. Although the history and physical examination are essential in the diagnosis of pericardial diseases, the frequency of associated symptoms and physical findings vary according to the severity of the disease and are not so highly specific as to be diagnostic by themselves. Therefore, echocardiography has an important complementary and additive diagnostic value to the history and physical examination for the detection and management of pericardial diseases.

## ACUTE PERICARDITIS

### Introduction

Visceral pericardial inflammation results from infection, surgical or nonsurgical trauma, autoimmunity, malignant infiltration, mediastinal irradiation, or bleeding. Inflammation of the pericardium results in a serous, serosanguineous, serofibrinous, hemorrhagic, chylous, cholesterol-laden, or purulent pericardial fluid; with persistence, it results in pericardial thickening and fibrosis, and uncommonly calcification. Any interference with myocardial venous and lymphatic drainage due to high central venous pressure augments pericardial fluid accumulation.

Acute "clinically diagnosed" pericarditis is the common garden variety of pericarditis in which there is no effusion, or any effusion is relatively small and clinically silent. It represents inflammation of the mesothelium of the pericardial sac with exudation of fibrin (1). The etiology is among the widest in all medicine. Any agent or process that affect the pericardium or its neighboring structures and organs may be involved. This covers the gamut of infectious agents, immunopathies (which may follow an infection in the pericardium or elsewhere), neoplasm, trauma, the vasculitides, metabolic disorders, and a large numbers of conditions of uncertain pathogenesis.

Specific prevalences and incidences are not firmly established, except that the vast majority of cases in western countries appear to be viral (including the immunodeficiency virus), whereas increasing numbers of bacterial (including tuberculous) pericarditis occur in immunocompromised patients (2–4). Parasitoses are not seen often, except in immigrants, and are much more common in countries where parasites are endemic. Biases in reported frequencies are due to particular patient populations, for example, hospitals with large numbers of oncology patients and referral centers that see the unusual cases that are difficult to diagnose and manage.

The natural history and prognosis depend on discovering the etiology, if possible, and whether the disease is appropriately diagnosed and managed, although the large majority of viral or "idiopathic" cases respond rapidly to nonsteroidal antiinflammatory agents and last only days to weeks (5,6).

## History

Onset may be abrupt or insidious, although certain varieties tend to be characterized by one or the other mode. Bacterial and viral forms often strike with dramatic symptoms, whereas uremic or tuberculous pericarditis may arrive unnoticed. Over the very large range of etiologies, pain is the most common single symptom, although frequently it is absent. Thus, rheumatoid pericarditis, which is very common in patients with rheumatoid arthritis, is nearly always silent, whereas most acute infectious pericarditis cases rarely lack pain. Pain in acute pericarditis may be sharp, "sticking," dull, aching, or pressurelike, with widely varying intensity. Typically it is sharp and pleuritic. It is relieved by sitting up and leaning forward.

Pain is basically precordial and can radiate in all distributions common to ischemic pain. This creates a problem in differential diagnosis when the pain either is not pleuritic or has a pressing quality, particularly with radiation to the jaw or one or both shoulders. *Practical Point: Pain perceived in the trapezius ridges, usually the left, is virtually pathognomonic for pericardial irritation* (in some patients it is perceived only in a trapezius ridge). Patients should be asked to point to the area, because patients *and most physicians* will describe it as "shoulder" or "neck" (7). Pain occasionally occurs in the mid-posterior thorax or below the left scapula. Nonproductive *cough* is common and exacerbates pleuritic pain. Productive cough occurs due to associated illness, such as pneumonia, lung cancer, or empyema. *Odynophagia* results from apposition of the esophagus to the posterior parietal pericardium. *Dysphagia* results from esophageal compression by pericardial effusion or when pericardial disease is due to the spread of esophageal inflammation, trauma, or malignancy. There is occasional nausea, anorexia, and even vomiting in the first few days; these tend to be self-limited. *Fever,* usually <39°C, is frequent and may precede the onset of chest pain. *Anxiety* is common in patients with a great deal of pain, particularly in those with preexisting heart disease. *Pallor* may be a clue to systemic illness.

### Physical Examination

*Blood pressure and arterial pulse* are unaffected in the absence of complications.

*Jugular veins* are unaffected in the absence of complications.

*Precordial examination* reveals no abnormalities, nor should *palpation,* unless the differential diagnosis involves a chest wall syndrome, which is suggested by local tenderness.

Upon *auscultation,* the heart sounds are not involved. There are no abnormal third (S₃) or fourth (S₄) heart sounds, and no murmurs, clicks, or ejection sounds except those caused by coexisting illness. The *pericardial rub* (friction sound), which is composed of one to three friction elements per cardiac cycle, is the *cardinal sign of pericarditis* (Fig. 15.1). Rubs may be transient or intermittent and often last hours to days; they rarely become chronic. They are considered to arise from friction between inflamed surfaces of the visceral and parietal pericardial mesothelium associated with absence of surfactant pericardial phospholipids that lubricate what would otherwise be hydrophilic surfaces (1). Pericardial friction rubs vary from relatively distant "scraping" sounds to loud, and occasionally palpable, harsh grating sounds synchronous with atrial systole, ventricular systole, and early ventricular diastole, any one or two of which may be missing. The loudest rub nearly always is the ventricular systolic rub and the weakest the ventricular diastolic rub. They are generally much louder in inspiration in the presence of some excess pericardial fluid, but inspiration alone makes nearly all rubs louder because of normal in-

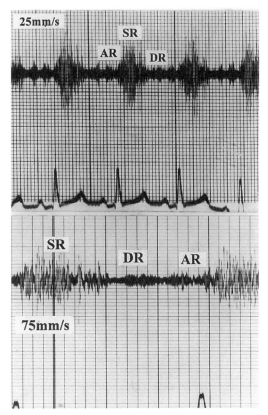

**FIG. 15.1.** Phonocardiogram at 25 mm/s (**top: electrocardiographic speed**) and analyzed further three times as fast showing typical triphasic pericardial friction. AR, atrial rub; Dr, ventricular diastolic rub; SR, ventricular systolic rub. (From Spodick DH. The pericardium: a comprehensive textbook. New York: Marcel Dekker, 1997, with permission.)

creased inspiratory filling of the right ventricle (RV), which is the anterior portion of the heart (Fig. 15.2). They differ from murmurs in that they often sound more "superficial" and do not follow the rules for location or radiation of murmurs, although fortuitously localized rubs may resemble murmurs. Eighty-nine of 100 rubs in an etiologically mixed series of acute pericarditis were loudest or only perceived at the left lower sternal border, where palpable rubs (common in uremic pericarditis) are nearly always appreciated. In addition to these typical *endopericardial*

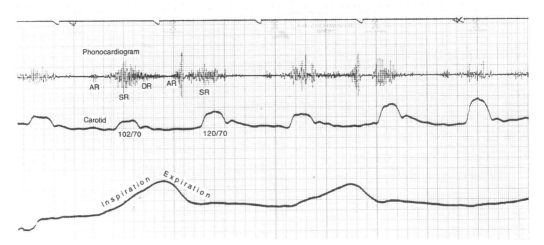

**FIG. 15.2.** Inspiratory amplification of rub. Phonocardiogram, carotid pulse, and respiratory thermistor output. Rub components increase during and at peak inspiration and decrease during expiration (the latter seen best at beginning and end of phonocardiogram). Patient has cardiac tamponade. Pressures obtained from brachial cuff. (From Spodick DH. The pericardium: a comprehensive textbook. New York: Marcel Dekker, 1997, with permission.)

*rubs*, occasionally there may be such severe inflammation that the parietal pericardium rubs against the adjacent pleura, chest wall (*exopericardial rub*), or both (*endoexopericardial rub*) (1).

## PERICARDIAL EFFUSION WITHOUT CARDIAC TAMPONADE

### Introduction

Pericardial effusion indicates an excess of liquid contents in the pericardium (i.e., more than the normal 15 to 35 mL of pericardial fluid) due to either irritation/inflammation or *hydropericardium* in fluid retention states (8). Effusions may remain entirely silent unless the fluid accumulates so fast or to such a great extent that it compresses the heart and produces cardiac tamponade. The prevalence is not well known, although some etiologies of acute pericarditis are more likely to produce effusions, whereas all fluid-retaining states (e.g., congestive heart failure, renal failure) seem to follow no rule in sometimes causing hydropericardium, the prognosis of which is that of the underlying disease.

### History

The history is that of the underlying disease, with the effusion often being discovered by accident, unless it is so large that compression of the lungs causes dyspnea, usually on exertion. However, some conditions (e.g., pericardial malignancies) may present as pericardial effusions.

### Physical Examination

*Blood pressure and arterial pulse* are not directly affected without tamponade.

*Jugular veins* are not distended without tamponade or concomitant heart disease.

*Precordial percussion* will reveal a dull to flat note over an enlarged cardiac silhouette with some postural shape change, but percussion is undependable unless the changes are gross.

*Abnormal heart sounds and murmurs* are not induced by nontamponading effusion, but existing sounds and murmurs may be made more distant. *Rubs* frequently persist despite effusion, suggesting that some rubbing surfaces are exopericardial.

## CARDIAC TAMPONADE

### Introduction

Cardiac tamponade is defined as significant compression (resulting from increased intrapericardial pressure) and impairment of filling of the heart by accumulating pericardial contents, including effusion fluids, pus, blood, clots, or gas, singly or in combination (9). Its diagnosis include (i) presence of a moderate to large pericardial effusion; (ii) increased intrapericardial pressure ≥3 mm Hg; (iii) increased and equalization of intrapericardial, right atrial (RA), pulmonary artery diastolic, and pulmonary capillary wedge pressures; and (iv) decreased cardiac output and blood pressure (with exaggerated pulsus paradoxus) and increased heart rate and systemic vascular resistance.

Because *tamponade is a pathophysiologic continuum,* patients may have mild to florid tamponade, the latter being a life-threatening emergency and the former a stage that can progress in that direction.

### Etiology

Cardiac tamponade is essentially the gamut of the many conditions that can cause pericardial inflammation (infectious or noninfectious), pericardial trauma, or bleeding. Among the most common causes of large pericardial effusions leading to cardiac tamponade are malignancy, uremia, acute or chronic idiopathic pericarditis, infection, anticoagulation, inflammatory connective tissue diseases, and, uncommonly, Dressler and postpericardiotomy syndromes (Table 15.1) (10–12).

Pericardial tumors usually resulting from metastasis from breast, lung, or skin malignancies manifest as large pericardial effusions (rather than isolated or multiple epicardial tumor masses) resulting in cardiac tamponade, effusive-constrictive pericarditis, or constrictive pericarditis. The effects of radiotherapy for breast or lung malignancies also can lead to pericardial inflammation, effusion, fibrosis, and similar clinical syndromes. Some etiologies, such as bacterial pericarditis, are especially likely to produce tamponade, although the possibility of tamponade should be anticipated in any patient with a pericardial lesion.

The natural history nearly always is one of steady progression, depending on the tempo of the inciting process. This is likely to be slow in many patients with cancer who do not bleed actively so that large effusions often accumulate before clinical tamponade. Active bleeding (including *hemopericardium),* however, speeds the evolution of any effusion. In all cases, relief (i.e., drainage) is the treatment, which will interrupt the natural history and reverse the prognosis, which is otherwise dismal.

### Pathophysiology

Normally and during inspiration, an increase in the negative intrathoracic and intrapleural pressure results in reduction of the intrapericardial pressure of >5 mm Hg; decrease in RA and RV pressures; and conse-

**TABLE 15.1.** *Common etiologies of cardiac tamponade*

| Etiology | Frequency % |
| --- | --- |
| Malignancy | 30–60 |
| Uremia | 10–15 |
| Idiopathic | 5–15 |
| Infection | 5–10 |
| Anticoagulation | 5–10 |
| Inflammatory connective tissue diseases | 2–6 |
| Dressler and postpericardiotomy syndromes | 0.5–2 |

Data from references 10–12.

quently increase in venous return to the right heart. Opposite hemodynamic changes occur simultaneously in the left atrium (LA) and left ventricle (LV). The reverse hemodynamic changes occur during expiration (Fig. 15.3). In cardiac tamponade during inspiration, there is still a mild decrease in intrapericardial pressure that results in increased venous return to the RV, which simultaneously limits LV filling due to the restraining pericardial effusion. In addition, during inspiration, decreased pressures in the pulmonary veins lead to a further decrease in left heart filling. These hemodynamic changes lead to de-

creased cardiac output, blood pressure, and pulse volume during inspiration (*pulsus paradoxus*).

### History

Overall, the history will be that of the inciting process, the appearance of tamponade often adding progressive dyspnea, at first on exertion. Yet, many patients may or may not have had recognizable antecedent acute pericarditis or systemic illnesses with potential pericardial components. Chest pain is variable, but dyspnea is almost invariable. Chest

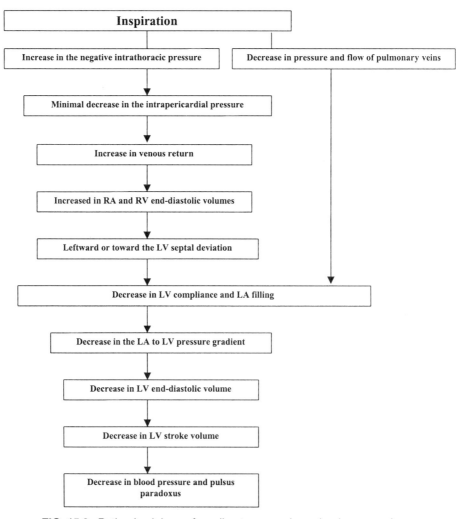

**FIG. 15.3.** Pathophysiology of cardiac tamponade and pulsus paradoxus.

trauma and bleeding diatheses should always raise a question of tamponade. Fluid retaining states *per se* induce hydropericardium without tamponade. Among these, however, acute or chronic renal failure also can provoke acute pericardial inflammation, whereas heart failure induces only a bland hydropericardium.

### Physical Examination

Physical findings in patients with cardiac tamponade vary according to the severity of the disease and the standard used for comparison. Also, the characteristic physical findings of cardiac tamponade are highly variable and commonly absent (Table 15.2) (10,13).

*Blood pressure and arterial pulse:* Systolic blood pressure tends to be low and progress to shock levels, although occasional patients with a large adrenergic drive will have normal to high blood pressures. The arterial pulse tends to be weak and thready in advanced stages. However, at any point, *pulsus paradoxus* usually is present, commonly defined as an inspiratory fall in arterial pressure of ≥10 mm Hg and frequently palpable in the radial pulse (14). *Note:* Muscular arteries are better than the elastic carotids to appreciate this phenomenon; indeed, pulsus paradoxus is a "pulsus"—*a pulse*— and originally was discovered by palpation. However, it is quantitated at the bedside by measuring blood pressure.

*Jugular veins:* Jugular veins will be distended unless the patient is hypovolemic (but they may be difficult to appreciate unless the patient has chronic tamponade, an uncommon situation). The Y descent will be absent. With blood loss (e.g., traumatic pericarditis during multiple trauma), jugular distention is not a reliable phenomenon because of hypovolemia.

*Precordial percussion and palpation:* This will be the same as for pericardial effusion. In addition, with large effusions there may be a Bamberger-Pins-Ewart sign, a zone of dullness and bronchial breathing between the tip of the left (rarely the right) scapula and the vertebral column (8).

*Auscultation:* Because of hemodynamic impairment, the first ($S_1$) and second ($S_2$) heart sounds tend to be of reduced intensity. $S_3$ tends to be suppressed because tamponade aborts the rapid filling phase of diastole and $S_4$ is variable, depending on the patient's age and condition prior to the lesion. There are no murmurs associated with tamponade, although a pericardial rub may persist.

*Other peripheral signs:* If the heart rate is not too fast and the patient has a "good" neck for inspection, distended jugular veins will show an X descent but absent or greatly attenuated Y descent, with the X descent appearing in mid systole (between $S_1$ and $S_2$). *These are not outward pulsations.* X and Y descents in compressive pericardial diseases

**TABLE 15.2.** *Physical findings in patients with cardiac tamponade*[a]

| Physical finding | Frequency (%) |
|---|---|
| Elevated jugular venous pressure | 40–100 |
| Sinus tachycardia | 50–75 |
| Pulsus paradoxus (≥20 mm Hg) | 17–75 |
| Hepatomegaly | 25–55 |
| Distant heart sounds | 25–35 |
| Systolic blood pressure <100 mm Hg | 15–35 |
| Pericardial rub | 25–30 |
| Peripheral edema | 20–30 |

[a]Lowest rates are reported in patients with echocardiographic findings suggestive of cardiac tamponade or in those with atypical forms of tamponade (i.e., after cardiac surgery) and highest rates in those with clinical evidence of tamponade.
Data from references 10–13.

are *collapses* from a high standing level that may be measurable but often are not, unless the patient is made to sit straight up. Scalp and retinal veins often are distended; occasionally the leg veins are distended.

## CONSTRICTIVE PERICARDITIS

### Introduction

Constrictive pericarditis is a form of cardiac compression caused by a rigid, fibrosed, or calcified pericardium with or without some residual fluid resulting in *decreased ventricular filling.* After reabsorption of pericardial fluid, the inflammatory process of the visceral and parietal pericardial layers leads to their fusion, fibrosis, and (with chronicity) calcifi-

cation. The scarring process is progressive and nearly always covers the whole heart. Constrictive pericarditis is hemodynamically characterized by restrained ventricular filling after the first third of diastole leading to rapid and marked elevation and equalization of ventricular end-diastolic and mean atrial pressures. This hemodynamic pattern forms the characteristic ventricular "square root sign" of pericardial constriction (Fig. 15.4). The end result is decreased ventricular end-diastolic volume, stroke volume, and cardiac output (15–17).

### Etiology

Etiology is virtually all the causes of acute pericarditis, with the curious exception of rheumatic carditis. The etiologic mix has varied considerably. In the United States, the most common etiology is idiopathic, presumably following viral infection, and postcardiac surgery (a form of traumatic pericarditis). In patients after cardiac surgery, manifestations of constriction can occur 1 to 5 years after the procedure (18). Tuberculosis, formerly relatively common, is seen today mainly in the immunocompromised population and in the Third World (15,19). Prevalence depends on the frequency and course of the inciting processes, which vary widely geographically. The natural history is one of progressive disability, although constriction exists in acute, subacute, and chronic forms. "Chronic constrictive pericarditis" as a blanket term has long been outmoded (19). Transient, clinically insignificant constriction frequently follows acute pericarditis for a few days and is recognizable by cardiographic methods (1,19).

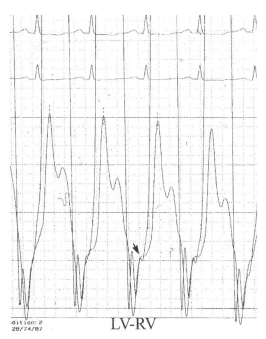

LV-RV

**FIG. 15.4.** Simultaneous left and right ventricular pressure tracing in a 54-year-old man with clinically suspected constrictive pericarditis. Note that the right and left ventricles demonstrate restrained ventricular filling after the first third of diastole leading to rapid elevation and equalization of their end-diastolic pressures (20 mm Hg) forming the characteristic "square root sign" of pericardial constriction *(arrow).*

### History

There may be no history of preceding illness, although the majority of patients have had some form of acute pericarditis or a condition, such as cardiac surgery or chest trauma, which could result in intrapericardial bleeding—the common substrate for eventual constrictive scarring (19). Pain is rare unless there has been chest trauma, including surgery. Most often there is progressive dyspnea beginning with dyspnea on exertion. Cardiothoracic surgery, other chest trauma, infective pericarditides, and the vasculitis-connective tissue disease group are familiar precursors, although numerous drugs (e.g., procainamide) occasionally induce constriction (19). Any hemopericardium, including those cases due to hemorrhagic disorders, should be considered as potentially constrictive if there has been pericardial trauma or inflammation (20).

### Physical Examination

*Systolic blood pressure* varies from low to normal to elevated, with corresponding strengths of arterial pulse. A definite pulsus paradoxus may be present but nearly always measures <15 mm Hg and most often is absent by sphygmomanometry.

*Jugular venous pulse:* Jugular veins nearly always are distended with a high pressure level, which may require sitting up to appreciate. Unlike tamponade, there are two definite collapses, the X descent in mid systole between $S_1$ and $S_2$ and the Y descent in early diastole (after $S_2$), with Y usually the deeper.

*Precordial percussion* usually is of no help. The abnormal $S_3$ may be palpable.

*Auscultation:* $S_1$ and $S_2$ nearly always are reduced in intensity because of the hemodynamic embarrassment. Sometimes the pulmonic valve component ($P_2$) is relatively accentuated (9). $S_4$ is variable but present regularly in the uncommon *elastic constriction* due usually to rubbery malignant tissue or an intrapericardial clot; $S_4$ is of little help diagnostically. *The cardinal physical finding is a loud and early $S_3$ occurring in well over half the cases* (19). It can be quite sharp and, at rapid rates, can resemble $S_1$ if it is the only loud sound. It often is palpable and sometimes may have a "knocking" quality, but this is seen less frequently, except in survivors of very chronic constriction. It does not arise from the pericardium itself, so the term "pericardial knock" is conceptually

flawed (19) but frequently used. *It is a special instance of the abnormal $S_3$* because it occurs at the sudden termination of the rapid filling period in early diastole, which is progressively brief and exceptionally rapid in constriction. Occasional systolic clicks are of uncertain origin but probably arise from the mitral apparatus, unrelated to constriction, unless (rarely) ventricular compression results in mitral or tricuspid prolapse. *Murmurs* occur if they had been previously present, if atrioventricular groove constriction involves one of the atrioventricular valves, or if one of the outflow arteries (pulmonary artery, aorta) undergoes ringlike compression. These murmurs mimic intrinsic disease at these locations. Rubs occasionally persist in patients who have constriction and may be exopericardial or due to imperfect envelopment of the heart by scar.

*Peripheral manifestations* include distention of veins in any extremity, ascites, and peripheral edema. In some cases, there may be conspicuous ascites without any peripheral edema (19). *Kussmaul sign*—inspiratory jugular venous distention or failure of jugular venous collapse during inspiration—replaces the normal inspiratory venous "collapse" and is common because the normal inspiratory acceleration of venous blood toward the heart occurs in the venae cavae but is resisted at the high-pressure RA, causing the neck veins to distend (19).

### EFFUSIVE CONSTRICTIVE PERICARDITIS

This condition is characterized by a mixture of previously discussed signs, depending on the relative degree of constriction versus effusion so that evidence of both conditions may be present simultaneously. For example, there may be an abnormal $S_3$ in the presence of a tamponading or nontamponading effusion because of underlying pericardial constriction that may only be revealed after drainage of pericardial fluid. Another clue is the Kussmaul sign during or after an effusion. Constriction with a pulsus paradoxus well over 10 mm Hg is a strong clue. If the jugular venous pulse can be well seen, an X descent larger than the Y descent is quite suggestive (19).

## ECHOCARDIOGRAPHY

### Introduction

Detection of pericardial diseases is one of the common applications of echocardiography. M-mode, two-dimensional (2-D), and Doppler echocardiography can accurately define the presence and size of a pericardial effusion; detect associated pericardial thickening (rarely calcification) or masses; and more importantly, determine their hemodynamic significance. Independent of its etiology, the extent and time of accumulation of a pericardial effusion as well as the extent of associated pericardial scarring will determine the echocardiographic manifestations of acute pericarditis, cardiac tamponade, and constrictive pericarditis.

### Acute Pericarditis with or without Pericardial Effusion

#### *M-Mode and Two-Dimensional Echocardiography*

The demonstration of pericardial effusion and/or pericardial thickening by these techniques confirms the diagnosis of pericarditis in a patient with a consistent clinical syndrome. A pericardial effusion is manifested by separation of the visceral from the parietal pericardium, by a decrease in the motion of the parietal pericardium, and when large by swinging of the heart.

A pericardial effusions is *small* (<100 mL) when it is localized posterior to the LV, is seen distal to the atrioventricular groove, and separation of the pericardial layers is <1 cm; *moderate* (100 to 500 mL) when fluid accumulates posteriorly and extends posterior to the LA, also is seen anteriorly, laterally, or apically, and pericardial separation is <1 cm; and

*large* (>500 mL) when fluid accumulates circumferentially, separation of the pericardial layers is >1 cm, and/or the heart swings in anteroposterior and mediolateral directions within the pericardial sac.

The absence of a pericardial effusion by echocardiography does not exclude the diagnosis of acute pericarditis. Pericardial effusion is not detected in at least one third of patients with clinically evident pericarditis and a pericardial friction rub. Similarly, the presence of a pericardial effusion does not establish the diagnosis of pericarditis. About one third of uremic patients have pericardial effusions (generally small) without pericarditis. In addition, echocardiography has limited sensitivity (40% to 60%) in detecting pericardial thickening >2 mm (21,22).

Although inflammatory pericardial effusions have some echocardiographic features that may separate them from those with a noninflammatory etiology, these characteristics are not specific enough to be diagnostic. Also, the sensitivity of echocardiography for detection of pericardial nodules or masses is low (<40%). However, the presence of intrapericardial strands or fibrous bands representing fibrin aggregates, thrombus, or rarely tumor is indicative of an inflammatory process. These bands extend from the visceral to parietal pericardium as partial or complete bandlike structures with linear, undulated, or hypermobile appearance (Fig. 15.5).

Two-dimensional echocardiography can identify loculated effusions, but its sensitivity is low, especially in patients after cardiac surgery. However, loculated pericardial effusions in patients with clinically suspected pericarditis are uncommon. Patients in the period immediately after cardiac surgery have a high incidence of loculated effusions or hematomas (most commonly in those who have undergone valve replacement). In these patients, transesophageal echocardiography (TEE) may be necessary due to the frequent technical difficulties in obtaining transthoracic images.

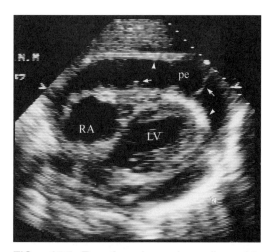

**FIG. 15.5.** Transthoracic echocardiographic subcostal four-chamber view in a 34-year-old man with infectious pericarditis demonstrates a large pericardial effusion (pe), significant parietal and visceral pericardial thickening *(arrowheads)*, and partial and complete fibrous bands extending from the visceral to the parietal pericardium *(arrows)*. LV, left ventricle; RA, right atrium.

The specificity of 2-D echocardiography for detecting pericardial effusions is compromised by the misinterpretation of epicardial fat. Subepicardial fat has a speckled or granular echo-reflectance compared to fluid. It is seen predominantly anterior to the heart, especially anteroapical to the RV and rarely (<7%) posteriorly. It is more common in the elderly, obese, diabetic, and in women. The prevalence of subepicardial fat increases with age (<1% in patients <30 years old and up to 15% in those >80 years old), but most of these deposits are small. Subepicardial fat is seen best in the long parasternal and subcostal views. Therefore, an echo-free space seen only anteriorly should not confirm the diagnosis of a pericardial effusion.

Two-dimensional echocardiography can differentiate a pericardial from a pleural effusion. A posteriorly located and large pericardial effusion extends anterior to the descending aorta and posterior to the LA. In contrast, a left pleural effusion will extend behind the descending aorta.

## Doppler Echocardiography

This technique is of complementary diagnostic value to M-mode and 2-D echocardiography in determining the presence or absence of cardiac tamponade or constrictive physiology in patients with pericarditis with or without pericardial effusions.

## Cardiac Tamponade

### Definition

Cardiac tamponade is defined on echocardiography as diastolic collapse of the right heart chambers (uncommonly of the left heart chambers), biatrial hypertension, and a significant increase in right heart stroke volume with a simultaneous decrease in left heart stroke volume with inspiration, all produced by a moderate to large pericardial effusion (small or moderate in acute hemorrhagic tamponade).

### Echocardiographic Diagnosis

The onset and severity of echocardiographic manifestations of cardiac tamponade are related to the rate and severity of fluid accumulation (global or localized); the patient's preexisting intravascular volume status (i.e., low-pressure cardiac tamponade if volume depletion is present); presence of underlying myocardial disease (i.e., absent chamber compression and pulsus paradoxus if high RV or LV end-diastolic pressure); and associated pericardial disease (effusive constrictive physiology if pericardial thickening or fibrosis present).

Although the traditional teaching is that cardiac tamponade is a clinical diagnosis, several series of patients with hemodynamic or frank echocardiographic evidence of cardiac tamponade have demonstrated that the characteristic clinical findings of tamponade (i.e., pulsus paradoxus) frequently are absent (Table 15.2) (10,11). In fact, the diagnosis of cardiac tamponade is more commonly suspected and appropriate workup pursued based on nonspecific clinical findings, such as tachycardia, hypotension, or jugular venous distention. On the other hand, no single echocardiographic parameter is pathognomonic for cardiac tamponade. In addition, patients with loculated pericardial effusions or hematomas can have atypical clinical, echocardiographic, and hemodynamic findings of cardiac tamponade. In these patients, echocardiography may have better diagnostic accuracy than clinical or hemodynamic data. Clinical evidence of cardiac tamponade generally identifies those patients with overt echocardiographic findings and significant hemodynamic derangement. In contrast, echocardiography frequently identifies those patients with minimal clinical or hemodynamic compromise, which allows for early diagnosis and therapeutic interventions. In conclusion, cardiac tamponade has a spectrum of severity rather than being an all-or-none phenomenon. Accurate diagnosis requires integration of clinical, echocardiographic, and commonly hemodynamic criteria.

Echocardiographic diagnosis of cardiac tamponade includes (i) a moderate to large pericardial effusion; (ii) RA diastolic compression at onset of systole; (iii) RV diastolic compression (23); (iv) uncommonly, compression of the left heart chambers; (v) RA hypertension manifested by persistent inferior vena cava plethora during inspiration and abnormal hepatic vein (or superior vena cava) outflow Doppler velocities (24); (vi) LA hypertension evidenced by abnormal pulmonary vein inflow Doppler velocities; and (vii) significant respiratory variability in the transmitral and tricuspid inflow Doppler velocities as a manifestation of the variable right and left heart stroke volumes (25,26). None of these findings is pathognomonic for cardiac tamponade, and their frequency is variable (Table 15.3).

## M-Mode Echocardiography

M-mode echocardiography can define better than 2-D echocardiography the presence, timing, and severity of RV diastolic collapse. Diastolic RV collapse occurs during early diastole and resolves in late diastole. Long- or short-axis parasternal and subcostal views are optimal (Fig. 15.6). Less specific signs resulting from decrease stroke volume during inspiration are decreased opening of the mitral valve and diminished E to F slope. M-mode imaging can define the extent of separation of pericardial layers and help to define the size of a pericardial effusion. The technique also can identify the presence of pericardial thickening, but with limited sensitivity and specificity.

## Two-Dimensional Echocardiography

This technique is more accurate than M-mode echocardiography in defining the size and hemodynamic compromise of a pericardial effusion. Similarly, this technique can define better than M-mode echocardiography the characteristics of right heart chamber diastolic collapse (Fig. 15.7 and Table 15.4).

**TABLE 15.3.** *Echocardiographic findings in cardiac tamponade*

| Finding | Frequency (%) |
| --- | --- |
| Moderate to large pericardial effusion | ≥95 |
| Right atrial diastolic compression | ≥90 |
| Right ventricular diastolic compression | ≥60 |
| Variable transmitral and tricuspid flow with respiration | ≥75 |
| Plethoric inferior vena cava | ≥60 |
| Abnormal hepatic vein flow patterns | ≥60 |
| Abnormal pulmonary veins flow patterns | ≥50 |
| Rarely, left atrial or left ventricular diastolic compression | ≤30% |

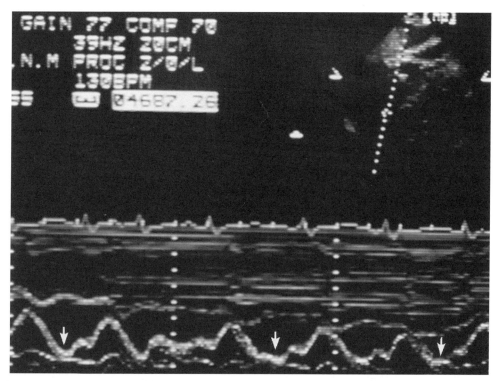

**FIG. 15.6.** M-mode echocardiogram of the posterolateral right ventricular wall in a 62-year-old man with a large malignant pericardial effusion and cardiac tamponade demonstrates significant right ventricular diastolic collapse *(arrow)*.

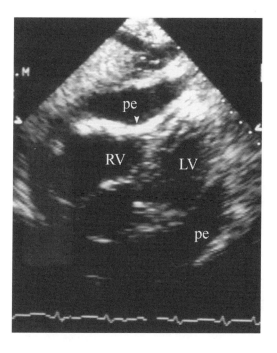

**FIG. 15.7.** Two-dimensional echocardiographic subcostal four-chamber view of the patient shown in Fig. 15.6 demonstrates a large pericardial effusion (pe) and significant right ventricular diastolic collapse *(arrowhead)*. Abbreviations as in previous figures.

**TABLE 15.4.** *Characteristics of right atrial and right ventricular diastolic compression in cardiac tamponade*

| Right atrial diastolic compression | Right ventricular diastolic compression |
|---|---|
| Most common and earliest finding | Occur after RA diastolic compression |
| Most sensitive (≥90%), but with low specificity (60%–80%) and positive predictive value (50%–60%)[a] | Lower sensitivity (≥60%), but with high specificity (≥90%) and positive and negative predictive values (about 80% for both) |
| Occurs when IPP is ≥4 mm Hg | Occurs at IPP ≥10 ± 4 mm Hg[b] |
| Occurs during late diastole/early systole and is worse during expiration or apnea | Occurs during early diastole. May be transient or last throughout early and mid diastole and disappear after atrial contraction. |
| Best noted on the mid portion of the RA lateral wall | Best seen on the RV anterior wall and infundibulum |
| Duration of at least one third or more of the cardiac cycle is more predictive of tamponade | Degree and duration of RV collapse do not correlate with severity of cardiac tamponade |
| Best seen on apical and subcostal views | Best seen on parasternal long- and short-axis views |

[a]Usually indicates equalization of intrapericardial and right ventricular (RV) pressures.
[b]RV diastolic compression indicates a drop in cardiac output of at least 20%.
IPP, intrapericardial pressure; RA, right atrial.

Two-dimensional echocardiography can suggest the etiology of a pericardial effusion, and the presence and degree of pericardial thickening and adhesions. An echolucent fluid may indicate a transudate and, therefore, a noninflammatory etiology. In contrast, a highly echogenic pericardial effusion with filamentous structures or fibrinous strands or bands suggests an inflammatory etiology (infectious, malignant, or hemorrhagic) (Fig. 15.5).

Cardiac tamponade most commonly is associated with a moderate or large sized pericardial effusion. However, in patients with acute bleeding into the pericardium (after heart surgery, coronary artery perforation during percutaneous coronary interventions, aortic dissection, and in blunt or penetrating chest trauma), cardiac tamponade can occur

with smaller or loculated pericardial effusions. In these patients, compression of the coronary sinus, LA, or LV by rapidly increasing pericardial pressure are common earlier signs of cardiac tamponade (27).

The diagnostic accuracy of 2-D echocardiography is higher in patients with large and circumferential pericardial effusions and in patients with clinical or hemodynamic evidence of cardiac tamponade. In patients with clinical findings of cardiac tamponade, RA or RV diastolic collapse is seen in about 90% of patients. In these patients, RA collapse is more common than RV diastolic collapse. However, in patients without clinical findings of tamponade, RA diastolic collapse is seen in one third of patients and RV collapse in 10%. Therefore, the sensitivity and negative predictive value of RA collapse are higher than

**TABLE 15.5.** *Sensitivity, specificity, and predictive values of right heart chamber collapse for detection of cardiac tamponade*

| Abnormality | Sensitivity (%) | Specificity (%) | Positive predictive value (%) | Negative predictive value (%) |
|---|---|---|---|---|
| RA collapse | 68 | 66 | 52 | 80 |
| RV collapse | 60 | 90 | 77 | 81 |
| RA and RV collapse | 45 | 92 | 74 | 76 |
| Any collapse | 90 | 65 | 58 | 92 |

RA, right atrial; RV, right ventricular.
Data from reference 12.

those of RV diastolic collapse. In contrast, the specificity and positive predictive value of RV diastolic collapse are higher than those of RA collapse (Table 15.5) (12).

Two-dimensional echocardiography plays a vital role in the rapid assessment and management of patients with blunt or penetrating chest trauma. In these patients, evidence of pericardial effusion with or without echocardiographic findings of tamponade is highly predictive of cardiac perforation, coronary artery laceration, or aortic rupture, and indicates the need for immediate open thoracotomy. A focused transthoracic echocardiogram or, less commonly, TEE is highly accurate in detecting pericardial effusions in these patients (28).

### Doppler Echocardiography

During respiration in patients with cardiac tamponade, there is an exaggerated increased in tricuspid early (E velocity) and late (A velocity) inflow velocities from >35% to >80% and >25% to >50%, respectively (normal variability ranges from 10% to 25%). Simultaneously, an exaggerated decrease of mitral inflow velocities of 30% to 50% is demonstrated (note that the effect on right-sided velocities is almost twice that of left-sided ones) (Fig. 15.8). Similar changes are seen in the pulmonic and aortic valves. A decrease in LA preload during inspiration leads to a decrease in the LA to LV pressure gradient and, therefore, to prolongation of the LV isovolumic relaxation time (IVRT; time elapsed from the closure of the aortic valve to the opening of the mitral valve) by >70% (usually >150 ms, normally ≤110 ms). The reverse phenomena occur during expiration, but the degree of decrease in right-sided velocities and increase in left-sided velocities are not as marked as during inspiration.

Doppler assessment of the flow patterns of the hepatic veins is of complementary diagnostic value in patients with cardiac tamponade. Normally, hepatic vein systolic flow ve-

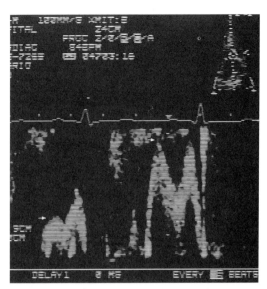

**FIG. 15.8.** Doppler inflow pattern of the mitral valve in a 43-year-old patient with cardiac tamponade demonstrates a marked increased (from 0.3 to 0.4 m/s to almost 0.8 m/s) of the early and late mitral valve velocities (E and A waves, respectively) from inspiration to expiration *(arrows)*. This respiratory variability of the mitral valve inflow resolved soon after pericardiocentesis.

locities are higher than the diastolic velocities, especially during inspiration. The systolic, diastolic, and atrial reversal velocities are minimal. In patients with cardiac tamponade, there is more marked predominance of systolic compared to diastolic velocities; reduction in the normal increase of flow during inspiration; and, during expiration, marked decrease or even reversal of diastolic flow. These changes are more marked after the first cardiac cycle during expiration. In patients with clinical findings of cardiac tamponade, the sensitivity and specificity of the hepatic vein flow patterns are 75% and 91%, respectively, but their diagnostic accuracy is lower in patients without clinical tamponade. The combination of these flow patterns with right heart chamber compression improves their specificity and positive predictive value for detection of cardiac tamponade (Table 15.6) (12).

**TABLE 15.6.** *Sensitivity, specificity, and predictive values of flow patterns of the hepatic veins for detection of cardiac tamponade*

| Abnormality | Sensitivity (%) | Specificity (%) | Positive predictive value (%) | Negative predictive value (%) |
|---|---|---|---|---|
| Abnormal venous flow | 75 | 91 | 82 | 88 |
| Abnormal venous flow and one right heart chamber collapse | 67 | 91 | 80 | 84 |
| Abnormal venous flow and two right heart chambers collapse | 37 | 98 | 90 | 75 |

Data from reference 12.

### Atypical Cardiac Tamponade

#### Cardiac Tamponade without Pulsus Paradoxus

Cardiac tamponade can occur without RV collapse and without pulsus paradoxus in patients with high RV or LV end-diastolic pressure. In these patients, RV to LV interdependence (septal deviation) and variability of stroke volume during respiration will be less accentuated or absent. Conditions associated with cardiac tamponade without pulsus paradoxus include positive-pressure breathing or ventilation; atrial septal defect; pulmonary hypertension with cor pulmonale; RV myocardial infarction; hypervolemia; LV systolic or diastolic dysfunction; and moderate or severe aortic regurgitation.

#### Low-Pressure Cardiac Tamponade

Low intravascular volume status leading to low end-diastolic pressures can be associated with RA, RV, or rarely LV diastolic collapse without clinical evidence of tamponade (29).

#### Acute and Subacute Localized Cardiac Tamponade

Patients with acute or subacute localized cardiac tamponade include those with blunt or penetrating chest trauma; patients with coronary artery perforation during percutaneous coronary interventions; patients with right heart chamber perforation after placement of a pacemaker, automatic implantable defibril-

lator, or central venous catheter; and patients after cardiac surgery. It occurs more commonly anterior and lateral to the RA and RV free wall. In these patients, the pericardial fluid appearance varies from an echolucent fluid collection to a highly reflective and irregular mass.

In patients after cardiac surgery and moderate to large pericardial effusions, anticoagulation is a contributor in >85% of patients (about 40% have undergone valve replacement), up to 30% of them have loculated effusions anteriorly or posteriorly, and postcardiotomy syndrome is the underlying cause in one third of patients. In these patients, sinus tachycardia, elevated jugular venous pressure, hypotension, and pulsus paradoxus are present in only 50%, 40%, 30%, and 20%, respectively. In these patients, the sensitivity of RV diastolic compression for cardiac tamponade is low (48% to 77%), and compression of left heart chambers due to localized hematomas is

**TABLE 15.7.** *Characteristics of atypical cardiac tamponade in patients after cardiac surgery*

Occurs within 3 d to 3 mo
Clinical signs of tamponade are absent in 50%–80% of patients
Equalization of pressures is seen in ≤50% of patients
Most common echocardiographic finding is isolated right atrial or right ventricular compression
Left atrial or left ventricular diastolic compression is common (up to 50% of patients)
Absence of anteriorly located effusion in 50% of patients
Pericardial effusions frequently loculated and small to moderate sized
Frequently misdiagnosed as heart failure, pulmonary embolism, sepsis, or myocardial infarction

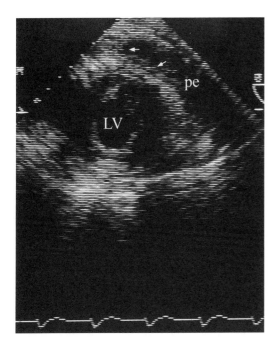

**FIG. 15.9.** Transesophageal echocardiographic transgastric short-axis view of the left ventricle (LV) in a 67-year-old man 2 days after uncomplicated coronary artery bypass surgery performed for unexplained cardiogenic shock and severe elevation of left atrial pressure. A technically limited transthoracic echocardiogram was unrevealing. Note a large and heterogeneously echo-reflectant *(arrows)* pericardial effusion located posterior and lateral to the LV. The patient was immediately taken to the operating room, and a large (400 mL) pericardial hematoma was evacuated. The patient subsequently had an uneventful clinical course.

seen more commonly (Table 15.7 and Fig. 15.9) (30). Echocardiography in these patients may have higher diagnostic accuracy for detection of cardiac tamponade than clinical or hemodynamic data (13).

*Pleural Effusion and Cardiac Tamponade*

Rarely, a large pleural effusion (infectious or hemorrhagic) can produce RV or LV diastolic compression and be associated with echocardiographic and clinical manifestations of tamponade.

### Echocardiography-Guided Pericardiocentesis

Echocardiography-guided diagnostic and therapeutic pericardiocentesis has proved to be a safe technique in patients with cardiac tamponade, especially in patients with acute or subacute (hemorrhagic) cardiac tamponade. Most (>60%) of these patients will rapidly develop severe hemodynamic compromise and have a high mortality unless promptly intervened. A rescue pericardiocentesis can be performed safely and successfully in >95% of these patients with guidance of 2-D echocardiography. Of importance, most of these patients (>80%) may not require further intervention other than percutaneous pericardiocentesis.

Echocardiography can define the distance that the pericardiocentesis needle should traverse from the subcutaneous tissue to the parietal pericardium; identify other interposing tissues or organs (stomach or liver from the subcostal approach or lung from apical approach); orient with regard to the best needle approach or puncture site (subxiphoid or left hemithorax); and localize the shaft of the needle as well as the draining catheter position. When the position of the needle or catheter is uncertain but blood has been aspirated, use of a small amount of saline contrast injected through the puncture needle can quickly opacify the pericardial space, identify the puncture needle or draining catheter, and accurately confirm the intrapericardial position of the needle (Fig. 15.10) (31–34).

Two-dimensional echocardiography can determine if the drainage of pericardial fluid was partial or complete; indicate whether the fluid reaccumulated before pulling out the pericardial drain; and determine the need for further intervention.

### Constrictive Pericarditis

#### Introduction

Echocardiography can play an important role in the diagnosis of constrictive pericardi-

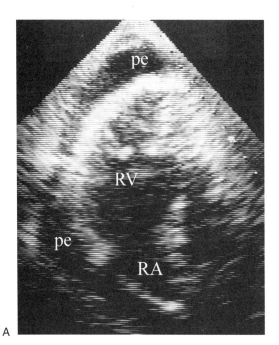 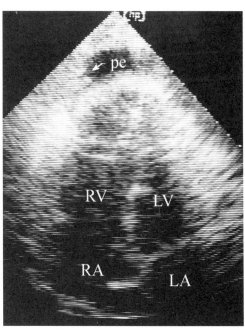

A                                                                          B

**FIG. 15.10. A:** Transthoracic echocardiographic apical four-chamber view in a 76-year-old man with cardiac tamponade and acute decompensation demonstrates a large pericardial effusion (pe) requiring an emergent echocardiography-guided pericardiocentesis that was successful. **B:** To confirm the intrapericardial location of the puncture needle, a small amount of saline contrast was injected. Note the pericardial space almost completely filled with saline contrast *(arrow)*.

tis. Although the echocardiographic manifestations of constriction are multiple, they are less sensitive and specific than those of cardiac tamponade. As with cardiac tamponade, there is no single echocardiographic finding pathog- nomonic for constrictive pericarditis. Therefore, the diagnosis of pericardial constriction requires integration of clinical, echocardiographic, hemodynamic, and, not uncommonly, surgical or histologic data (Fig. 15.11).

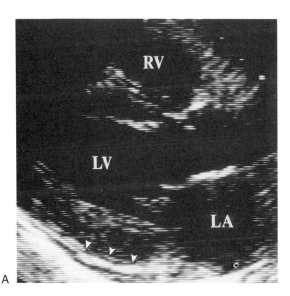

**FIG. 15.11. A:** Parasternal long-axis view in a 43-year-old woman with systemic lupus erythematosus and heart failure symptoms demonstrates at least moderate thickening and hyperreflectance of the visceral pericardium *(arrowheads)*. Constrictive pericarditis was suspected by Doppler echocardiography. **B,C:** Cardiac catheterization demonstrated elevation of right atrial pressure (14 mm Hg) with prominent Y descent *(arrows)* as well as elevation (16 mm Hg) and equalization of the right and left ventricular end-diastolic pressures *(arrows)*.

A

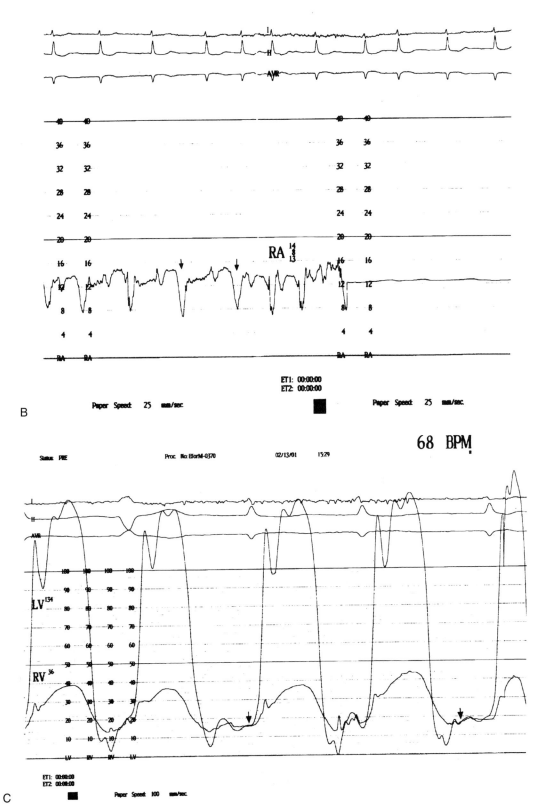

**FIG. 15.11.** *Continued.*

### Diagnosis

Echocardiographic findings of pericardial constriction include (i) pericardial thickening and/or sclerosis (hyperreflectance) and rarely calcification; (ii) no or mild atrial enlargement; (iii) usually normal sized ventricles with normal wall thickness and systolic function; (iv) abnormal septal diastolic motion; (v) premature opening of the pulmonary valve; (vi) abnormal RV and LV filling patterns accentuated by respiration; and (vii) LA and RA hypertension with restricted filling as assessed by Doppler inflow velocity patterns of the pulmonary veins and hepatic veins, respectively (35–37). There is no echocardiographic finding pathognomonic for constriction (Table 15.8).

### General Considerations

Increased echo-reflectance of the posterior visceral or parietal pericardium suggests pericardial thickening. With progression of pericardial thickening and fibrosis, the space between the epicardial and pericardial layers becomes echo dense, and the visceral and parietal layers manifest decreased and parallel motion indicative of adhesion (no separation or sliding motion during systole). Pericardial calcification also can be detected, but it is uncommon and nonspecific because it can occur in the absence of constriction. However, the presence of calcification denotes a chronic etiology and is an independent predictor of perioperative mortality (38). Pericardial calcification or thickening can be patchy or diffuse. The sensitivity of echocardiography for detecting mild degrees of pericardial thickening is poor, but it is improved in the presence of pericardial fluid. Moderate or severe degrees of pericardial thickening are identified more accurately, but precise pericardial thickness measurements are limited. Computed tomography (CT) and magnetic resonance imaging (MRI) may be more accurate than echocardiography for identifying the presence and severity of pericardial thickening. Finally, TEE may provide more accurate assessment of pericardial thickness than transthoracic echocardiography (36,39).

### M-Mode Echocardiography

The normal pericardial thickness as determined by TEE M-mode echocardiography is 1.2 ± 0.8 mm. M-mode imaging can detect pericardial thickening and calcification in 53% to 76% of patients with surgically proven constriction. A thickened pericardium is identified more easily anterior to the RV free wall. TEE is superior to transthoracic echocardiography for detection of pericardial thickening, and its correlation with CT is within 1 mm. Using a pericardial thickness cutoff value of 3 mm, the sen-

**TABLE 15.8.** *Echocardiographic findings in constrictive pericarditis*

| Characteristic | Frequency (%) |
| --- | --- |
| Pericardial thickening | 30–40 |
| Pericardial calcification | <10 |
| Pericardial effusion[a] | 25–30 |
| Normal or mildly enlarged atria | ≥75 |
| Abnormal septal diastolic motion | ≥70 |
| Constrictive Doppler pattern of mitral or tricuspid valve inflow worsened by inspiration | ≥90 |
| Restrictive Doppler pattern, especially of mitral valve inflow | <10 |
| Left atrial hypertension | ≥95 |
| Abnormal pulmonary vein Doppler inflow pattern | ≥95 |
| Plethoric inferior vena cava | ≥70 |
| Abnormal hepatic veins Doppler outflow pattern exacerbated by expiration | ≥75 |

[a]These patients commonly have effusive constrictive pericarditis.

sitivity and specificity of pericardial thickening for detection of constrictive pericarditis are 95% and 86%, respectively (39).

The atria may be enlarged, and the posterior wall of the LV shows abrupt flattening at mid and late diastole secondary to abrupt cessation of LV filling. Other M-mode findings include a steep or rapid E to F slope of the mitral valve; early closure of the mitral valve due to decreased filling and increased LV end-diastolic pressure; premature opening of the pulmonic valve due to increased RV end-diastolic pressure; exaggerated posterior motion (toward LV notch septal displacement) or early interventricular septal diastolic notch due to transseptal pressure differences during the early filling of ventricles; and atrial systolic notch (transient posterior or toward the LV septal displacement after atrial activation) followed by an anterior or toward the RV displacement. Although M-mode abnormalities lack specificity and therefore are not diagnostic of constrictive pericarditis, a normal M-mode echocardiogram suggests that pericardial constriction is unlikely.

### Two-Dimensional Echocardiography

Although this technique can detect pericardial thickening, its sensitivity and specificity are limited. Measurements of pericardial thickening by 2-D imaging correlate modestly at best with autopsy findings. In addition, the correlation of pericardial thickening with hemodynamic evidence of constriction is <40%, probably due to the frequent occurrence of irregular, localized, or patchy pericardial thickening. Also, 2-D echocardiography can demonstrate the abnormal septal motion patterns associated with constriction (early septal diastolic bounce, atrial systolic notch, and early diastolic notch), but this technique is less precise than M-mode echocardiography.

Two-dimensional echocardiography can identify the absence of normal sliding motion of the parietal and visceral pericardium, seen best on the RV free wall in the long parasternal and subcostal views. Finally, 2-D imaging demonstrates the commonly associated inferior vena cava and hepatic vein dilation.

### Doppler Echocardiography

Doppler echocardiography in patients with constrictive pericarditis can demonstrate abnormalities similar to those seen in cardiac tamponade. Because of the rigid pericardium, the degree of inspiratory flow increase to the right heart is of lesser degree than in cardiac tamponade. As for cardiac tamponade, alterations in flow during respiration are a continuum and reciprocal between the right and left heart. The pressures of all cardiac chambers are elevated; consequently, chamber filling is decreased throughout the cardiac cycle and respiration.

During inspiration, decrease in the negative intrathoracic pressure leads to decrease in pressure of the pulmonary veins; decrease in pressure gradient from the pulmonary veins to the LA during systole and diastole; decrease in gradient between the LA and LV; and decrease in pulmonary venous peak systolic and predominantly diastolic velocities; as well as increase in atrial reversal velocity and duration. A marked decrease in the mitral early (E wave) and late (A wave) velocities is noted. An increase in IVRT is demonstrated. Opposite changes occur during expiration (35–37).

Although a decrease in negative intrathoracic pressure during inspiration does not lead to a decrease in intrapericardial pressure as in cardiac tamponade, it still leads to increased venous return to the right heart chambers. This increase in venous return, in conjunction with the decrease in the LV filling, allows a reciprocal increase in tricuspid valve inflow and hepatic vein outflow Doppler velocities.

Therefore, a characteristic constrictive mitral Doppler inflow pattern is seen in most patients (>90%). During expiration, the E peak velocity is predominant and usually <90 cm/s; E deceleration time is short (<160 ms); A peak velocity is one third to one half of E wave velocity (<50 cm/s); E/A ratio is ≥1.5; and IVRT usually is <80 ms. A small proportion of patients (about 10%) will show a restrictive filling pattern in which E peak velocity again is predominant; E deceleration is short (<120 ms); A wave velocity is <25% of E velocity; and E/A ratio is ≥2 (37). A characteristic pulmonary vein Doppler flow pattern during expiration consists of low peak systolic velocities (usually <50 cm/s); predominance of diastolic velocities (<70 cm/s); systolic to diastolic ratio of <1; and peak atrial reversal of <20 cm/s (40).

A change from expiration to inspiration consisting of a >30% fall in mitral E velocity and a 20% to 30% fall in the systolic and predominantly of the diastolic peak velocities of the pulmonary veins inflow; reciprocal increase of >40% in tricuspid inflow velocity; and 50% increase of IVRT have a sensitivity of >85% and a specificity of >90% for constrictive pericarditis.

The hepatic vein Doppler flow velocities show a characteristic "W" pattern produced by a decrease in systolic and diastolic flows and an increase in the corresponding late systolic and diastolic flow reversals. During expiration, the diastolic reversal increases by >50%, and the systolic and diastolic forward flow velocities decrease >25% and >50%, respectively (37). This pattern has a sensitivity of 68% and a specificity of 100%.

Some patients with constrictive pericarditis and marked LA hypertension may have blunted or absent respiratory variation of Doppler mitral E velocity. Repeated Doppler recording of mitral inflow after head-up tilt or sitting positions to decrease LV preload unmasks the characteristic respiratory variation of the mitral E velocity in most patients (40).

### Effusive Constrictive Pericarditis

This is an uncommon clinical syndrome, generally is subacute, and is characterized by the presence of a moderate to large pericardial effusion, pericardial thickening, and Doppler echocardiographic features suggestive of cardiac tamponade. The diagnosis is confirmed when intracardiac pressures remain elevated after pericardiocentesis. The causes of this condition are similar to those for cardiac tamponade and constrictive pericarditis. The M-mode, 2-D, and Doppler echocardiographic features of this condition are indistinguishable from those of cardiac tamponade or constriction alone (41).

### Differentiation of Constrictive Pericarditis from Restrictive Cardiomyopathy

The clinical, echocardiographic, and hemodynamic differentiation of constrictive pericarditis from restrictive cardiomyopathy is difficult. Doppler echocardiography plays an important role in their differentiation, but not a single finding is specific enough of each condition to rely exclusively on echocardiography to make such a distinction (35,37,42). These two conditions can be differentiated in the majority of patients by the integration of clinical, hemodynamic, Doppler echocardiography, and CT or MRI data (37,42–45). The diagnosis is established in a few patients only after surgery (Table 15.9) (16,40,45,46).

### SUMMARY

### Diagnostic Value of History and Physical Examination

Chest pain is the most common and characteristic symptom of acute pericarditis. It typically is sharp, pleuritic, and relieved by sitting up and leaning forward. *Pain perceived in the trapezius ridges, usually the left, is virtually pathognomonic for pericardial irritation.*

The *pericardial rub* (friction sound), which is composed of one to three friction elements per cardiac cycle, is *the cardinal sign of pericarditis,* but it may be transient or intermittent and often last hours to days. Sinus tachycardia, jugular venous distention, and pulsus paradoxus with variable frequency rates are the cardinal physical findings of cardiac tamponade. Similarly, jugular venous distention, pulsus paradoxus, and a loud, early abnormal $S_3$ are consistent with constrictive pericarditis.

**TABLE 15.9.** *Differentiation of constrictive pericarditis from restrictive cardiomyopathy*

| Distinctive feature | Constrictive pericarditis | Restrictive cardiomyopathy |
|---|---|---|
| Clinical | 1. Previous cardiac surgery<br>2. Radiation therapy | Chronic systemic disease |
| M-mode or two-dimensional echocardiography | 1. Pericardial thickening >3 mm<br>2. Posterior wall diastolic flattening<br>3. Normal appearance and thickness of myocardium<br>4. Normal LV cavity | 1. Normal pericardium (<2 mm)<br>2. Abnormal appearance and increased myocardial thickness<br>3. Small LV cavity |
| Doppler echocardiography | 1. Constrictive pattern of mitral inflow in >90% of patients<br>2. >30% decrease of mitral E peak and pulmonary vein systolic and diastolic velocities from expiration to inspiration<br>3. Pulmonary vein systolic/diastolic ratio ≥0.65<br>4. >50% increase of the isovolumic relaxation time from expiration to inspiration<br>5. During expiration, >50% increase in hepatic vein diastolic reversal and decrease of systolic and diastolic forward flow velocities of >25% and >50%, respectively | 1. Restrictive pattern of mitral inflow in >90% of patients<br>2. <15% decrease of mitral E peak and pulmonary vein systolic and diastolic velocities from expiration to inspiration<br>3. Pulmonary vein systolic/diastolic ratio ≤0.40<br>4. Predominant forward hepatic vein flow during diastole; increase in systolic and diastolic reversals during inspiration |
| Hemodynamics | 1. LVEDP-RVEDP ≤5 mm Hg[a]<br>2. PASP <55 mm Hg<br>3. RVEDP/RVSP >1/3[b]<br>4. LV or RV dip and plateau filling | 1. LVEDP-RVEDP >5 mm Hg<br>2. PASP >55 mm Hg<br>3. RVEDP/RVSP <1/3 |

[a]This parameter has 60% sensitivity and 71% specificity for constrictive pericarditis (45).
[b]This parameter has 93% sensitivity and 57% specificity for constrictive pericarditis (45).
LVEDP, left ventricular (LV) end-diastolic pressure; PASP, pulmonary artery systolic pressure; RVEDP, right ventricular (RV) end-diastolic pressure; RVSP, RV systolic pressure.

## Limitations of History and Physical Examination

1. The etiology and frequency of symptoms and physical findings are notoriously variable in all pericardial diseases. Ascertainment biases exist in institutions with emphasis on referred patients with unusual causes or due to specialization in specific causes. For instance, in institutions with large oncology, rheumatology, or cardiovascular disease services, pericardial diseases related to malignancies, immunopathies, or after cardiac surgery, respectively, will yield large ranges for incidences and prevalence. These data clearly are not representative of a general population.

2. History of almost any kind of pericardial disease varies from absence of symptoms to florid expression.
3. A large variability in reported bedside data compels keeping in mind all of the possibilities and that many, if not most, may be absent in any case at any time.

## Diagnostic Value of Echocardiography

Echocardiography plays an essential complementary, frequently additive, and uncommonly primary diagnostic role in patients with acute pericarditis, cardiac tamponade, or constrictive pericarditis. Thus, specific indications for echocardiography in these patients have been delineated by the American College of Cardiology and the American Heart Association (Table 15.10) (47).

Echocardiography can define the presence and size of a pericardial effusion; detect pericardial thickening (rarely calcification); and determine their hemodynamic significance. However, the time and extent of accumulation of a pericardial effusion and/or pericardial scarring will determine the presence and severity of echocardiographic manifestations.

Demonstration of pericardial effusion and/or thickening by echocardiography confirms the diagnosis of pericarditis in a patient with a consistent clinical syndrome.

Clinically suspected cardiac tamponade frequently is based on nonspecific symptoms and physical findings, with the exception of a pericardial rub or pulsus paradoxus of ≥20 mm Hg. Echocardiography frequently identifies patients with cardiac tamponade and minimal clinical or hemodynamic compromise, which allows for early therapeutic interventions. In patients with clinically evident cardiac tamponade, echocardiography generally demonstrates significant hemodynamic derangement and can assist in an urgent pericardiocentesis. Echocardiography is of important diagnostic value in patients with loculated pericardial effusions or hematomas and frequent atypical clinical and hemodynamic findings of cardiac tamponade. Finally, echocardiography is of important complementary diagnostic value in patients with suspected constrictive pericarditis.

**TABLE 15.10.** *Indications for echocardiography in pericardial diseases*

1. Patients with suspected pericardial effusion, tamponade, constriction, or effusive constriction
2. Patients with suspected bleeding into the pericardial space
3. Follow-up study to evaluate recurrence of effusion or to diagnose early constriction
4. Patients with acute myocardial infarction and persistent pain, hypotension, and a friction rub
5. Follow-up study to detect early signs of tamponade in the presence of large or rapidly accumulating effusions[a]
6. Echocardiographic guidance and monitoring of pericardiocentesis[a]

[a]Class IIa indication.

## Limitations of Echocardiography

1. Echocardiography does not detect pericardial effusions in one third of patients with clinically evident pericarditis, and one third of uremic patients have small pericardial effusions without pericarditis.
2. Echocardiography has limited sensitivity (<60%) in detecting pericardial thickening.
3. Echocardiography cannot accurately differentiate types of pericardial fluid (blood, exudate, or transudate); its sensitivity for detection of pericardial nodules or masses is low (<40%), and its specificity can be decreased by misinterpretation of epicardial fat as an effusion.
4. No single echocardiographic parameter is pathognomonic for cardiac tamponade, and this technique is less specific in the diagnosis of atypical forms of tamponade. Therefore, its final diagnosis requires integration of clinical, echocardiographic, and, frequently, hemodynamic data.
5. Flow patterns of hepatic veins cannot be assessed in one third of patients with suspected cardiac tamponade or constriction. These patterns are less reliable in patients with atrial fibrillation or significant tricuspid regurgitation, and in those on positive-pressure ventilation.
6. Echocardiography is less sensitive and specific for detection of constrictive pericarditis than for cardiac tamponade. Therefore, the ultimate diagnosis of constriction is based on typical hemodynamic findings and confirmation of pericardial thickening by CT or MRI.
7. Echocardiography has poor sensitivity for detection of patchy, localized, or mild pericardial thickening or calcification (<75% detection in patients with surgically proven constriction) and is unreliable for measurement of pericardial thickness (<50% correlation with hemodynamic or autopsy evidence of constriction).
8. Echocardiographic detection of pericardial calcification is nonspecific for the diagnosis of constriction.

9. Patients with constrictive pericarditis and marked LA hypertension may have blunted or absent characteristic respiratory variation in the mitral Doppler E velocity.

10. Doppler flow patterns of the hepatic veins in patients with constriction can be masked by a holosystolic reversal in patients with significant tricuspid regurgitation and by a limited diastolic flow during sinus tachycardia.

## REFERENCES

1. Spodick DH. Acute, clinically noneffusive ("dry") pericarditis. In: Spodick DH. The pericardium: a comprehensive textbook. New York: Marcel Dekker, 1997: 94–113.
2. Moreno R, Villacastin JP, Bueno H, et al. Clinical and echocardiographic findings in HIV patients with pericardial effusion. Cardiology 1997;88:397–400.
3. Zayas R, Anguita M, Torres F, Gimenez D, et al. Incidence of specific etiology and role of methods for specific etiologic diagnosis of primary acute pericarditis. Am J Cardiol 1995;75:378–382.
4. Foster E. Pericardial effusion: a continuing drain on our diagnostic acumen. Am J Med 2000;109:169–170.
5. Sagrista-Sauleda J, Angel J, Permanyer-Miralda G, et al. Long-term follow-up of idiopathic chronic pericardial effusion. N Engl J Med 1999;341:2054–2059.
6. Spodick DH. Diagnosis and management of acute noneffusive pericarditis. Cardiol Board Rev 1994;11: 13–16.
7. Spodick DH. Pitfalls in the recognition of pericarditis. In: Hurst JW, ed. Clinical essays of the heart. New York: McGraw-Hill, 1985:95–111.
8. Spodick DH. Pericardial effusion and hydropericardium without cardiac tamponade. In: Spodick DH. The pericardium: a comprehensive textbook. New York: Marcel Dekker, 1997, 126–152.
9. Spodick DH. The normal and diseased pericardium: current concepts of pericardial physiology, diagnosis and treatment. J Am Coll Cardiol 1983;1:240–251.
10. Levine M, Lorell B, Diver D, et al. Implications of echocardiographically assisted diagnosis of pericardial tamponade in contemporary medical patients: detection before hemodynamic embarrassment. J Am Coll Cardiol 1991;17:59–65.
11. Sagrista-Sauleda J, Merce J, Permanyer-Miralda G, et al. Clinical clues to the causes of pericardial effusions. Am J Med 2000;109:95–101.
12. Merce J, Sagrista-Sauleda J, Permanyer-Miralda G, et al. Correlation between clinical and Doppler echocardiographic findings in patients with moderate and large pericardial effusion: implications for the diagnosis of cardiac tamponade. Am Heart J 1999;138: 759–764.
13. Tsang T, Barnes M, Hayes S, et al. Clinical and echocardiographic characteristics of significant pericardial effusions following cardiothoracic surgery and outcomes

14. Spodick DH. Pulsus paradoxus. In: Spodick DH. The pericardium: a comprehensive textbook. New York: Marcel Dekker, 1997:191–199.
15. Mayers RBH, Spodick DH. Constrictive pericarditis: clinical and pathophysiologic characteristics. Am Heart J 1999;138:219–232.
16. Henein MY, Rakhit RD, Sheppard MN, et al. Restrictive pericarditis. Heart 1999;82:389–392.
17. McCully RB, Higano ST, Oh JK. Diagnosis of constrictive pericarditis. Circulation 1999;99:2476.
18. Dardas P, Tsikaderis D, Ioannides E, et al. Constrictive pericarditis after coronary artery bypass surgery as a cause of unexplained dyspnea: a report of five cases. Clin Cardiol 1998;21:691–694.
19. Spodick DH. Constrictive pericarditis. In: Spodick DH. The pericardium: a comprehensive textbook. New York: Marcel Dekker, 1997:214–259.
20. Spodick DH. Bloody pericardial effusion: clinically significant without intrinsic diagnostic specificity. Chest 1999;116:1506–1507.
21. Hinds S, Reisner S, Amico A, et al. Diagnosis of pericardial abnormalities by 2D-echo: A pathology-echocardiography correlation in 85 patients. Am Heart J 1992;123:143–150.
22. Auer J, Berent R, Eber B. Pitfalls in the diagnosis of pericardial effusion by echocardiography. Heart 1999;82:613.
23. Ball JB, Morrison WL. Cardiac tamponade. Postgrad Med J 1997;73:141–145.
24. Himelman RB, Kircher B, Rockey DC, et al. Inferior vena cava plethora with blunted respiratory response: a sensitive echocardiographic sign of tamponade. J Am Coll Cardiol 1988;12:1470–1477.
25. Appleton CP, Hatle LK, Popp RL. Cardiac tamponade and pericardial effusion: respiratory variation in transvalvular flow velocities studied by Doppler echocardiography. J Am Coll Cardiol 1988;11:1020–1030.
26. Burstow DJ, Oh JK, Bailey KR, et al. Cardiac tamponade: characteristic Doppler observations. Mayo Clin Proc 1989;64:312–324.
27. Steiner MA, Marshall JJ. Coronary sinus compression as a sign of cardiac tamponade. Cathet Cardiovasc Diagn 2000;49:455–458.
28. Chan D. Echocardiography in thoracic trauma. Emerg Med Clin North Am 1998;16:191–207.
29. Dwivedi SK, Saran R, Narain VS. Left ventricular diastolic collapse in low-pressure cardiac tamponade. Clin Cardiol 1998;21:224–226.
30. Dardas PS, Tsikaderis DD, Makrigiannakis K, et al. Complete left atrial obliteration due to localized tamponade after coronary artery perforation during PTCA. Cathet Cardiovasc Diagn 1998;45:61–63.
31. Salem K, Mulji A, Lonn E. Echocardiographically guided pericardiocentesis—the gold standard for the management of pericardial effusion and cardiac tamponade. Can J Cardiol 1999;15:1251–1255.
32. Tsang TS, Freeman WK, Barnes ME, et al. Rescue echocardiographically guided pericardiocentesis for cardiac perforation complicating catheter-based procedures. The Mayo Clinic experience. J Am Coll Cardiol 1998;32:1345–1350.
33. Muhler EG, Engelhardt W, Von Bernuth G. Pericardial effusions in infants and children: injection of echo contrast medium enhances the safety of echocardiographi-

of echo-guided pericardiocentesis for management. Chest 1999;116:322–331.

cally-guided pericardiocentesis. Cardiol Young 1998;8: 506–508.

34. Tsang TSM, Freeman WK, /Sinak LJ, et al. Echocardiographically guided pericardicentesis: evolution and state-of-the-art technique. Mayo Clin Proc 1998;73: 647–652.
35. Cheng TO. Doppler features of constrictive pericarditis. Circulation 1997;96:3799–3800.
36. Chandraratna PA. Echocardiography and Doppler ultrasound in the evaluation of pericardial disease. Circulation 1991;84:I-303–I-310.
37. Oh JK, Hatle LK, Seward JB, et al. Diagnostic role of Doppler echocardiography in constrictive pericarditis. J Am Coll Cardiol 1994;23:154–162.
38. Ling LH, Oh JK, Breen JF, et al. Calcific constrictive pericarditis: is it still with us? Ann Intern Med 2000; 132:444–450.
39. Ling LH, Oh JK, Tei C, et al. Pericardial thickness measured with transesophageal echocardiography: feasibility and potential clinical usefulness. J Am Coll Cardiol 1997;29:1317–1323.
40. Oh JK, Tajik AJ, Appleton CP, et al. Preload reduction to unmask the characteristic Doppler features of constrictive pericarditis. A new observation [see comments]. Circulation 1997;95:796–799.

41. Woods T, Vidarsson B, Mosher D, et al. Transient effusive-constrictive pericarditis due to chemotherapy. Clin Cardiol 1999;22:316–318.
42. Lein AL, Cohen GI, Pietrolungo JF, et al. Differentiation of constrictive pericarditis from restrictive cardiomyopathy by Doppler transesophageal echocardiographic measurement of respiratory variations in pulmonary venous flow. J Am Coll Cardiol 1993;22:1935–1943.
43. Hatle LK, Appleton CP, Popp RL. Differentiation of constrictive pericarditis from restrictive cardiomyopathy by Doppler echocardiography. Circulation 1989;79: 357–370.
44. Mancuso L, D'Agostino A, Pitrolo F, et al. Constrictive pericarditis versus restrictive cardiomyopathy: the role of Doppler echocardiography in differential diagnosis. Int J Cardiol 1991;31:319–328.
45. Hurrell D, Nishimura R, Higano S, et al. Value of dynamic respiratory changes in left and right ventricular pressures for the diagnosis of constrictive pericarditis. Circulation 1996;93:2007–2013.
46. Mehta A, Mehta M, Jain A. Constrictive pericarditis. Clin Cardiol 1999;22:334–344.
47. Cheitlin MD, Alpert JS, Armstrong WF, et al. ACC/AHA guidelines for the clinical application of echocardiography. Circulation 1997;95:1686–1744.

# Subject Index

Page numbers followed by f indicate figures; those followed by t indicate tables.

## A

A₂ (aortic component of second heart sound), 17–18, 18f, 19f

Abdominal compression test, 10–11, 10f

Abscess, due to infective endocarditis
anatomy and physiology of, 266–267
echocardiography of, 274f, 275, 275f, 277–278, 277t
epidemiology of, 266
location of, 270

Acceleration time, 142–143

Acceleration zone, 148

Acute myocardial infarction (AMI). *See also* Myocardial infarction (MI)
auscultation in, 76–79, 78f
blood pressure and arterial pulse in, 73–74
clinical history of, 70–71, 70t, 71t
diagnosis of, 83–84
echocardiography of
during hospital stay, 84–86
with mechanical complications, 86–90, 87f–89f, 91f, 92f
posttreatment, 90–93, 92t
resting, 81, 81t, 82f, 82t
stress, 81–83, 83t
suspected, 83–84
general appearance in, 72–73
heart murmurs in, 77–78, 77f
heart sounds in, 76–77
Killip classification of, 77
natural history and prognosis with, 67–68, 68t
pericardial friction rub in, 78–79
physical examination for, 71–79, 72t
physical examination in
diagnostic value of, 95–96
limitations of, 96–97
precordial examination in, 74–76, 75f
risk stratification for, 84, 90–93, 92t
venous pulse in, 74

Acute neurologic ischemic syndromes. *See* Stroke
etiology of, 287, 287f

Adenosine echocardiography, of coronary artery disease, 93, 94t

Aliasing velocity, in mitral regurgitation, 181

AMI. *See* Acute myocardial infarction (AMI)

Anacrotic notch, 5f

Aneurysm(s)
aortic, 237f
atrial septal, 58
systemic embolization from, 293–294, 293f
left ventricular
in coronary artery disease, 75–76, 75f, 85
with thrombus, 290, 290f
mycotic, in infective endocarditis, 267, 270
pseudo-
after myocardial infarction, 90, 92f
valve, 275, 276f, 277–278, 277t

sinus of Valsalva, 239f

Angina
in aortic stenosis, 203
classification of, 70t
decubitus, 69
first-effort (warm-up), 69
fixed threshold, 67t, 69
increasing (crescendo), 67t, 70
mixed, 67t
new-onset, 67t, 70
nocturnal, 69
postinfarction, 67t
rest, 67, 67t, 69
spontaneous, 67t
stable (exertional), 67t
clinical history of, 69–70
unstable, 67t
clinical history of, 70
echocardiography after treatment of, 90–93, 92t
risk stratification with, 68t, 90–93, 92t
variable threshold, 67t, 69
variant or Prinzmetal, 67t
Anginal "equivalent," 69

Angle of Louis, 9

Ankylosing spondylitis, and aortic regurgitation, 238f

Anorexia, in congestive heart failure, 105t, 106

Antibiotic prophylaxis, for infective endocarditis, 283

Aorta
ascending, 48
coarctation of. *See* Coarctation of the aorta
descending, 48, 60t
echocardiography of, 47–48
tubular, 48

Aortic aneurysm, 237f

Aortic arch
in coarctation of the aorta, 319–320, 320f
echocardiography of, 48, 60t

Aortic area, 27

Aortic atheroma, systemic embolization from, 292–293, 292f

Aortic component of second heart sound (A₂), 17–18, 18f, 19f

Aortic dissection, during pregnancy, 330, 332

Aortic ejection click, 206–207, 207f, 231

Aortic ejection sound, 21f

Aortic regurgitation (AR), 225–248
acute, 226, 234–236, 235t
aortic valve replacement for, 244–245, 244t
appearance in, 235
arterial and carotid pulses in, 227f, 228, 228f
blood pressure in, 227–228, 227f, 235t, 236, 245
chronic, 226, 235t
degenerative, 237, 240f–241f
differential diagnosis of, 234
echocardiography of, 236–245
after aortic valve replacement, 245
for aortic valve replacement, 244–245, 244t
color Doppler, 47, 60t, 236–237, 241, 242f–243f, 248
continuous wave Doppler, 239–241, 240f–241f
diagnostic value of, 247, 247t